T0265021

BIOSENSOR TECHNOLOGY

FUNDAMENTALS AND APPLICATIONS

edited by

RICHARD P. BUCK
WILLIAM E. HATFIELD
University of North Carolina
Chapel Hill, North Carolina

MIRTHA UMAÑA
Private Consultant
Chapel Hill, North Carolina

EDMOND F. BOWDEN
North Carolina State University
Raleigh, North Carolina

MARCEL DEKKER, INC. NEW YORK AND BASEL

ISBN 0-8247-8414-6

This book is printed on acid-free paper.

MARCEL DEKKER, INC.
270 Madison Avenue, New York, New York 10016

Current printing (last digit):
10 9 8 7 6 5 4 3 2 1

PRINTED IN THE UNITED STATES OF AMERICA

Preface

The availability of new technology and better communications among engineers, physicists, biologists, and chemists has set the stage for rapid and important advances in the development of biosensors. This new biosensor technology has allowed new applications of classical ideas for biosensors by permitting use of new structures and input functions to probe the transfer functions of systems (contributions by physicists and electrical engineers), development and use of new materials (contributions by chemists), development of specialized and unusual chemistry (contributions by immunologists), and development of new formats for sensors especially for in vivo applications (contributions by physiologists). Those who use the new technologies are stimulating the new research on biosensors.

Although sensors have been used in biological applications for centuries, it was after the discovery of the prototype chemically sensistive semiconductor device that electrical engineers and solid state physicists took up the chemical sensor field and continued the physical sensor developments. Their contributions have been decisive in microminiaturization, especially fabrication of small versions of already practical devices. Similarly, the contributions of physicists in designing quartz crystal piezoelectric devices have expanded the chemical sensor field greatly.

Optical physics has been employed advantageously in sensors. An example is the development of optical absorbance change or luminescence sensors interrogated by probe beams and read by emitted light through optical wave guides such as optical fibers of plastic or glass. Sensors using specially coated optical wave guides, including those that modulate the evanescent wave depending on chemical reactions with the exterior coating, are another development of advanced technology.

Contributions by physiologists and clinical chemists are not so clearly recognized, but they are very important when judged in terms of commercialization by both large and start-up companies. These contributions include the in vivo optical sensors, the microencapsulated pH sensing dyes called optodes, and the closely related optrodes. Conversion and specialization of conventional electrochemical sensors into physiologically useful sensors has been a technological triumph. Prior to studies by electrochemists of carbon fiber microelectrodes, microfabricated dots, hemispheres and lines, electrophysiologists had already made 0.1 μm tip capillaries as junction-type reference electrodes and ion exchanger-filled tips for ion assays within single cells.

Symposia and conferences are exceptionally important in a field that employs such a diverse group of scientists. This book contains the proceedings of the International Symposium on Biosensors: Fundamentals and Applications, which was held on the campus of the University of North Carolina at Chapel Hill on September 7-9, 1989. The program was designed to emphasize the physics, engineering, analytical chemistry, and biochemistry (including immunochemistry) as they exist now, and as they may make contributions to sensors technology in the 1990s. Fundamental issues of sensitivity and selectivity were emphasized wherever possible.

The initial session of the symposium was devoted to tutorials on fundamentals of electrochemical, microelectronic, optical and piezoelectric devices. The presentations included:

Richard P. Buck "Electrochemical Sensors and Biosensors; Some Connections with Optical Chemical Sensors"

Jay N. Zemel "Microfabricated Chemical Sensors"

Raymond E. Dessy "Swords into Plowshares - the Way Waveguide, SAW, and Piezoelectric/Pyroelectric Sensors Work"

In addition to the tutorial lectures mentioned above, the program included a number of invited lectures and contributed poster presentations. Manuscripts accompanying many of these constitute these proceedings, although some authors did not elect to submit manuscripts. All of the manuscripts that were received were read by impartial reviewers, and the authors of acceptable manuscripts had the opportunity to make revisions and corrections in view of the comments by the reviewers. The editors wish to thank the reviewers for their help.

The book consists of four sections. Following an introduction to the field of biosensor technology, there are four chapters devoted to microelectrodes and microelectronic devices. The next section consists of ten chapters on modified electrodes, amperometric, and potentiometric sensors, and the final section of fourteen chapters deals with optical and acoustic wave-based sensors.

The symposium was generously supported by the NC Section ACS, the North Carolina Biotechnology Center,[1] the United State Army Research Office,[2] the North Carolina Microelectronics Center, and Akzo Corporate Research America. The NC Section ACS and the participants in the symposium wish to thank these organizations for their support and for the opportunity to assemble many of the leaders in research on biosensors for presentations of the most recent results on the fundamentals and applications of biosensors.

The editors and symposium organizers also wish to thank Drs. Steve Bobbio, Jack Buchanan, Len Geddes, and Susan Schiffman for their valuable assistance. We also wish to express our especial appreciation and gratitude to Mrs. Linda Caulder for her dedicated efforts which led to a successfully organized symposium and a promptly edited book containing the proceedings of the symposium.

Richard P. Buck

William E. Hatfield

Mirtha Umaña

Edmond F. Bowden

---

[1] Any opinions, findings, conclusions, or recommendations expressed in this publication are those of the author(s) and do not necessarily reflect the views and policies of the North Carolina Biotechnology Center.

[2] The views, opinions, and/or findings contained in this report are those of the author(s) and should not be construed as an official Department of the Army position, policy, or decision, unless so designated by other documentation.

Contents

*Invited speakers are indicated by bold letters.

I

Introduction

1

Sensor Issues for the 1990s: An Introduction to the North Carolina Section American Chemical Society Symposium on Biosensors

RICHARD P. BUCK, Department of Chemistry, University of North Carolina, Chapel Hill, NC 27599-3290

WHY SENSORS NOW?

Analytical chemists have done research on, made and used sensors for years. Ion-sensitive and redox- sensitive electrodes have been known and used for 100 years...since the days of Nernst. Membrane-based glass electrodes were invented in 1906; rudimentary ion selective membrane electrodes appeared soon after synthetic, polymer-based ion exchanging materials were invented in 1935. Continuous electrolytic (coulometric) gas analyzers for SO_2 were made by 1949. Practical amperometric sensors have been around at least since the Keidel Cell Moisture Monitor (continuous electrolytic water monitor of the 1950s). The Clark amperometric ambient and dissolved oxygen partial pressure sensor has been known, commercialized and adapted to various biochemical and clinical analyses for many years.

High temperature, solid state electrochemical cells have been known from the detailed analyses of Wagner in the 1950s, and applications of defect, ion conducting oxide cells to fuel cells and the sensing of ambient oxygen have been known equally long. Optical chemical sensors (color-forming or bleaching reactions, shifts of absorption maxima by dielectric change or stabilizing reactions with ground or excited states) were made as soon as inexpensive spectrophotometers became available in the late 1930s and especially 1940s. Practical, small physical sensors for temperature, strain, acceleration, velocity and much more, were available during and after World War II.

So...why sensor research now? The answer is compounded from availability of new technology (not specifically chemical) and better communications among engineers, physicists, biologists and chemists than ever seemed possible before.

PRINCIPAL ROLE OF NEW TECHNOLOGY

New technology drives interest in, and development of sensors. Only secondarily have specific needs driven development. New technology has allowed many new embodiments of classical ideas for sensors by permitting use of new structures and new input functions to probe the transfer functions of systems (contributions of physicists and electrical engineers), development and use of new materials (contributions by chemists), development of specialized and unusual chemistry (contribution of immunologists), and development of new formats especially for *in vivo* applications (contributions by physiologists). Practitioners of the new technologies are pushing sensor research. After 1970 and the discovery of the prototype (Bergveld) chemically sensitive semiconductor device, electrical engineers and solid state physicists took up the chemical sensor field and continued the physical sensor developments. Their contributions have been decisive in microminiaturization, especially fabrication of small versions of already practical devices. Applications of the field effect-based sensors *per se* in microfabricated devices seems very much less important than once thought. Similarly the contributions of physicists in designing quartz crystal piezoelectric devices have expanded the chemical sensor field greatly, although the concept of mass sensors for ambient adsorb- and absorb-able gases using the change in resonant frequency of a bulk quartz crystal was exploited some 20 years ago. The forms of devices: thick crystal bulk wave (conventional gas analyzer or film thickness monitor), thick crystal shear wave (quartz microbalance), SAW delay time (Rayleigh wave along surface of a relatively thick crystal exposed to gases or liquids), SAW resonant frequency excited from the under side of the crystal, and very thin quartz films oscillating in complex ways (Lamb waves) are parts of the emerging technology for applications to gas and to liquid samples. Materials with crystals in the 21 space groups without a center of symmetry show changes of dimension with application of an electric field. Conversely, application of electric fields induces dimensional changes and acoustic waves.

On the same side of the irreversible thermodynamic equation is the pyroelectric effect in which a thermal gradient induces a field and a measureable voltage drop. This latter effect is presently used in the dc mode in contrast with the piezoelectric devices that use ac mode. Many of the same materials show both pyro- and piezoelectric effects. However the rules for selecting materials requires knowledge of crystal symmetry. These new devices are exceedingly sensitive to thermal gradients (heat flux) and seem, at this early date, to be a most profitable direction for chemical sensors using thermal effects: adsorption-desorption, solution-dissolution, simple bond formation (of all types)-dissociation enthalpies. This statement does not intend a criticism of temperature sensors such as thermistors whose physics and chemistry remain an interesting field for research on mechanisms of charge conduction and material properties.

The role of optical physics cannot be underestimated for the development of optical absorbance change or luminescence sensors interrogated by probe beams and/or read by emitted light through optical wave guides: through transparent optical fibers of plastic or glass. Sensors using specially coated optical wave guides, including optical fibers and films that modulate the evanescent wave depending on chemical reactions with the exterior coating, are another development from advanced technology. The latter technology is not familiar to many conventionally trained chemists because a new parameter: the refractive index of materials. It is as important in sensor design of as the chemistry of the absorbing or reacting layer.

Contributions by physiologists and clinical chemists are not so clearly recognized, but very important if judged in terms of commercialization by large companies and several start-up companies. In vivo optical sensors, the microencapsulated pH sensing dyes called optodes, were conceived and developed at the Max Planck Institute for Systemic Physiology by Lubbers and coworkers. Later a very closely related concept, optrodes, was developed at Livermore Labs by Hirschfeld and coworkers. Conversion and specialization of conventional electrochemical sensors into physiologically useful sensors has been a technological triumph. Prior to studies by electrochemists of carbon fiber microelectrodes, microfabricated dots, hemispheres and lines, electrophysiologists had already made 0.1 μm tip capillaries as junction-type reference electrodes (for net membrane potential measurements) and ion exchanger-filled tips for ion assays within single cells. One must also mention the role of physiologists and clinical chemists in pointing out the special analytical problems of clinical, intensive care, doctors' offices, and *in vivo* measurements.

A logical combination of 1) the interfacial potential difference (pd) at an electrolyte/membrane interface (whether generated by faradaic or non-faradaic charge separation processes) and 2) the well known solid state physical generation of electron/hole pairs in Si by irradiation by energetic photons, leads to a new kind of device. The notion is 'light addressable potentiometry'. Whatever the interfacial pd is, it can be perturbed and in some sense measured by generation of charge that partially cancels the local field.

THE PRESENT ROLE OF CHEMISTRY

For about 20 years many of the current ideas of sensor chemistry have been known and exploited. These include use of chemically modified redox electrode surfaces as ion selective electrodes

(Michael Sharp radical salt electrodes); use of enzymes in reactive layers to generate from neutral charge substrate, species that can be sensed (potentiometric enzyme electrodes); use of enzymes in amperometric sensors (modifications of Clark oxygen electrodes); use of enzymes and mediators in amperometric sensors (glucose sensors since 1960s); use of mediators in redox reactions, formerly called 'secondary intermediates' in early 1950s (Br_2-Br^- for oxidation of electrochemically inert SO_2, or $Mn^{+2/3}$ for NO_2); use of selective reagents to generate response specificity (crown ethers and natural and synthetic ionophores in monovalent and divalent ion sensors since 1965); and use of selective layers to extract or partition species into surface layers on sensors (King quartz crystal mass sensors in mid 1960s), to name but a few examples.

The new technology, contributed by chemists in recent years, has frequently been a perturbation on existing classical ideas, formats or systems. Electronic-conducting electrodes with surfaces modified with pure ion conductors cannot serve as sensors for non-redox ions since the membrane/electrode interface is blocked (capacitively coupled). However, in the same way that mercury films can accumulate trace metals prior to anodic stripping, ion exchange films can accumulate trace ionic redox species that could be subsequently determined by either anionic or cathodic stripping. Electronic-conducting electrodes, modified with mixed conductors, can be sensors of organic gases that dissolve and increase ion or electron mobilities in a reproducible way.

More importantly, mixed conductor films may selectively catalyze the surface redox reactions of species that are not themselves electroactive in rapid, reversible ways. Redox enzymes involving coenzymes NAD, FAD, and certain quinones need this catalysis by 'promoter' films. Or, enzyme/coenzymes can be incorporated in mixed conductor films with exciting applications to amperometry of electrochemically inert substrates such as glucose and ethanol. At this time, the question of just how effective the enzyme system can be made remains unanswered. How many turns-over can the enzyme system: mediator/promoter/enzyme combination sustain? Layered systems of electrode, electron transfer promoter layer (NMPTCNQ-type, ferrocene and other covalently attached layers with different degrees of flexibility in penetrating to the enzyme active site), enzyme/coenzyme reaction layer, dialysis stabilizing layer, may be less effective than mixed or wired systems. In the latter, covalently attached electron transfer reagents are used to modify the enzyme which is imbedded in a mixed conductor polymer. An unmodified enzyme/coenzyme system can be at least partially 3-D wired by mixing with it a saturated organic solution of promoters. Extensive literature has accumulated on variations of glucose oxidase chemistry at electrodes. Because the principles are general, applications of discoveries for the glucose sensor may be found in many other sensors for neutral species attacked by redox enzymes.

Design of open chain and cyclic ionophores for selective extraction of particular ions has been a major achievement in the synthetic part of chemical sensor research. Not only have new ion-dipole compounds been made (with controlled locations of ether oxygens, carbonyl oxygens and nitrogen centers), but carriers with reversible covalent bond formation have been discovered. The major thrust has been to remove ordinary electrostatic (simple ion exchange) selectivity as the main operating principle that leads to the usual Hofmeister series. Instead selective interactions are emphasized to produce sensors that deviate from the Hofmeister sequence to permit analysis of phosphate and bicarbonate, for example, and Li^{+} and Mg^{+2} among the cations.

Design of optical sensors has lagged behind trial and error development. It is clear now that color forming reactions and related classical technology can be adapted to wave guide technology. It is clear that colored hydrophobic complexes and organic dyes change their absorption coefficients and wavelength of maximum absorption upon changing the composition of the membrane phase through absorption of substances to be detected. However the microscopic design of systems to accomplished a selective color reaction seems to be lacking.

THE CONSUMER ROLE: BIOTECHNOLOGY AND MEDICINE AS AN EXAMPLE

New applications of sensors in biotechnology and in medicine give visibility to the sensor field because the applications may be important, e.g. blood gas analyzers, blood parameters for critical care settings, critical level drug monitors, and for doctor's offices (pH, pK^+, pNa^+, pCa^{2+}, pCl^-, $pHCO_3^{-2}$, BUN, glucose, and hematocrit). But relatively few, if any, new principles for sensors have come <u>from</u> these fields. Instead, the applications to these fields have served to broaden the knowledge of sensor developers, especially in the direction of microsensors, and *in vivo* sensors. Problems such as biocompatibility bring new dimensions to the analytical chemists. Awareness of materials science has had a surprising impact on sensor design that has moved the entire field from conventional 'dip' style sensors to much more sophisticated products. For example, microfabricated sensors allow better measurements under conditions that 'smaller is better', and when low output impedance is necessarily better than high, for example.

On the other hand, different technologies, just because they are new, do not necessarily demand changes in products and processes that are already satisfactory and successful. For example, it is merely interesting to apply 'fast' ion conductors of Na^+ or reconstituted protein Na^+-conducting channels in lipid bilayers to construction of sodium ion sensors. The operating principle is simply that a material is selected that has rapid, reversible interfacial ion exchange and ideal permeability (transference number of unity). Glass polymeric silicate-aluminate membranes and passive plasticized membranes containing synthetic neutral carriers or ion exchangers are already satisfactory, stable, rugged, and generally useful.

THE EDUCATION - COMMUNICATION ROLES: Chemists and Other Disciplines

Discovery of new principles seems to have little to do with the present widespread interest in sensors. Virtually all of the principles of new sensors have been known from classical notions of electrostatics, thermodynamics and transport (in the case of electrochemical sensors), physical optics, energy schemes of optical transitions for absorption and emission, effects of local environment and reactions on transition energies (in the case of optical sensors), and coupled mechanical-electrical-thermal effects (in the case of mass and thermal flux and other physical sensors). Analytical chemists, especially, have realized the need for sensors and detectors. It has been a subsection of analytical chemical science for many years.

The problem has been, and still is, one of organizing the technologies and corresponding specialists. Developing sensors is largely a communication problem. Communication of technology is one part, but communication of basic chemical materials science has been another. The difficulty has been communications of chemical, electrochemical, and analytical spectroscopic ideas to engineers and some physicists. However, the barriers are largely down through the aid of workshops, symposia, personal communications and collaborations. The next barrier is the biochemical and immunoscience interface with analytical chemistry. Progress has been made almost exclusively by bioanalytical chemists who are already conversant with theory and practice of these important fields. In devising the program for this Symposium, tutorials on fundamentals of electrochemical, microelectronic, optical and piezoelectric devices were presented.

THE CHEMICAL SENSOR FIELD

Chemical sensors make up the majority of new sensors. Chemical, including environmental, biochemical, biotechnological, clinical, and medical applications dominate the field. Yet, microfabrication, microstructure, and microelectronic technology is, at least partially, driving research at the present. It should be an important aim of chemists to maintain control of this field since it is the chemistry that provides the recognition processes, while the size, shape, and structure of the device are merely parts of the transduction and/or amplification. Otherwise chemical sensors will be relegated to the eighth volume of a series on solid state sensors!

PROPOSED DEFINITIONS:PHYSICAL, CHEMICAL AND MIXED TRANSDUCER DEVICES

An arrangement that generates a measurable material property is a chemical transducer device. It incorporates a recognition process that is characteristic of the material at the molecular, chemical level, and it incorporates a transduction into a useful signal. A pure physical transducer device generates and transduces a parameter that does not depend on the chemistry *per se*, but is a result of the system responding as aggregates of point masses or charges. There must also be some gray areas that defy these categories. The transduction into 'a useful signal' requires external measurement, and may require a perturbation, i.e. an optical absorption change requires a probing light beam. A resistance change requires an applied ac voltage, etc. A voltage generated by a chemical system, a membrane cell or a battery, is clearly a chemical sensing device. A thermistor temperature measurement of an arbitrary phase does not reflect the chemistry and so is physical. A thermocouple voltage measurement could conceivably be either chemical or physical: to determine an alloy composition at constant temperature, or to measure temperature with a known or calibrated alloy. Certain measurements: vibration, force, displacement, velocity, acceleration, flow rate, volume, time, and 3-D structure are most often physical. However chemical effects on displacement or vibration are the basis of piezoelectric devices. Temperature changes from background, optical transmission, absorption, refraction, emission and scattering changes, magnetic permeability changes, voltage, current, resistance, and capacitance changes are most often the transduction part of chemical sensor devices.

PROPOSED DEFINITIONS:CHEMICAL SENSORS AND BIOSENSORS

Chemical sensors are those that use chemical processes in the recognition and transduction steps. Biosensors are a subsection of chemical sensors that use biological recognition processes. Both are intrinsically 'chemical'.

SENSORS VS SYSTEMS: SELECTIVITY, SENSITIVITY, AMPLIFICATION

Selectivity is a measure of a sensor's ability to discriminate among species of similar chemical character. It is connected with the sensors primary 'recognition' function. On the other hand, the inherent transduction provides some amplification which is further enhanced by the measuring circuit. Thus, sensitivity which is the measure of low level detectability is connected with amplification. Smart sensors have the amplification 'on board'. But as soon as one attempts to improve selectivity or sensitivity, by additional separation steps or addition hardware, the sensor becomes a system. Once again there can be gray areas when distinguishing sensors from sensor systems. Often it is perfectly clear, e.g. when a whole chromatographic system contains a sensor at a distinguishable point.

SENSORS, DETECTORS, ACTUATORS AND DOSIMETERS

Sensors are chemically reversible devices. When an ambient is presented to the sensor, the interfacial processes are rapid and reversible. Ideally, a response to a step up in measured quantity reaches a steady state value as soon as the external surface concentration reaches the bulk value by usual transport processes. A step down returns the response to a lesser value or to baseline. Continuous cycling of steps up and steps down, of various magnitudes, should develop a steady state calibration response. Some level of hysteresis must be expected and a slow move of base line response may be tolerated and corrected by sequential standard samples. Some sensors are not reversible and, in the worst case, are one-time detectors that self destruct or become insensitive after a single measurement. Actuators are sensors or detectors combined with an active output. Dosimeters are virtually unsaturable irreversible detectors that continue to accumulate a one directional input signal.

II

Microelectrodes and Microelectronic Devices

2
Solid State Potentiometric Sensors

Jiri Janata

Center for Sensor Technology
University of Utah, Salt Lake City
Utah, 84112, U.S.A.

1. Introduction

It is more than fifteen years ago since the first integrated solid state electrochemical sensors have been described [1,2]. These were ion-sensitive field effect transistors (ISFET) which belong to the group of electrochemical sensors, specifically potentiometric sensors. Since then, other solid state electrochemical and non-electrochemical sensors have appeared and the ISFETs themselves have reached the state of maturity which now brings some of them close to commercialization. This is quite remarkable if we realize that only a relatively few researchers have been working in this area, certainly as compared to the related ion selective electrodes. The obstacles which had to be overcome have been both of the conceptual and practical nature originating from the fact that these devices are the product of integration of two seemingly diverse technologies: solid state device physics and electrochemistry. Soon after the initial explorations of the ISFETs, transistors utilizing enzymatic selectivity [3] and potentiometric solid state sensors based on

This paper was originally presented at the Electrofinn Analysis Conference, Turku, Finland June 6-9, 1988.

chemical modulation of electron work function [4] have appeared. The purpose of this paper is to review the present state of development of these devices both from a theoretical and practical point of view.

2. Ion Sensors

The ion selective membrane can be used in two basic configurations (Fig.1). If the solution is placed on either side of the membrane such arrangement is

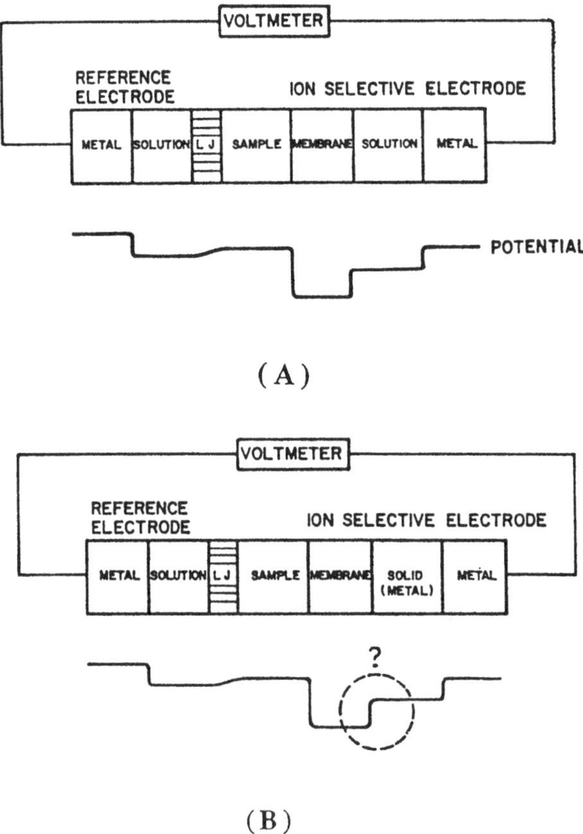

Fig. 1 Schematic representation of the (A) symmetrical and (B) asymmetrical arrangement of ion selective membrane.

called symmetrical. It is found in conventional ion selective electrodes in which the internal electrical contact is provided through the solution in which an internal reference electrode is immersed. In the non-symmetrical arrangement one side of the membrane is contacted by the sample (usually aqueous) while the other side is contacted by some solid material. An example of this type are coated wire electrodes and ion sensitive field effect transistors.

In a conventional ion selective electrode the membrane is placed between the sample and the internal reference solution. The composition of the internal solution can be optimized with respect to the membrane and the sample solution. In the interest of symmetry it is advisable to use the same solvent inside the electrode as is in the sample. This solution also contains the determinand ion in the concentration which is usually in the middle of the dynamic range of the response of the membrane. The ohmic contact with the internal reference electrode is provided by adding the salt which contains the appropriate ion to form a fast reversible couple with the solid conductor. In recent designs gel-forming polymers have been added into the internal compartment. They do not significantly alter the electrochemistry but add some convenience in handling.

The obvious advantage of the symmetrical arrangement is that the processes at all internal interfaces can be well defined and that most non-idealities at the membrane/solution interface tend to cancel out. Because the volume of the internal reference compartment is typically a few milliliters the electrode does not suffer from exposure to electrically neutral compounds which would penetrate the membrane and change the composition of this solution. This type of potentiometric ion sensor has been used in a majority of basic studies of ion selective electrodes and most commercial ion selective electrodes are also of this type. The drawbacks of this arrangement are also related to the presence of the internal solution and to its volume. Mainly for this reason it is not conveniently possible to miniaturize it and to integrate it into a multi-sensor package.

The general tendency to miniaturize chemical sensors and to make them more convenient has led to the development of potentiometric sensors with solid internal contact. These sensors include coated wire electrodes (CWE), hybrid sensors and ion sensitive field-effect transistors (ISFET). The contact can be a conductor, semiconductor or even an insulator. The price which has to be paid for the convenience of these sensors is in the more restrictive design rules which have to be followed in order to obtain a sensor with performance comparable to the conventional symmetrical ion selective electrode.

The key issue in these sensors is the interface between the ion selective membrane and the contact. The most convenient way to present this problem is in the form of the equivalent electrical circuit in which the resistances and capacitances have their usual electrochemical meaning (Fig. 2). It is necessary to include the

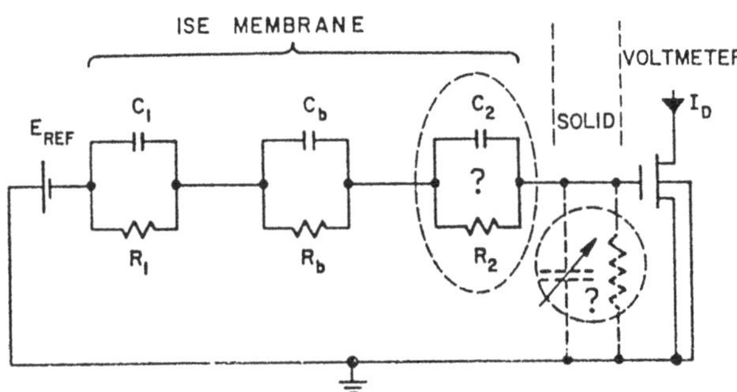

Fig. 2 Equivalent electrical circuit of a coated wire electrode and an ISFET.

electrometer (or at least its input stage) in the analysis of these sensors. In most modern instruments the amplifier is an insulated gate field-effect transistor (IGFET) which has an input dc resistance of greater than 10^{14} Ω and an input capacitance on the order of picofarads.

The internal contact between the membrane and the preamplifier represents a parasitic impedance. Let us consider two limiting cases concerning the values of the equivalent resistances in Fig. 2. A good ion selective electrode has high exchange current density and therefore low value of the charge transfer resistance R_1 ($i_o = 10^{-3}$ A cm^{-2}, i.e. $R_{ct} = 25\ \Omega$ cm^2). This means that at least one charged species can transfer easily between the sample and the membrane and establish the potential difference according to one of the mechanisms discussed above. The bulk membrane resistance R_b can be as high as $10^6\ \Omega$ cm^2. However, because no net current passes through the membrane, the potential in the bulk of the membrane is uniform, i.e. there is no electric field inside the membrane. In a conventional symmetrical ISE arrangement the composition of the internal solution can be always chosen in such a way that the interfacial charge transfer resistance R_2 is comparable to R_1. Thus, a well established potential profile exists throughout this structure. On the other hand if the R_2 is high, the input capacitor together with the interfacial capacitance C_2 and the (variable) parasitic capacitance form a (variable) capacitive divider. In such a case the voltage which appears at the input capacitor of the electrometer depends not only on the electrostatic potential of the membrane but also on the undefined parasitic impedance of the connector, and the electrode exhibits unstable characteristics.

The simplest example of a potentiometric ion sensor with solid internal contact is a coated wire electrode (CWE) in which the internal wire is covered with an ion selective polymeric membrane thus forming a compact and inexpensive ion sensor [5]. Noble metal internal wires were used in the early designs of the CWE, mainly for the reasons of their chemical stability. Such electrodes often exhibited unacceptable drift. The high value of the internal charge transfer resistance at the membrane/wire interface has been recognized as being the cause of this problem [6]. It is not surprising if we realize that the typical electrode reactions at noble metals are of the redox type, i.e. the charge transferring species is the electron. On the other hand in most ion selective membranes the charge conduction is done by ions. Thus, a mismatch between the charge transfer carriers can exist at the noble metal/membrane interface. This is particularly true for polymer based membranes which are invariably ionic conductors. On the other hand solid state membranes which exhibit mixed ionic and electronic conductivity such as chalcogenide glasses, perovskites, and silver halides form good contact with noble metals.

Several solutions of the problem of the conducting internal contact have been suggested. The most direct approach involves the interposition of a thin layer of aqueous gel which contains the fixed concentration of the salt of the primary ion. This approach, which has met with only a limited success, can be seen as the miniaturization of the conventional ISE structure. The main reason for its failure is the fact that water can permeate through the membrane and establish its own activity inside the sensor structure according to its chemical potential in each individual phase. In other words, the water permeating through the membrane reaches its osmotic equilibrium according to the concentration of the solutes present in the gel. This can lead not only to the significant change of the internal activity of the primary salt inside the gel but often to a catastrophic failure of the whole structure when the osmotic pressure inside the gel exceeds the limits of the mechanical stability of the membrane. This problem cannot be avoided because the osmolality of the sample is not known a priori and cannot be controlled during the experiment. The second problem relates to the Severinghaus effect (vide infra). In principle this problem can be avoided by establishing an electrochemical reaction with as high exchange current density as possible at the internal interface, by interposing a thin layer of Ag/AgCl between the membrane and the insulator [7] with the hope that the chloride ion exchange will dominate the internal interfacial potential. Using this strategy ISFETs without the Severinghaus interference have been prepared. In principle the same effect can cause problems in a conventional ISE, however, mainly due to the relatively large volume (e.g. 3-5ml) of the internal solution it is not observed in practice.

In summary, it is possible to design well behaved CWEs and to expect that their electrochemical performance will be comparable to the conventional ISEs. However, the design of the membrane/solid interface has to be done with the understanding of the electrochemical processes which take place at that interface. If the final resistance is high then the problems such as drift become directly proportional to the length of the internal contact, specifically to the magnitude of the parasitic capacitance and resistance. Consequently, these problems can be minimized by decreasing the distance between the ion selective membrane and the amplifier. The logical stage in progression in the evolution of these sensors are then a hybrid ion sensor [8] and ion sensitive field effect transistor [9] .

The close integration of the ion selective layer with the amplifier, as it occurs in an ISFET, offers some unique sensing possibilities but also creates its own problems. The problem areas of the ISFETs with polymeric membranes are shown in Fig. 3. They have been recognized as the encapsulation (1), adhesion (2) of the

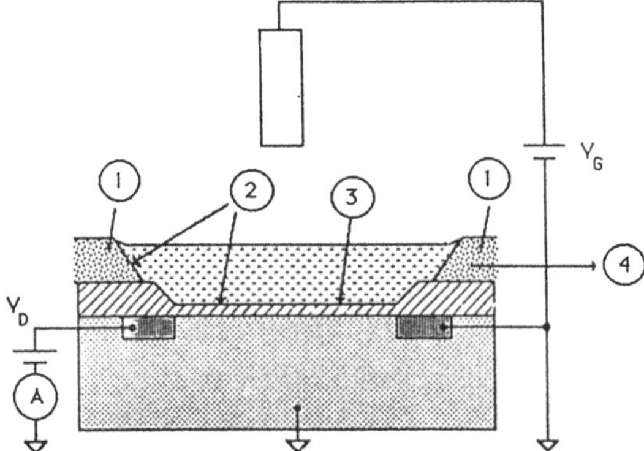

Fig. 3 Problem areas of ISFET: (1) Encapsulation; (2) Membrane adhesion; (3) Acidobasic interference; (4) Crosstalk.

membrane to the chip and to the encapsulation [9], and the acidobasic interference (3) at the membrane/transistor interface [10]. Moreover, the early attempts to deposit several different membranes in close proximity of each other is difficult due to the cross-contamination (4) of these membranes [11]. Most of these problems have now been solved.

It has been found [10] that in some situations electrically neutral species can penetrate through the polymeric membrane of the ISFET and change the value of the interfacial potential at the insulator/membrane interface. This applies especially to the acidobasic species such as CO_2, lower carboxylic acids, ammonia, etc. when the pH of the solution is far from their pK and they exist essentially in undissociated form. In other words, the ion selective membrane of the ISFET cannot reject electrically neutral species.

There have been several attempts to solve the problem of the adhesion of the membrane to the chip surface and to the surrounding encapsulation. The simplest approach has been to silanize the chip prior to the encapsulation step [9]. However, that improves only the adhesion of the encapsulant and of the membrane to the chip surface, but does not prevent the development of the electrical shunt between the membrane and the encapsulant. A much more elaborate solution has been the construction of a suspended polymeric mesh which holds the membrane down [12]. Although it has improved the performance of the individual ISFET it has not solved the problem of preparation of a multiple-membrane ISFET sensor.

A major step forward in encapsulation and multiple membrane deposition has been made recently by using ionophore doping of the generic membrane [13] in combination with some other, previously reported techniques. It is known [14] that plasticized PVC can be made ion selective by doping it with ionophores. It is also known that the optimum performance is obtained from the ISFET if the ion-selective membrane forms a continuous envelope around the encapsulated chip [15]. This eliminates the interface between the encapsulant and the membrane which causes the electrical shunt. Because the distances between the individual ion-selective gates of a multisensing chip are short, it is essential that the lateral diffusion of the electroactive ingredients of the individual membranes is minimized. The new plasticizer, bis-(2-ethylhexyl)sebacate used in these membranes [16] decreases the lateral diffusion 100 fold as compared with the conventional plasticizers. The final contribution to this development came from the use of photolithographically produced encapsulation most of which is done at the wafer level [17]. The result is a dual-gate ISFET in which the long term drift is < 0.05 mV hr^{-1} and with the usable lifetime of approximately 2 months. Clearly there is a room for further improvement. Thus, the encapsulation process will further benefit from the recently developed electrochemical encapsulation [18]. The primary adhesion of the membrane to the chip can be further improved by using carboxylated PVC [19]. The high concentration of the carboxylic group also has a beneficial effect on the electrochemical properties of the membrane, particularly on the rejection of the anions due to the Donnan failure [20]. Therefore, the optimum configuration is an ISFET with a continuous carboxylated PVC membrane which is individually doped with a suitable ionophore over the respective gate areas. The gates themselves contain a thin layer of Ag/AgCl which eliminates the interference from the neutral species.

Finally a few words about the pH ISFET. We must remember that field effect transistor is basically a charge-sensing device. From the very beginning [1,2] of the research of this device, it has been known that the FET with a bare gate insulator exposed to the solution responds to changes of pH. Because pH is such an important parameter to measure a very considerable amount of research and speculation has been devoted to the explanation of the mechanism of this response. Clearly, there is a pH-dependent charge at the solution/transistor interface. The slope of this response has been found to vary between 50% of theoretical for SiO_2 to 92% for silicon nitride. Other materials such as Al_2O_3 or Ta_2O_5 and other oxides have been reported to yield nearly theoretical responses. It is necessary to pause here and to realize that all these materials are very good bulk insulators. Therefore, they could not be used as pH-sensing membranes in a conventional ISE configuration. However, in an ISFET configuration these materials are the part of the input gate capacitor, and their use is possible.

It is quite adequate to accept the fact that the pH-dependent charge resides somewhere at the insulator "surface" and that the corresponding image charge in the transistor channel affects the transconductance. Let us now invoke the basic electrochemical characteristics of the interface, the distinction between the non-polarized (resistive) and polarized (capacitive) interface. The argument about the location of the pH-dependent charge has revolved around this distinction: one school of thought has been that the charge is located in one plane, at the surface of the insulator and that the interface behaves as a capacitor at which the charge is generated by the de-protonation/protonation of the surface bound sites. This is the basis of so called "site-binding theory" (SBT). In this theory it is assumed that there are ionizable binding sites present at the surface of the insulator which determine the distribution of the compensating charge in the adjacent layer of solution. This distribution is the result of the interplay between the thermal forces and electrostatic forces originating in the fixed pH-dependent charge at the surface as governed by the Poisson-Boltzmann distribution. It leads to the Gouy-Chapman model of the diffuse layer which is formally identical with other models of space charge distribution. The potential decays exponentially from its surface value ψ_0

$$\psi_x = \psi_0 \exp(-\kappa x) \qquad (1)$$

with the effective thickness κ^{-1} of the space charge region being defined as

$$(8\pi C_0 z^2 e_0^2/\varepsilon kT)^{1/2} = \kappa \qquad (2)$$

where ε is the dielectric constant, C_0 is the bulk concentration and e_0 is the charge of electron.

The other model postulates the existence of the hydrated layer of finite thickness within which the de-protonated/protonated sites are situated. Clearly, in the limit of zero thickness of the hydrated layer the two theories merge. It is obvious that the SBT models the interface as a capacitor with one plate located at the surface and the other at the average distance κ^{-1} in solution. In other words the interface is considered to be ideally polarized. On the other hand the hydration layer model allows penetration of at least one type of ion through the interface and thus considers this interface to be non-polarized. How much non-polarized depends on the value of the exchange current density of the communicating ion(s). The equivalent electrical model is, of course, a parallel capacitor/resistor combination. From the point of view of the response it is obvious that the interface described by the capacitive model (SBT) would respond to adsorption of any charged species inside the space charge region. On the other hand, adsorption would have little or no effect on the potential difference at the interface described by the hydration layer model because that potential difference is uniquely and unequivocally given by the Nernst equation. Of course the complicating factor in a real situation would be the existence of the mixed potential at the interfaces which have low total exchange current density.

The common ground to accommodate both models has been proposed by Sandifer [21] who has shown that the sub-Nernstian response of some materials and the presence of troublesome adsorption and stirring effects can be rationalized by considering the number of available binding sites and the thickness of the hydrated layer. The magnitude of the exchange current density depends on the concentration of the binding sites inside the hydrated layer. For the glass electrode this is estimated to be 3.2M [22]. As the number of binding sites decreases from 3 to 0.1M the interfacial potential of a 10Å thick layer is increasingly affected by adsorption (Fig. 4) and the response deviates more from theoretical. On the other hand, both the adsorption effects and the sub-Nernstian behavior vanish if the thickness of the hydrated layer is allowed to exceed the thickness of the space charge layer inside the membrane Fig.5. This model goes a long way towards explaining some

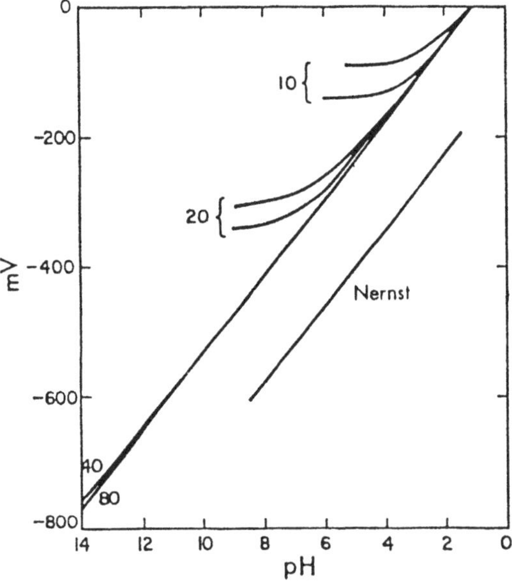

Fig. 4 Effect of adsorption on ISFET surface. The thickness of the hydrated layer (in angstroms) is shown as parameter. The upper curve in each bracketed set corresponds to the absence of adsorption, the lower curve shows the adsorption of 100 mM adsorbate (Reprinted from Ref. 21 with permission of J. Sandifer).

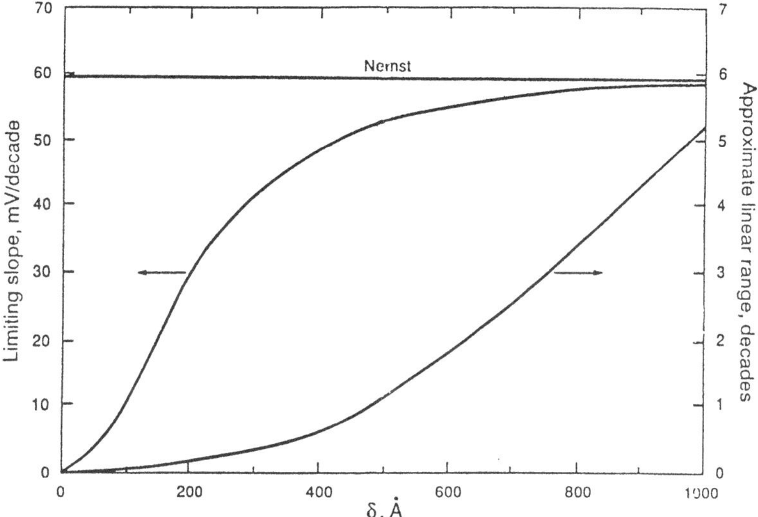

Fig. 5 Effect of thickness of the hydrated layer on slope and dynamic range for the assumed concentration of binding sites C_0 = 0.1 mM. (Reprinted from Ref. 21 with permission of J. Sandifer).

experimental results reported in the literature for ISFETs with oxide or nitride surfaces. Unfortunately, the properties of these materials prepared in different laboratories differ substantially. It is known that silicon nitride forms an oxygen-rich layer at the surface whose thickness depends on the deposition conditions. This "passivation" layer seems to form rapidly but is very stable even under continuous exposure to aqueous electrolyte solutions [9]. The hydration of this layer seems to fit the requirements and predicted behavior of the Sandifer model. The ISFETs which have been exposed to solution for more than one hour show no adsorption effects as would be expected from Sandifers, in contrast with the SBT model.

3. Potentiometric Enzymatic Sensors

Enzymatic reactions combine substrate specificity with the high amplification factor. From that viewpoint they are ideal selective layers for chemical sensors, including potentiometric sensors. However, they are not specifically part of the information acquisition/processing scheme in the Nature. Their exclusive role is to lower, highly selectively, the activation energy barrier of certain reactions, thus acting as regulators. Because of this, their use in various sensing schemes may suffer from the problems related to the mode of coupling with the transducer.

A schematic diagram of an enzymatically coupled potentiometric sensor is shown in Fig. 6. Its basic operating principle is simple: an enzyme (a catalyst) is

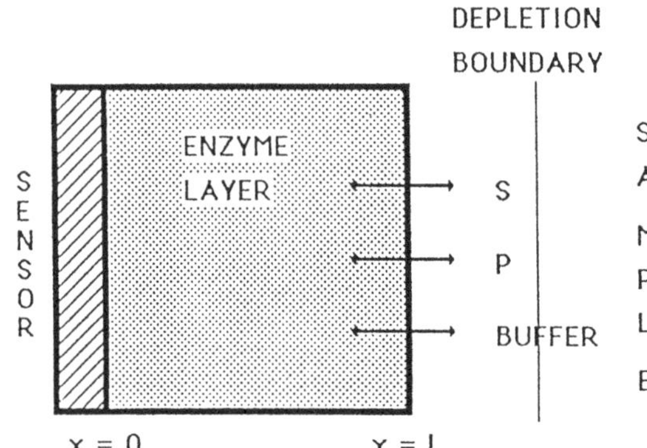

Fig. 6 Potentiometric enzyme sensor.

immobilized inside a layer into which the substrate(s) diffuse. As it does, it reacts according to the Michaelis-Menten mechanism and the product(s) diffuse out of the layer, into the solution. Any other species which participate in the reaction must also diffuse in and out of the layer. Because of the combined mass transport and chemical reaction this problem is often referred to as diffusion-reaction mechanism. It is quite common in electrochemical reactions where the electroactive species which undergo chemical transformation at the electrode, participates in some coupled chemical reactions. Mathematically this case is described by a set of second-order partial differential equations which are usually solved numerically. Because enzymes operate only in an aqueous environment the immobilization matrices are gels, specifically hydrogels.

The general diffusion-reaction equation for species i in one direction (x) is

$$\frac{\partial C_i}{\partial t} = + D_i \frac{\partial^2 C_i}{\partial x^2} \pm R(C_i) \quad (3)$$

When the pH-dependent Michaelis-Menten equation is substituted for the reaction term R (C_i) we obtain for substrate S

$$\frac{\partial C_S}{\partial t} = D_S \frac{\partial^2 C_S}{\partial x^2} - \frac{V_m C_S}{\Re(pH)(C_S + K_m)} \qquad (4)$$

It is convenient to normalize the variables in Eq.4 with respect to the gel layer thickness, bulk concentrations and characteristic diffusional time. The normalized diffusion-reaction equation is then

$$\frac{\partial C_S}{\partial t} = D_S \frac{\partial^2 C_S}{\partial x^2} - \frac{\phi^2 C_S}{1 + C_S} \qquad (5)$$

where ϕ is so called Thiele modulus.

$$\phi = L\,[V_m/K_m D_S\,\Re(pH)]^{1/2} \qquad (6)$$

This transformation is done for all variables. For $\phi > 10$ the mechanism is diffusion controlled. Conversely, for small values of the Thiele modulus the process is reaction controlled, which means that the diffusional fluxes of all species participating in the reaction (Eq. 5) are greater than the reaction term.

The actual solution of this problem depends on the initial and boundary conditions. These, in turn, depend on the approximations chosen for the model. Let us now review briefly the approximations which have been made for the enzymatically coupled potentiometric sensors and rank them in approximate order of seriousness.

(1) linear diffusion gradient inside the enzyme layer
(2) no partitioning of reactants and products between the gel and the sample
(3) no depletion layer at the gel/sample boundary
(4) no effect of mobile buffer capacity
(5) no effect of fixed buffer capacity
(6) no pH dependence of K_m
(7) no Donnan potential at the gel/sample boundary
(8) rates of protonation reactions are fast

Approximation (1) is a bad one despite the fact that it leads to a simple mathematical solution: The concentration profiles are not linear. The partitioning of species between the gel and the sample (2) is also related to the existence of the Donnan potential (7) but it is a problem even for electrically neutral species (e.g. oxygen). If the solution is stirred the effect of the depletion layer at the gel/membrane interface is negligible (3). However, it could be a problem in stationary solutions. Approximations (4) through (6) would be the most serious for enzymatic sensors in which the output is related to the change of pH, because then the buffer capacity would have to be low. However, for sensors which use some other reactants/products than hydrogen ion a large excess of buffer would make the effects due to these assumptions negligible. Finally, rates of (almost) all protonation reactions (8) are extremely fast and they can be safely assumed to be instantaneous on the time-scale of all the other processes.

With these assumptions in mind we will now complete the outline of the solution of the diffusion-reaction problem as it applies to the most difficult case, the pH based enzymatic sensors. We assume only that there is no depletion layer at the gel/solution boundary (3), there is no fixed buffer capacity (5) and that the protonation reactions are very fast (8). The objective of this exercise is to find out the optimum thickness of the gel layer which is critically important for all zero-flux-boundary sensors.

As a rule, hydrogen ion is involved not only in the pH-dependency of the reaction term (Thiele modulus) but also as the actively participating species involved in the acid-base equilibrium of the substrates, reaction intermediates, and products. Furthermore, enzymatic reactions are always carried out in the presence of a mobile buffer. By mobile we mean a weak acid or a weak base which can move in and out of the reaction layer, as opposed to immobile buffer represented by the gel (and the protein) itself. Thus, we have to include the normalized diffusion- reaction equation for hydrogen ion and for the buffer species. These equations have to be coupled with the buffer dissociation equilibrium.

Next we have to define the boundary and the initial conditions. For so called "zero flux" sensors there is no transport of any of the participating species across the sensor/enzyme layer boundary. Such condition would apply to e.g. optical, thermal or potentiometric enzyme sensors. In that case the first space derivatives of all variables at point x are zero. On the other hand, amperometric sensors would fall into the category of "non-zero-flux sensors" by this definition and the flux of at least one of the species (product or substrate) would be given by the current through the electrode.

The lack of the depletion layer at the gel/solution boundary (x=L) is guaranteed by stirring of the sample. Under those conditions the concentration of all species at that boundary is equal to the bulk values, and the initial conditions correspond to the situation in which all species except the substrate are initially present inside the enzyme layer.

This is a system of stiff, second-order partial differential equations which can be solved numerically to yield both transient, and steady state concentration profiles within the layer. Comparison of the experimental calibration curves and of the time response curves with the calculated ones provides the verification of the proposed model from which it is possible to determine the optimum thickness of the enzyme layer. Because the Thiele modulus is the controlling parameter in the diffusion-reaction equation, it is obvious from Eq. 6 that the optimum thickness L will depend on the other constants and functions included in the Thiele modulus. Because of this, the optimum thickness will vary from one kinetic scheme to another.

Another important observation is related to the detection limit, dynamic range and sensitivity. For the expected values of the diffusion coefficient (in the gel) of approximately 10^{-6} cm^2 s^{-1} and substrate molecular weights about 300, the detection limit is approximately 10^{-4}M. This is due to the fact that the product of the enzymatic reaction is being removed from the membrane by diffusion with approximately the same rate as it is being supplied. The dynamic range of the sensor depends on the value of the K_m and V_m (which depends on the enzyme loading). Generally speaking, higher loading should extend the dynamic range at the top concentration range. It is often stated incorrectly that "the sensor has close to theoretical dependence" or a "nernstian response" which means that a one-decade change of the bulk concentration of the substrate is expected to yield a one-decade change of the surface (x=0) concentration. In the case of potentiometric enzyme sensors it would yield the slope of approximately 60 mV/decade. It is not intuitively obvious, but clearly evident from the comparison of the experimental and calculated response curves that there is no "general theoretical" slope, each enzymatic sensor having its own depending on the mechanism and on the conditions under which it operates. We must remember, that decade/decade slope would occur only if a constant fraction of the product would reach the x=0 interface. The upper limit of the dynamic range depends on the value of the ratio $V_m/K_m D_S \Re(pH)$ in the Thiele modulus. It can be increased by enzyme loading but, obviously, only up to a point. Normally the dynamic range is approximately between 10^{-4} and 10^{-1}M.

The verification of the proposed model has been done on enzymatic field effect transistors for a diffusion-reaction mechanism involving the oxidation of ß-D-glucose catalyzed by glucose oxidase (GOD)/catalase system [23]

$$\text{GLUCOSE} + E_O \Leftrightarrow [E_O\text{-GLU}] \Rightarrow E_R + \text{GLUCONATE} + H^+$$

$$+$$

$$O_2$$

$$\Updownarrow$$

$$E_O + H_2O_2 \Leftarrow E_R\text{-}O_2$$

$$\Updownarrow \text{ CATALASE}$$

$$H_2O + 1/2\, O_2$$

and for hydrolysis of penicillin catalyzed by ß-lactamase [24]. In both cases hydrogen ion is the species detected by the transistor surface. As has been pointed out earlier, the agreement between the predicted and experimental responses verifies the validity of the model and allows us to plot the concentration profiles inside the gel layer. The required thickness has been found to be approximately 150µ for the glucose sensor and 20µ for the penicillin. From these profiles we can see that the thinner membranes or directly immobilized enzymes would produce a reduced sensitivity. On the other hand, the thicker the enzyme layer the slower the response. Thus, we can trade the time response for the signal-to-noise ratio by adjusting the thickness of the enzyme containing layer.

Other parameters which affect the response characteristics of these sensors are the partitioning coefficients and the diffusion coefficients of all species, and the parameters related to the enzyme activity itself, such as the enzyme concentration, K_m and V_m. They are in turn affected by the preparation of the enzyme layer, e.g. by the degree of crosslinking, by the degree of the inactivation of the enzyme etc.. It is therefore not surprising to find that these devices have generally widely diverse lifetime, time response, detection limits and sensitivity. The value of the experimentally verified model is then mainly in establishing the design parameters not only for potentiometric, but also, for other zero-flux boundary enzymatic sensors. It should be mentioned here that the above analysis of the potentiometric enzyme sensors has been done for ENFETs but that it is equally applicable for other types of enzymatic potentiometric sensors.

Because each enzyme sensor has its own unique response, it is necessary to construct the calibration curve for each sensor separately. The obvious way to reduce interferences is to use two sensors in differential mode. It is possible to prepare two identical enzyme sensors and either omit or deactivate the enzyme in one of them. This sensor then acts as a reference device. If the calibration curve is constructed by plotting the difference of the two outputs as the function of concentration of the substrate the effects of variations in the ambient composition of the sample as well as temperature and light sensitivity can be substantially reduced.

4. Work Function Sensors

The macroscopic device analogous to a solid state potentiometric work function sensor is the vibrating capacitor or so called Kelvin probe [25]. The chemical modulation of the electron work function is a relatively new principle applied to chemical sensing. It relies on the fact that the two principal components of the electron work function, the Fermi level and the surface potential, of an organic layer change when a chemical species is adsorbed on or absorbed in such a layer. In order to make use of this effect we have developed a suspended gate field-effect transistor (SGFET) into which the organic polymer is introduced by electrochemical deposition (Fig. 7). An advantage of this type of sensor is that a wide variety of organic semiconductors with different selectivity can be applied and used in a well controlled manner. This is particularly important for the fabrication of multisensors [26,27]. Furthermore, because this is a potentiometric (equilibrium) sensor, there is no special requirement on the conductivity of the organic layer. The only pre-requisite is that it makes an electronic contact with the suspended metal gate, the condition which is easily satisfied for electrodeposited layers.

The origin of the chemical signal can be expressed in thermodynamic terms.

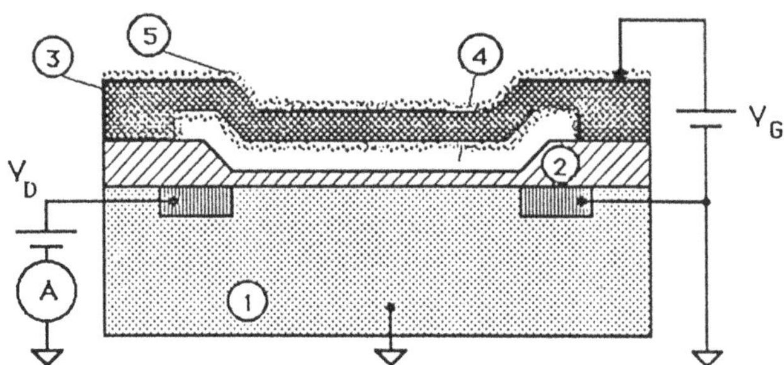

Fig. 7 Diagram of the suspended gate field-effect transistor. 1- substrate; 2- insulator; 3- suspended metal gate; 4- gap; 5- chemically selective layer.

At equilibrium the number of moles, n, of all species and their chemical potentials, μ, in a phase (e.g. in a chemically selective layer) are related through the Gibbs-Duhem equation according to which if a new species enters the organic layer the chemical potentials of all species in that layer must change. These include the change of the electrochemical potential of the electron - the Fermi level and therefore the electron work function.

The graphical representation of the situation in the gate of SGFET is shown in Fig. 8 where the energy band diagram of the chemically selective layer is shown. In this figure the material is considered to be a p-type semiconductor. The position of the energy level for the dopant and thus the position of the Fermi level in the whole phase depends on the position of the intrinsic Fermi level of the pure material, E_{FI}, on the electron donor / acceptor properties of the dopant and, if the dopant is charged, on the occupational density of the donor states E_D. Therefore, for a n-type material the dopant energy level (donor) would be located close to the conduction band edge, E_C, and the Fermi level would be closer to that edge accordingly. In Fig. 8 the acceptor molecules (i.e. p-type semiconductor) are considered to be charged and therefore their distribution depends on their occupancy. This fact is shown by the symbol for a distribution ($\succ$) in Fig. 8.

The electrochemical potential of an electron can be expressed as the sum of the chemical potential and electrostatic energy, $e\phi_G$

$$\mu = \mu - e\phi_G \tag{7}$$

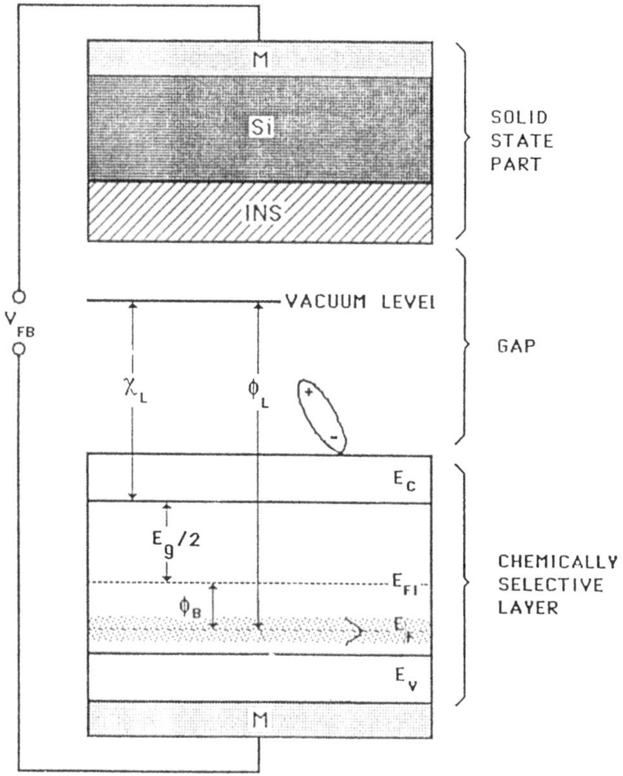

Fig. 8 Energy band diagram of the gate of SGFET.

where ϕ_G is the bulk (Galvani) potential of the phase. Because this energy is referenced against vacuum level, it consists of the energy contributions resulting from the bulk potential $\psi = (\phi_B + Eg/2)$ and from the surface (dipole) potential χ. Thus,

$$\mu' = \mu' + e\chi + e\psi \qquad (8)$$

The work function of the chemically sensitive layer ϕ_L is then

$$-\phi_L = \mu_L - e\chi_L \qquad (9)$$

From Eq. 9 we see that the chemical modulation of the work function can originate from two effects: action of the guest molecule on the energy state distribution in the bulk of the phase, i.e. by the absorption term μ_L in Eq.9 or by modulation of the surface potential χ_L , i.e. by adsorption. These two terms have different dependence on the activity of the guest molecule. The chemical potential follows the logarithmic law while the surface concentration depends on the type of the applicable adsorption isotherm. This may, in fact, create some problems in resolving the two types of contributions to the overall change of the work function because the relative degree of their contribution is not known *a priori.*

An example of an organic layer which changes its work function due to chemical modulation is electrochemically deposited polypyrrole. Because of its strong hydrogen bonding properties, it binds water, alcohols, acetonitrile, etc. [26,27]. It can be deposited under a variety of conditions such as different deposition potential, different electrolyte, different solvents and additives. The result is a spectrum of materials which show different affinity to different chemical species.

5. Summary

Modern potentiometric sensors rely on the close integration of the high impedance pre-amplifier with the chemically selective part of the device. The rules under which this integration has to be done are well understood and solutions to most practical problems have been developed. Because of the convenience of their use and the possibility to group them into multisensors, these sensors can be seen as a logical replacement for traditional ion-selective and enzyme electrodes. The possibility of using the chemical modulation of electron work function represents a new general principle for potentiometric sensing in gases and dielectric fluids.

Acknowledgement

The financial assistance for presentation of this paper provided by the Humboldt Stiftung is gratefully acknowledged.

REFERENCES

1. P. Bergveld, *IEEE-Trans. BME-19*, 70 (1970).

2. T. Matsuo, M. Esashi and K. Inuma, *Digest of Joint Meeting of Tohoku Sections of IEEE* (1971).

3. S. Caras and J. Janata, *Anal. Chem.*, **52**, 1935 (1980).

4. I. Lundstrom and C. Svensson in *Solid State Chemical Sensors*, (J. Janata and R. J. Huber, eds.), Academic Press, 1985.

5. H. Freiser, Coated Wire Ion Selective Electrodes, Chapter 2, Ion-Selective Electrodes in *Analytical Chemistry,* Vol. 2 (H. Freiser, ed.), Plenum Press, New York, 1980.

6. M. Trojanowicz, Z. Augustowska, W. Matuszewski, G. Moraczewska and A. Hulanicki, *Talanta*, **29**, 113 (1982).

7. X. Li, M. J. Verpoorte and D. J. Harrison, *Anal. Chem.*, **60**, 493 (1988).

8. T. A. Fjeldy and K. Nagy, *J. Electrochem. Soc.*, **127**, 1299 (1980).

9. J. Janata and R. J. Huber, in *Ion Selective Electrodes in Analytical Chemistry*, Vol. 2 (H. Freiser, ed.),1983.

10. E. J. Fogt, D. F. Untereker, M. S. Norenberg and M. E. Meyerhoff, *Anal. Chem.*, **57**, 1995 (1985).

11. R. B. Brown, R. J. Huber and J. Janata, *Proc. Transducers*, Philadelphia, June 1985.

12. G. F. Blackburn and J. Janata, *J. Electrochem. Soc.*, **129**, 2580 (1982).

13. K. Bezegh, A. Bezegh, J. Janata, U. Oesch, Aiping Xu and W. Simon, *Anal. Chem.*, **59**, 2846 (1987).

14. E. J. Fogt, P. T. Calahan, A. Jevne and M. A. Schwinghammer, *Anal. Chem.*, **57**, 1155 (1985).

15. P. T. McBride, J. Janata, P. A. Comte, S. D. Moss and C. C. Johnson, *Anal. Chim. Acta*, **101**, 239 (1978).

16. U. Oesch, A. Xu, Z. Brzozka, G. Suter and W. Simon, *Chimia*, **40**, 351 (1986).

17. N. J. Ho, J. Kratochvil, G. F. Blackburn and J. Janata, *Sensors and Actuators*, **4**, 413 (1983).

18. K. Potje-Kamloth, M. Josowicz and J. Janata, Anal. Chem. 1988 submitted.

19. T. Satchwill, and D. J. Harrison, *J. Electroanal. Chem.*, **202**, 75 (1986).

20. E. Lindner, E. Graf, Z. Niegreisz, K. Toth, E. Pungor and R. P. Buck, *Anal. Chem.*, **60**, 295 (1988).

21. J. R. Sandifer, *Anal.Chem.*, **60**, 1553 (1988).

22. G. Eisenmann "Glass Electrodes for Hydrogen and Other Cations", Marcel Dekker, New York ,1967.

23. S. D. Caras, D. Petelenz and J. Janata, *Anal. Chem.*, **57**, 1920 (1985).

24. S. D. Caras and J. Janata, *Anal. Chem.*, **57**, 1924 (1985).

25. M. Josowicz and J. Janata, in *Chemical Sensor Technology*, Vol 1, (T. Seiyama, ed.), Kodansha Ltd., 1988.

26. Josowicz, M., and Janata, J., *Anal.Chem.*, **58**, 514 (1986).

27. Josowicz, M., Janata, J., Ashley, K. and Pons, S., *Anal. Chem.*, **59**, 253 (1987).

3

Voltammetric Detection of Neurotransmitter Release

R. MARK WIGHTMAN UNIVERSITY OF NORTH CAROLINA
CHAPEL HILL, NORTH CAROLINA

To understand more about the structure and function of the brain is one of the largest challenges for modern science. In the early 1970's Ralph Adams proposed that electroanalytical techniques could aid in this endeavor by providing a selective way to monitor the concentration of the catecholamines and serotonin, neurotransmitters of considerable importance in the brain. The early work of Adams and his coworkers (1) established techniques such as liquid chromatography with electrochemical detection (LCEC) that are now widely used in a number of different neuroscience laboratories. The topic of this review, in vivo voltammetric measurements of dopamine, also originated in his laboratory. Today, several voltammetric approaches are available for reliable in vivo use, especially for the study of dopamine, the subject of our research. At the same time, our increased understanding of the brain environment has led to the definition of a series of new questions that require improved in vivo methods. This review is intended to show some of the ways in which these questions have been approached.

Dopamine was first considered to be a neurotransmitter in the late 1950's (2,3). Using a fluorescence assay, neuroscientists were able to show that this compound is found in high amounts (50 nmoles/gram) in a region of the brain known as the caudate nucleus. In the 1960's it was shown that patients with Parkinson's disease show an almost complete depletion of dopamine in this region. The pathways of dopamine-containing neurons have been mapped in the rat brain making it an ideal species for the further characterization of this system. Dopamine neurons in the caudate nucleus were demonstrated to have the capability to uptake dopamine from the surrounding fluid which can inactivate dopamine neurotransmission. It was further shown that drugs of abuse such as cocaine and amphetamine could inhibit this uptake process, and this cellular action correlates with the behavioral changes induced by these drugs. A correlation also exists between the binding of antipsychotic drugs to dopamine receptors and their efficacy in controlling the symptoms of schizophrenia. Thus, the interest in dopamine neurotransmission is far reaching, as it seems that the proper regulation of this process is required for normal functioning and behavior.

The ability to monitor dopamine neurotransmission directly could provide useful insights into this process, and this fundamental information may in turn be beneficial in the design of therapies for disease states associated with dopamine systems. For example, microelectrodes have been used to monitor the capability of cell transplants to release catecholamines (4). This procedure tests the viability of these cells to release catecholamines before and after transplant and can provide information necessary for the evaluation of the efficacy of this approach. While our investigations are on a more fundamental level, they should lead to an increased understanding of dopamine function in the brain.

1. Methods to Sample Compounds in the Extracellular Space of the Brain.

Several approaches have been taken to sample the chemical species found in the extracellular space of the brain. Among the first was the push-pull perfusion cannula which consists of two concentric tubes through which physiological fluid is simultaneously infused (pushed) and withdrawn (pulled) (5,6). In this way the compounds in the brain are removed and can be analyzed using any technique suitable for use with small volumes. Radiolabelled substances were used in early studies because of the low amounts present. The high sensitivity of LCEC makes it ideal for these analyses (7,8).

An improvement in the push-pull method is the dialysis perfusion cannula first devised by Ungerstedt (9). This is similar to the earlier device with the flow of perfusion fluid now enclosed within a dialysis membrane. Small molecules present in the external medium can diffuse across the membrane and be removed from the brain. For example, a miniaturized design incorporates small diameter fused silica tubes inserted into a dialysis hollow fiber of 300 μm O.D. (10). The small internal volume of this cannula allows the use of very slow perfusion flow rates (ca. 100 nL/min). With this approach, the low basal concentration of dopamine (~30 nM) in the ECF of the caudate nucleus can be detected (11,12). The change in the concentration of dopamine following a pharmacological stimulus known to exert profound behavioral changes can also be detected with the dialysis methods (13). Thus, dialysis perfusion coupled to smallbore LCEC provides a method capable of quantitative determinations of ECF dopamine levels without the interference of other electroactive substances on a time scale of minutes.

The high sensitivity and selectivity of the dialysis technique have established it as an important tool for the measurement of changes in brain chemistry. Its use will continue to grow because it can be used to sample any compound which can cross the membrane and for which suitable analytical techniques exist. For example, it could be used to measure the rate of penetration of pyschoactive drugs from the bloodstream into the brain. Thus, the development of other <u>in vivo</u> sensors should be aimed at providing complementary measurements. The dimensions of dialysis devices are typically large, on the order of millimeters.

While this makes them applicable to large regions of the rat brain such as the caudate, smaller regions cannot be easily studied. Smaller sensors will provide complementary information on more local concentration changes. Dialysis probes sample on a minute time scale. This is adequate for characterizing pharmacological effects that may occur on a time scale of several minutes to hours. Other forms of _in vivo_ sensors should be capable of faster measurements to provide complementary information related to more rapid methods of neural stimulation.

Voltammetric electrodes meet many of these requirements and have been used for many years to sample chemicals in the brain. Leland Clark was the first to show that this approach could be used to measure oxygen levels and ascorbate concentrations in the mammalian brain (14). In early work, Adams' group showed that the fate of species injected in the brain could be monitored (15), and that homovanillic acid could be monitored in the lateral ventricles following stimulation of dopaminergic pathways (16). Gonon showed that electrochemical surface modification could be used to resolve various compounds (17). However, some of the early work with carbon electrodes was flawed by problems in identification of the detected species (18). This has been the subject of a recent review and most of the problems are now clearly recognized (19).

2. Recent Progress in In Vivo Voltammetry.

To understand the process of neurotransmission more clearly, and to learn about the processes which modulate these events, we would ideally like to monitor chemical dynamics in the synaptic cleft with millisecond time resolution. The probe should be highly selective for the species of interest and capable of measuring the low concentration of neurotransmitters present in the ECF of the brain. The results of dialysis perfusion experiments clearly define the selectivity and sensitivity requirements for an electrode suitable for _in vivo_ detection of dopamine in the caudate nucleus. Furthermore, the probe should provide a stable response so that it can be used for long periods of time. None of these requirements have been totally met to this date, but considerable information can be obtained with methods already developed.

To achieve the small size necessary for in vivo measurements, many investigators have adopted the use of carbon-fiber electrodes (20-22). In the design that we employ, the carbon fiber is sealed inside a glass capillary and bevelled to a sharp tip (23). The sensing area of this device is an ellipse with a minor radius of 5 μm and a major radius of 35 μm. This probe is sufficiently small that considerable information can be obtained concerning the spatial variations in neurotransmitter release in vivo (24). The uncoated electrode can be used to detect a number of neurochemicals including catecholamines and their acid and alcohol metabolites, ascorbic acid, uric acid, and 5-hydroxytryptamine.

To increase selectivity for catecholamines, a perfluorinated ion-exchange membrane (Nafion) is coated on the electrode surface (25). Nafion is a cation-exchange material and improves selectivity because the amine-side chain of dopamine is protonated at physiological pH and thus it can be accumulated at a Nafion coated electrode. In contrast, ascorbate and DOPAC (both weak acids) are anions at this pH, and tend to be excluded, resulting in an approximate 200-fold greater sensitivity for dopamine as compared to these substances. Furthermore, if the coating is sufficiently thin, dopamine can penetrate through the film on a subsecond time scale (26).

The Nafion coating has other advantages besides selectivity. The coated electrodes show less deterioration than bare electrodes when implanted in the brain, and continuous use for up to eight hours is commonplace. Because of the low value of the diffusion coefficient in Nafion ($D = 1x10^{-9}$ cm^2 s^{-1}) the diffusion layer (the region perturbed by electrolysis) is restricted to the interior of the film. This has two advantages--the dopamine-o-quinone, a potential neurotoxin produced by the electrolysis of dopamine, is generated for a brief period of time and is restricted to the interior of the film. In addition, the diffusion layer region is the same in the brain and in solutions in which the electrode is calibrated after the experiment.

To increase the time resolution of the technique, several rapid electrochemical techniques have been employed. Chronoamperometry, a technique in which a potential step is applied to the electrode sufficient to electrolyze the species of interest, has been used by several investigators (27). We have adopted the procedure of fast-scan cyclic voltammetry, a procedure originally developed for _in vivo_ use by Millar et al. (28). In this technique the potential of the electrode is first ramped to a value sufficient to oxidize dopamine and then returned to its initial value in a time of ~ 10 ms. The current measured during this time interval results from oxidation of dopamine and other species adjacent to the electrode as well as background processes which are associated with the electrode surface. The resultant current-voltage curves (voltammograms) obtained in this way are subtracted from one another to provide information on the species which changed in concentration over the time interval of the measurement. Therefore, this method is best suited to determine rapid concentration changes in which the subtraction procedure gives the voltammogram of the species which has changed in concentration. The voltammograms are repeated at 100 ms intervals which is the time scale for dopamine penetration through the film. Thus, these electrodes give an almost instantaneous concentration readout. The advantage of this technique is that voltammograms provide a "fingerprint" for identification because the shapes of the voltammograms for DOPAC, ascorbate, serotonin, and other interferences are quite different from that of dopamine (29).

In vivo voltammetry has been used in several different applications to observe neurotransmitters in the brain. With electrochemically modified electrodes basal concentrations of dopamine in the striatum can be measured (30). However, the waves for DOPAC and dopamine overlap at the electrochemically treated electrode and this procedure is only effective following inhibition of monoamine oxidase. Nafion-coated, electrochemically modified electrodes have been used for the detection of basal concentration of serotonin (31). However, this procedure is not sufficiently selective for dopamine (32). Several investigators have used local potassium injections in the striatum (33-36) to elicit dopamine release. In addition, electrical stimulation of the ascending dopaminergic fibers (27, 37-41) causes dopamine overflow detectable by voltammetry. In both cases the measured changes in signal are unequivocally caused by dopamine. The use of direct neuronal stimulation has been successful for dopamine determination even with electrodes which are only partially selective for dopamine because the stimulus and measurement of dopamine are synchronized (42).

3. Stimulated Dopamine Release.

Stimulation of the medial forebrain bundle has long been used as a method to probe brain function. For example, behavioralists have examined the phenomena of self-stimulation of freely moving rats that can control the stimulation to the brain (43), as well as circling behavior induced by electrical stimulation (44). The use of this technique in neurochemical studies of dopamine in the striatum has been reviewed (3). Roth and coworkers have used this technique to study synthesis regulation, especially in the case of autoreceptor regulation (45). Thus, there is a broad body of work to support the use of stimulation of dopaminergic cell processes to learn more about their chemical aspects. A major thrust of our ongoing research is to use this paradigm to understand more about dopaminergic processes, and at the same time to approach the condition where the natural firing rate of the neuron is used to trigger dopamine release.

In our experimental paradigm, stimulating electrodes are implanted in the medial forebrain bundle, the location of a large group of dopamine axons. Constant-current, biphasic pulses are used to activate these neurons. Electrophysiological studies show that the stimulation conditions employed directly activate dopamine neurons (46). Voltammetric electrodes in the striatum are used to simultaneously monitor the evoked release of dopamine. When the stimulus is initiated, a chemical change is detected within 100 ms. The observed concentration, which depends on the stimulus frequency, rapidly increases during the stimulation, and then returns to the original baseline within a few seconds after cessation of the stimulation (Figure 1A).

The rapid time scale of the concentration changes make it clear that the subsecond time resolution is required to observe these events.

The detected substance is voltammetrically identical to dopamine (Figure 1B). In our laboratory we have adopted five

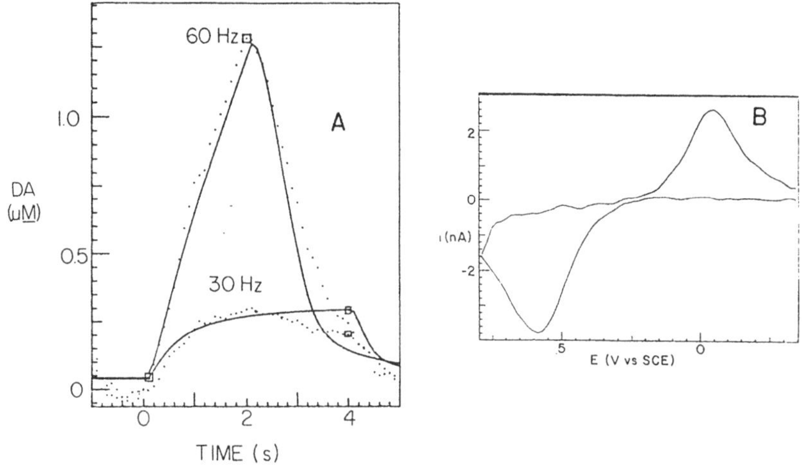

Figure 1. Dopamine concentration in the caudate nucleus during medial forebrain stimulations of different frequency. (A). Temporal changes in response to 30- and 60-Hz stimulations. Dots are experimental points and solid lines are from the model (vide infra). The measured current has been converted to concentration based on post-calibration curves.

(B). Cyclic voltammogram of dopamine obtained <u>in vivo</u>.

criteria which we believe must be met to identify the compound detected with _in vivo_ electrochemistry (47). The criteria for identification are:

1) Voltammetric identity of the monitored and authentic compound.

2) Chemical verification by an independent means.

3) Anatomical specificity of the observed response.

4) Response to stimuli which concurs with the known physiology.

5) Response which concurs with the known pharmacology.

We have used these criteria to identify dopamine in the caudate nucleus and nucleus accumbens following electrical stimulation of the medial forebrain bundle (37b,48). Several other laboratories have adopted our stimulation protocol and have confirmed our results. For example, it has been confirmed that DOPAC is formed on a much slower time scale than seen in Figure 1 (49). In our original work (37), we employed stimulation frequencies of 60 Hz only. In part this was because our limit of detection for dopamine was sufficiently high so that the lower concentrations which are a result of lower stimulation frequencies were difficult to detect. As a result of instrumentation improvements and data processing we are now capable of detecting the 100 nM concentration that occurs as a result of 10 Hz stimuli. Recently, others have reported the detection of 40 nM using our instrumentation and approach (50).

4. Interpretation of the In Vivo Results.

The results in Figure 1 are satisfying at first glance--the goal of detecting dopamine concentration changes in the brain as a result of stimulated neuronal activity has been achieved. But, at the same time, the results raise several questions. The first two that we have tried to answer are:

1. What is the diffusional environment at the electrode tip? Where is the electrode with respect to the synapse?

2. What does the observation of a neurotransmitter mean with respect to neurotransmission?

Since the electrode is much larger than a synapse, the measurements must be of dopamine which "overflows" from the synaptic region into the extracellular space and diffuses to the electrode tip. However, the distance over which dopamine can diffuse during a 4-s, 30-Hz stimulation is relatively small ($l = (Dt)^{1/2}$) and thus the dopamine must come from nerve terminals within a radius of less than ~50 μm from the electrode. We find that movement of the electrode small distances (100 μm) inside the striatum can drastically alter the amplitude of the measured response, further supporting the view that we are sampling from a small, heterogeneous population of nerve terminals (24). Although single unit recordings show that neuronal activity ceases at the end of the stimulation, we often find that dopamine overflow appears to continue past this time. As we have shown, this is also evidence for the diffusion of dopamine from the release site to the electrode surface (40,51). This process can be modeled by a convolution procedure which requires a knowledge of the diffusion coefficient of dopamine and an estimate of the diffusion distance. Such modeling fits well to diffusion distances of 5-10 μm.

In a series of papers we have demonstrated that a neurochemical model can be constructed which, when combined with the diffusion processes described above, has all of the features of the measured <u>in vivo</u> data obtained during medial forebrain stimulation (40,52,53). In this model the measured overflow is expressed as a combination of the kinetic processes of release and uptake. The rate equation is:

$$\frac{d\,[DA]}{dt} = [DA]_p f - \frac{V_{max}}{[K_m/[DA]] + 1}$$

where [DA] is the instantaneous concentration of dopamine and f is the stimulus frequency. The second term on the right describes uptake which we have shown is best described in the striatum by a single component (54) with a K_m value of 200 nM. The V_{max} term can be determined directly *in vivo* after high frequency stimulations because dopamine concentrations can exceed the K_m by 10-fold. The first term on the right characterizes release in terms of $[DA]_p$, the amount of dopamine released per stimulus pulse, and estimates of this parameter can be obtained from the experimental data. The following features of the experimental data obtained in the caudate nucleus are predicted with the integrated form of this model:

1. For stimulus durations up to 5 s, 60-Hz stimulations result in a linear increase in dopamine concentration in the ECF (40).
2. The maximal concentration of dopamine decreases with decreasing frequency of stimulation over the range 60 to 10 Hz (40).
3. At stimulus frequencies of 30 Hz and below, dopamine concentration reaches a new steady-state value within 1 s of stimulation (40).
4. For typical, experimentally derived, values of the kinetic parameters ($[DA]_p$ = 60 nM, K_m = 200 nM, and V_{max} = 2 μM/s) the model predicts a concentration of dopamine in ECF of 30 nM for physiological rates of firing, a value in good agreement with estimates from dialysis experiments (55).
5. Competitive uptake inhibitors result in an increase in the stimulated overflow of dopamine with the biggest change observed at low frequencies (50). This is modeled by a change in the apparent value of K_m without a change in the other kinetic parameters from their predrug values.

6. Agents which increase dopamine synthesis (L-DOPA (50), D-2 antagonists (53)) also increase the amount of stimulated overflow, but with a distinctively different dependence on the frequency of the stimulation than competitive uptake inhibitors. Such changes are modeled by a change in the apparent value of $[DA]_p$ without a change in the other kinetic parameters from their predrug values.
7. Overflow curves obtained in the nucleus accumbens also are described by the model. The kinetic parameters employed are the same as in the caudate nucleus except that the value of V_{max} is smaller (53).

Thus, this model describes stimulated release over a broad range of conditions. The model is both useful and practical because it is simple and describes the measured events in three easily defined kinetic constants. However, the model is not applicable under all conditions, such as when release processes fatigue or other extreme situations. Such conditions can be described by a more sophisticated mathematical model of the nerve terminal region published by Justice (39b, 56). The combined used of quantitative measurements and sophisticated models should allow a more complete understanding of the neurotransmission process.

BIBLIOGRAPHY

1. Adams, R.N., Anal. Chem. 48, 1126A-1138A (1976).

2. Cooper, J.R., Bloom, F.E., Roth, R.H., The Biochemical Basis of Neuropharmacology, Oxford University Press, Oxford (1986).

3. Westerink, B.H.C., Horn, A.S., Korf, J., The Neurobiology of Dopamine, Academic Press, London (1979).

4. (a) Rose, G., Gerhardt, G., Strmberg, I., Olson, L., Hoffer, B., Brain Res. 341, 92-100 (1985).
(b) Stromberg, I., Almqvist, P., Bygdeman, M., Finger, T.E., Gerhardt, G., Granholm, A.-Ch., Mahalik, T.J., Seiger, A., Hoffer, B., Olsen L., Proc. Natl. Acad. Sci., U.S.A. 85, 8331-8334 (1988).

5. Myers, R.D., Methods in Psychobiology, Vol. II, Academic Press, London, pp 169-211 (1972).

6. Nieoullon, A., Cheramy, A., Glowinski, J., J. Neurochem. 28, 819-828 (1977).

7. Zetterstroem, T., Sharp, T., Marsden, C.A., Ungerstedt, U., J. Neurochem. 41, 1769-73 (1983).

8. Justice, J.B., Jr., Wages, S.A., Michael, A.C., Blakely, R.D., Neill, D.B., J. Liq. Chromatogr. 6, 1873-96 (1983).

9. Neurochemical Analysis of the Conscious Brain: Voltammetry and Push-Pull Perfusion, Annals of the New York Academy of Sciences 473, (1987).

10. (a) Wages, S.A., Church, W.H., Justice, J.B., Anal. Chem. 58, 1649-1656 (1986).
(b) Church, W. H., Justice, J. B., Anal. Chem. 59, 712-716 (1987).

11. Church, W.H., Justice, J.B., Byrd, L.D., Eur. J. Pharm. 139, 345-348 (1987).

12. Zetterstroem, T., Sharp, T., Ungerstedt, U., Eur. J. Pharm. 106, 27-37 (1984).

13. Church, W.H., Justice, J.B. and Neill, D.B., Brain Res. 412, 397-399 (1987).

14. Ray, C.D., Bickford, R.G., Clark, L.C., Jr., Russert, W.E., Mayo Clin. Proc. 40, 781-790 (1965).

15. McCreery, R.L., Dreiling, R., Adams, R.N., Brain Res. 73, 23-33, (1974).

16. Wightman, R.M., Strope, E.R., Plotsky, P., Adams, R.N., Nature 262, 145-146 (1976).

17. (a) Gonon, F., Buda, M., Cespuglio, R., Jouvet, M., Pujol, J.R., Nature 286, 902-904 (1980).
(b) Gonon, F.G., Fombarlet, C.M., Buda, M.J., Pujol, J.F., Anal. Chem. 53, 1386-1389 (1981).

18. Stamford, J.A., J. Neurosci. Meth. 17, 1-29 (1986).

19. Marsden, C.A., Joseph, M.H., Kruk, Z.L., Maidment, N.T., O'Neill, R.D., Schenk, J.O., Stamford, J.A., Neurosci. 25, 389-400 (1988).

20. Ponchon, J.-L., Cespuglio, R., Gonon, F., Jouvet, M., Pujol, J.F., Anal. Chem. 51, 1483-1486 (1979).

21. Fox, K., Armstrong-James, M., Millar, J., J. Neurosci. Meth. 3, 37-48 (1980).

22. Dayton, M.A., Brown, J.C., Stutts, K.J., Wightman, R.M., Anal. Chem. 52, 946-950 (1980).

23. Kelly, R., Wightman, R.M., Anal. Chim. Acta 187, 79-87 (1986).

24. May, L.J., Wightman, R.M., Brain Res. 487, 311-320 (1989).

25. (a) Gerhardt, G.A., Oke, A.F., Nagy, G., Moghaddam, B., Adams, R.N., Brain Res. 290(2), 390-395 (1984).
(b) Nagy, G., Gerhardt, G.A., Oke, A.F., Rice, M.E., Adams, R.N., Moore, R.B., Szentirmay, M.N., Martin, C.R., J. Electroanal. Chem. 188, 85-94 (1985).
(c) Brazell, M.P., Kasser, R.J., Renner, K.J., Feng, J., Moghaddam, B., Adams, R.N., J. Neurosci. Meth. 22, 167-172 (1987).

26. Kristensen, E.W., Kuhr, W.G., Wightman, R.M., Anal. Chem. 59, 1752-1757 (1987).

27. Justice, J.B., Voltammetry in the Neurosciences, Humana Press, Clifton, NJ, pp 3-102 (1987).

28. Millar, J., Stamford, J.A., Kruk, Z. L., Wightman, R.M., Eur. J. Pharm. 109, 341-348 (1985).

29. Baur, J.E., Kristensen, E.W., May, L.J., Wiedemann, D.J., Wightman, R.M., Anal. Chem. 60, 1268-1271 (1988).

30. Gonon, F.G., Navarre, F., Buda, M.J., Anal. Chem. 56, 573-575 (1985).

31. Crespi, F., Martin, K.F., Marsden, C.A., Neurosci. 27, 885-896 (1988).

32. Wiedemann, D., Tomusk-Basse, A., Wilson, R.L., Rebec, G.V., Wightman, R.M., manuscript in preparation.

33. Ewing, A.G., Wightman, R.M., Dayton, M.A., Brain Res. 249, 361-370 (1982).

34. Rice, M.E., Oke, A.F., Bradberry, C.W., Adams, R.N., Brain Res. 340, 151-155 (1985).

35. Gerhardt, G.A., Rose, G.M., Hoffer, B.J., J. Neurochem. 46, 842-850 (1986).

36. Schenk, J.O., Bunney, B.S., Voltammetry in the Neurosciences, Justice, J.B., Ed., Humana Press, Clifton, NJ, pp 139-160 (1987).

37. (a) Ewing, A.G., Bigelow, J.C., Wightman, R.M., Science 221, 169-171 (1983).
(b) Kuhr, W.G., Ewing, A.G., Caudill, W.L., Wightman, R.M., J. Neurochem. 43, 560-569 (1984).
(c) Ewing, A.G., Wightman, R.M., J. Neurochem. 43, 570-577 (1984).

38. (a) Gonon, F.G., Buda, M.J., Neurosci. 14, 765-776 (1985).
(b) Gonon, F.G., Neurosci. 24, 19-28 (1988).

39. (a) Michael, A.C., Ikeda, M., Justice, J.B., Brain Res. 421, 325-335 (1987).
(b) Nicolaysen, L.C., Ikeda, M., Justice, J.B., Neill, D.B., Brain Res. 460, 50-59 (1988).

40. Wightman, R.M., Amatore, C., Engstrom, R.C., Hale, P.D., Kristensen, E.W., Kuhr, W.G., May, L.J., Neurosci. 25, 513-523 (1988).

41. (a) Stamford, J.A., Kruk, Z.L., Millar, J., Br. J. Pharmac. 94, 924-932 (1988).
(b) Stamford, J.A., Kruk, Z.L., Millar, J., Brain Res. 454, 282-288 (1988).
(c) Stamford, J.A., Kruk, Z.L., Palij, P., Millar, J., Brain Res. 448, 381-385 (1988).

42. Kuhr, W.G., Wightman, R.M., Brain Res. 381, 168-171 (1986).

43. Wise, R.A., The Neurobiology of Opiate Reward Processes, Smith, R., Lane, R., Eds, pp 405-437 (1983).

44. Van Der Heyden, J.A.M., Pharm. Biochem. Behav. 21, 567-274 (1984).

45. Roth, R.H., Annals of the N. Y. Acad. of Sciences 430, 27-54 (1984).

46. Kuhr, W.G., Wightman, R.M., Rebec, G.V., Brain Res. 418, 122-128 (1987).

47. Wightman, R.M., Brown, D.S., Kuhr, W.G., Wilson, R.L., Voltammetry in the Neurosciences, Justice, J.B., Ed., Humana Press, Clifton, NJ, pp 103-138 (1987).

48. Kuhr, W.G., Bigelow, J.C., Wightman, R.M., J. Neurosci. 6, 974-982 (1986).

49. Michael, A.C., Justice, J.B., Neill, D.B., Neurosci. Lett. 56, 365-369 (1985).

50. Rice, M.E., Nicholson, C., Anal. Chem., submitted.

51. Engstrom, R.C., Wightman, R.M., Kristensen, E.W., Anal. Chem. 60, 652-656 (1988).

52. May, L.J., Kuhr, W.G., Wightman, R.M., J. Neurochem. 51, 1060-1069 (1988).

53. May, L.J., Wightman, R.M., J. Neurochem., in press.

54. Near, J.A., Bigelow, J.C., Wightman, R.M., J. Pharmacol. Exp. Ther. 245, 921-927 (1988).

55. Wightman, R.M., May, L.J., Michael, A.C., Anal. Chem. 60, 769A-779A (1988).

56. Justice, J.B., Nicolaysen, L.C., Michael, A.C., J. Neurosci. Meth. 22, 239-252 (1988).

4

Application of Field Effect Electro-Osmosis to Separation-Based Sensors

KIUMARS GHOWSI and ROBERT J. GALE Chemistry Department, Louisiana State University, Baton Rouge, Louisiana 70803

INTRODUCTION

One area of great promise in microcolumn separations is their use for analysis of discrete biological systems. The direction of research in this area is toward development of capillary electrophoresis with smaller capillary diameters for use as chemical sensors. The low volume capability, sensitive detection schemes, and use of electro-osmotic flow for low-volume injection schemes make this a powerful approach to developing sensors for small biological environments. The principle of the sensor is selectivity by separation (capillary electrophoresis) and sensitivity by detection (electrochemical) (1).

Capillary electrophoresis places a buffer-filled capillary between two buffer reservoirs and a potential field is applied across this capillary. The electric field creates an electro-osmosis flow of buffer toward the cathode. The electric field also causes electrophoretic flow of ionic solutes, which move against the electro-osmotic flow. This causes separation due to different mobilities, since the electrophoretic flow is less than the electro-osmotic flow and the solutes go toward the cathode, where they can be detected. The two fundamental equations describing the response time and the resolution are given as follows (2),

$$t = \frac{L^2}{\bar{\mu}_s V} = \frac{L^2}{(\bar{\mu}_E + \mu_{EO})V} \qquad [1]$$

$$R_s = \frac{\mu_{E,A} - \mu_{E,B}}{\bar{\mu}_s} \frac{N^{1/2}}{4} = \left(\frac{\mu_{E,A} - \mu_{E,B}}{(\bar{\mu}_E + \mu_{Eo})^{1/2}}\right)\left(\frac{V^{1/2}}{4\sqrt{2}\,D^{1/2}}\right) \qquad [2]$$

where $\bar{\mu}_s$ is the average migration mobility of the solute, μ_E is the electrophoretic mobility, $\mu_{E,A}$ and $\mu_{E,B}$ are the electro-phoretic mobilities for the two solutes, $\bar{\mu}_E$ is the average electrophoretic mobility, μ_{EO} is the electro-osmosis mobility, V is the applied voltage across the capillary, and L is the length of the capillary. It can be seen from eq.[2] that the best resolution will be obtained when the electro-osmosis mobility just balances the electrophoretic mobility.

$$\mu_{EO} = -\bar{\mu}_E$$

In this condition the analysis time (equation 1) goes to infinity.

ELECTROKINETIC FIELD EFFECT DEVICE BASED ON CAPILLARY FIELD EFFECT ELECTRO-OSMOSIS

We have postulated a novel phenomenon called capillary field effect electro-osmosis (3). This effect combines the metal-insulator-electrolyte system with capillary electro-osmosis. Through field effect electro-osmosis, we should like to control the electro-osmotic flow in a capillary covered with a metallic coating at its outside surface. This control is done by an applied, perpendicular electric field, generated by a voltage, V_G, as shown in figure 1. By changing V_G the voltage drop across the double layer changes. This change includes the change in zeta potential, ζ, which in turn causes a modification in the electro-osmotic flow. By field effect electro-osmosis, it should be possible to change the zeta potential very easily, or it can be tuned to a certain value by applying the appropriate external voltage V_G. A schematic of a metal-insulator-electrolyte-electrokinetic field effect device (MIEEKFED) is shown in figure 2. This device should be able to control the flow of an electrolyte by two voltages, V_d, the voltage applied across the capillary and the gate voltage, V_G. It has been shown that the zeta potential is a complex function of V_G (3)

$$\zeta = f^{-1}(V_G) \text{ for } V_d = 0 \qquad [3]$$

The zeta potential has been plotted versus V_G (the voltage across the metal-insulator-electrolyte) in figures 3 and 4. In these figures the effects of concentration and pH on the zeta potential are illustrated.

Since for MIEEKFED, V_d also is applied across the capillary, then the voltage perpendicular to the capillary wall is not constant nor equal to V_G. The new voltage at any point across the capillary, at the distance X from the cathode is $V_G - V_d \cdot \frac{X}{L}$, where L is the length of the capillary. Now the zeta potential as

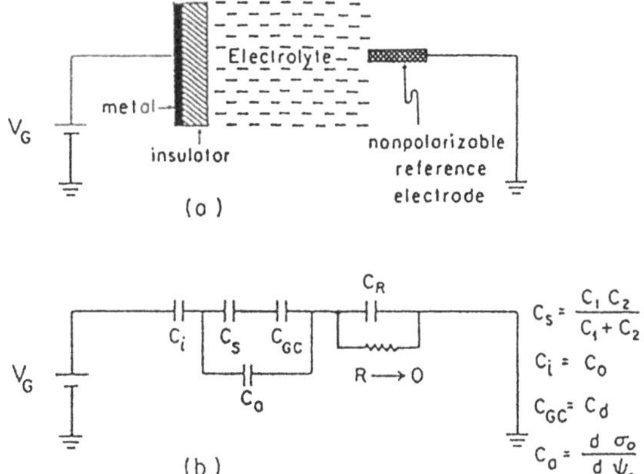

FIGURE 1. a) Metal-Insulator-Electrolyte and reference electrode structure

b) Circuit diagram of a MIE

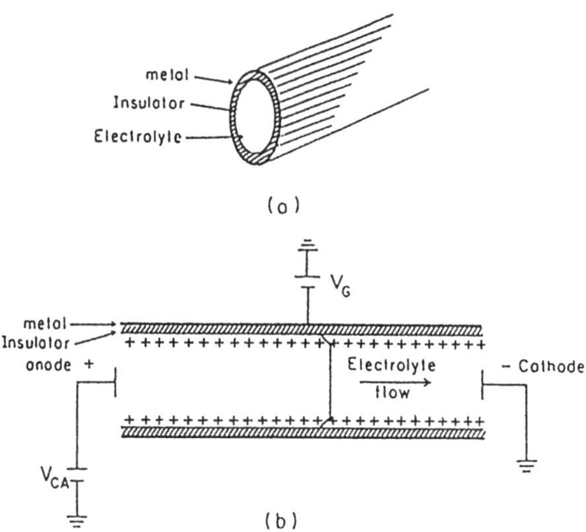

FIGURE 2. a) A capillary covered with metallic coating
b) Cross section of Metal-Insulator-Electrolyte Field Effect Device (MIEEKFED)

a function of X is $\zeta(X) = f^{-1}(V_G - V_d \cdot \frac{X}{L})$. The following design, shown in figure 5, is proposed for constant zeta potential across the capillary. The capillary is coated with a resistive layer. By connecting one side of the resistive layer on the capillary to V_G and the other side to ground, the voltage across the length of the capillary is $V_G \cdot X/L$ (figure 5B). The resistive layer should have high resistance because the current passes through this layer and less heat will be generated. The two voltages of V_d and $V_c = V_d - V_G$ are connected to the anode and the cathode, respectively, as shown in figure 5A. As illustrated in figure 1B, this circuit topology creates a constant voltage ($V_d - V_G$) between the resistive layer and the electrolyte. The zeta potential across the capillary is

$$\zeta - f^{-1}(V_d - V_G)$$

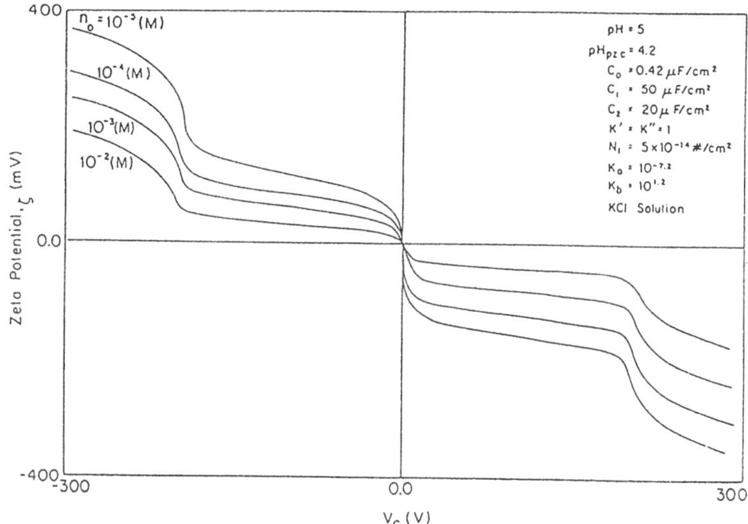

FIGURE 3. Change in zeta potential as a function of V_G for various concentrations using the site binding model for nonideal case.

and the electro-osmosis mobility is proportional to the zeta potential.

$$\mu_{EO} \propto \zeta$$

The voltage between the cathode and the anode is V_G when $V_G \neq 0$ and $V_c \neq 0$.

POTENTIAL APPLICATION FOR SEPARATIONS BASED SENSORS

Suppose there is a sample with three negatively charged solutes A, B, and C. Each one has an electrophoretic mobility in the buffer solution used for analysis. The mobilities are μ_A, μ_B, and μ_C, respectively, such that $|\mu_A| < |\mu_B| < |\mu_C|$. For analysis using MIEEKFED, 1) The sample is injected to the microcapillary by

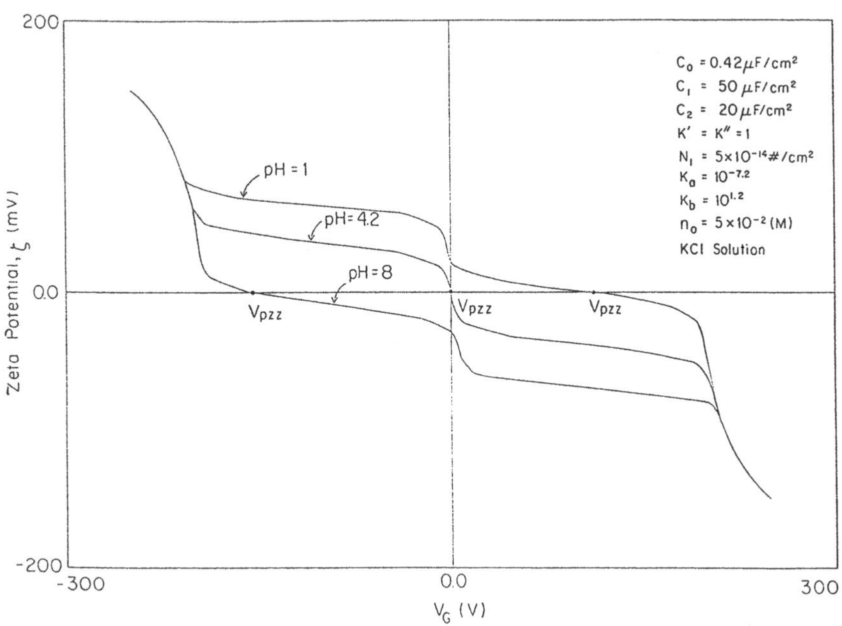

FIGURE 4. Change in zeta potential ζ as a function of V_G for different pH and constant concentration.

electromigration. In this step, $V_G = 0$, $V_C = 0$ and V_d is applied across the capillary between the cathode and anode. 2) Keep $V_G = 0$, $V_C = 0$, and apply V_d for a period of time such that the sample reaches almost to the middle of the capillary (fig 6). 3) V_G and V_C are set such that the electro-osmosis mobility magnitude becomes the same as the electrophoretic mobility of solute B. In this condition, the migration velocity of B is zero and the migration velocity of A and C are negative and positive. Maintaining this trapping position for a while causes the separation of A, B AND C in the capillary. Since the separation is done at zero migration velocity the length of capillary could be reduced. 4) In this step the electro-osmosis mobility could be increased such that all the solutes are drifted toward the cathode and they are detected there.

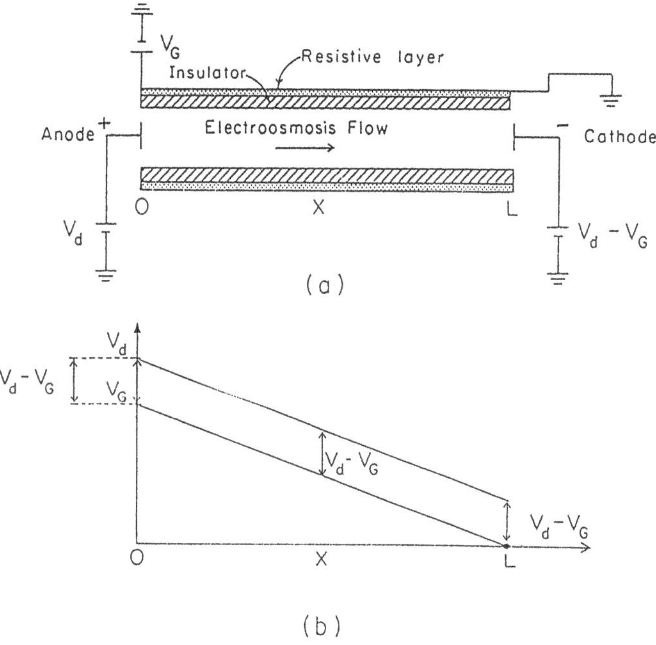

FIGURE 5. a) The schematic of MIEEKFED with the constant zeta potential across the capillary.
b) The voltage perpendicular to the wall of the capillary versus X.

ACKNOWLEDGMENTS

Kiumars Ghowsi is grateful to the Chemistry Department, LSU, for a teaching assistantship and Dr. R. J. Gale extends thanks to Professor R. C. Mohanty for partial support from the Army Research Office through Southern Research Institute of Pure and Applied Sciences, Southern University and LSU.

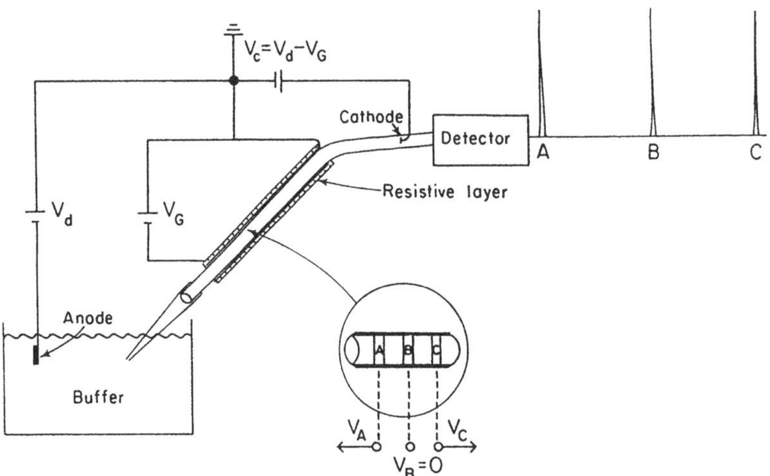

FIGURE 6. The MIEEKFED is used as the separation based sensor for detection of solute B

REFERENCES

1) A. G. Ewing, R. A. Wallingford and T. M. Olefirowicks, "Capillary Electrophoresis," Anal. Chem., 61, 292A-303A (1989).

2) J. Jorgenson and K. D. Lukacs, Anal. Chem., 53, 1298-1302 (1981).

3) K. Ghowsi and R. J. Gale, Manuscript submitted to the IEEE Transactions on Electron Devices.

5

Serotonin-Sensing Properties of Identified Invertebrate Neurons

RODNEY S. SKEEN, WILLIAM S. KISAALITA, and BERNARD J. VAN WIE, Department of Chemical Engineering, Washington State University Pullman, Washington

SIMON J. FUNG, and CHARLES D. BARNES, Department of Veterinary and Comparative Anatomy, Pharmacology and Physiology, Washington State University, Pullman, Washington

1 ABSTRACT

Results in the development of a chemical sensor, for the neurotransmitter serotonin, which will use living neurons as the primary transducer are reported. The exposure of identified neurons from the visceral ganglia of the pond snail *Limnea stagnalis* to serotonin has revealed a reversible, concentration dependent increase in the rate of spontaneous action potential generation, over a concentration range of four orders of magnitude. Data are also presented which indicate that after exposure to serotonin the neuron undergoes a desensitizing process. These findings are discussed in relation to the development of a neuron based chemical sensor.

2 INTRODUCTION

A major problem for all disciplines that work with biological systems is the lack of fast, accurate, and reusable sensing devices. For example, antibody electrodes, affinity binding sensors, and chemiluminescence fiber optic probes rely heavily on competitive binding between a marked ligand and the substance of interest at receptor sites (1). Because of this, their response time is slow since the sensor must reach equilibrium before producing an accurate signal. Chemical sensitive field effect transistors which measure pH changes caused by enzymatic reactions (2), are highly specific, but are limited to measuring compounds for which a suitable enzyme can be isolated. In addition, enzymes are expensive and are unstable over long periods of time. Other techniques use immobilized whole cells or microorganisms and measure electrical potential changes caused by a metabolic by-product of the analyte of interest (3). These sensors tend to be less specific (4) and are limited by the slow diffusion rate of the chemical to the microbial cell, metabolism of the substance and subsequent diffusion of the metabolite to the electrode.

In recent years, it has been demonstrated that isolated antennae dissected from the crab *Callinectes sapidus* can be used for chemical sensing (5-6). By monitoring random afferent axons of the antennae, both a concentration dependent response to compounds such as γ-aminobutyric acid, 3-oxyo-hexanedioic acid, glutaric acid, 2-aminoethanol, L-alanine, isonicotinic acid, thiamine, phospho(enol)-pyruvate, glutamate, glutamine, adenosin diphosphate, and adenosin 5′-monophosphate, and desirable sensing characteristics such as a fast response time. repeatability, selectivity, and a wide sensitivity range has been shown (5). The use of intact nervous tissue for sensing also demonstrates the capability of using electrically excitable tissue to convert binding events into digital electrical signals. The generation of digital signals is advantageous since they are less prone to noise and interference than the analog signals produced by most biosensing devices (7). Besides, the availability of reliable digital signals has been cited by Bignell (8) and Koelman and Regtien (9) as an important factor required for future development of microsensors because such responses are microprocessor compatible, and can be easily applied in bus-organized data acquisition systems. Excitable tissue has an inherent digital output because as the analyte interacts with the tissue it triggers changes in the transmembrane potential, either through secondary messengers, or directly, which are then amplified by ionic channels that are voltage dependent, to produce discrete voltage spikes or action potential (AP) events. A typical AP lasts only a few milliseconds and is tens of millivolts in amplitude. Because of their large amplitude, APs are easy to monitor. In addition, it has been shown that the concentration of the detected chemical is encoded in the frequency at which APs occur.

This paper reports representative results from a systematic study of the effects of the neurotransmitter, serotonin, on identified neurons from the visceral ganglia of the pond snail *Limnea stagnalis*. The *Limnea* neurons were chosen as a model system because of their large size, the ease in which they can be identified, and their ability to withstand intracellular recording for extended periods of time. Serotonin, was chosen for this study since it is present in a wide range of species. and both its distribution and effects have been extensively studied in invertebrates (10). Furthermore, a sensor for serotonin would have potential significance in both clinical medicine and physiological studies since this neurotransmitter has been linked to disorders such as Parkinson's disease (11), and some forms of depression (12).

3 METHODS

The circumoesophageal nerve ring was dissected from an adult *Limnea stagnalis* snail and placed in a dish of *Limnea* saline made up of 50 mM Na^+, 2.5 mM K^+, 4 mM Ca^{2+}, 4 mM Mg^{2+}, 10 mM glucose, 68.5 mM Cl^-, and buffered to a pH of 7.4 with 10 mM HEPES (Sigma, St. Louis, MO). The visceral ganglia was then separated from the cluster, transferred by pipette to a Sylgard 184 (Dow Corning, Midland, MI) lined 35 mm petri dish, and pinned down using a minute dissecting pin (Fine Science Tools, Belmont, CA). The orientation of the ganglia after pinning allowed the visual identification of the giant visceral ventral neurons VV1 and VV2 (13). To soften the protective sheath the ganglia was soaked for 30 minutes in the petri dish containing a 0.2 % solution of trypsin (Sigma type III).

The recording chamber for these experiments was a Sylgard lined 35 mm petri dish, fitted with inlet and outlet flow lines and surrounded by a water jacket. Water from a temperature controlled bath was circulated through the chamber housing and an insulated water jacket around the feed line to maintain the chamber at a temperature between 27° C to 29° C. Serotonin solutions between 10^{-8} M and 10^{-2} M were made fresh before each experiment by first dissolving serotonin creatinine sulfate complex (Research Biochemicals Inc., Natick, MA) in *Limnea* saline to make a stock solution. The stock solution was then diluted in 10 fold increments and each of these solutions were placed in separate burettes. Each solution was introduced to the ganglia by opening the corresponding burette stopcock. The addition and removal of fluid from the recording chamber was accomplished by using a ten roller peristaltic pump (Rainin Instrument Co., Woburn, MA) on both the inlet and outlet lines. Inlet flow was introduced at the bottom of the chamber while the outlet port was suspended near the upper one-third of the dish. Consequently, there was constant inlet flow and pulsating outlet flow as the liquid rose to the outlet port and was drawn off, thus, lowering the level until it dropped below the port. The volume of fluid in the chamber fluctuated between 2.6 ml and 4.3 ml. Tracers studies showed the chamber had complete solution turnover in 4 minutes at the 4.0 $ml/minute$ feed rate used in all experiments.

Impalement of the VV1 and VV2 cells with a glass microelectrode, filled with 3 M KCl, was done under a dissecting microscope using a hydraulic micromanipulator (Narishige USA, Inc., Greenvale, New York). Electrode resistance ranged between 20 to 30 $M\Omega$. Intracellular signals were conducted by a silver wire (A-M Systems Inc., Everett, WA) from the microelectrode to a Dagan 8700 amplifier (Dagan Corporation, Minneapolis, MN). The spontaneous activity from the impaled neuron was monitored continuously on an oscilloscope (Tektronix Corp., Beaverton, OR), stored on a modified VCR recorder (Vetter Co., Rebersburg, PA), and sent to an on-line data processing system.

Healthy cells were selected for analysis based on their ability to generate repetitive APs greater than 50 mV. On-line data analysis was accomplished

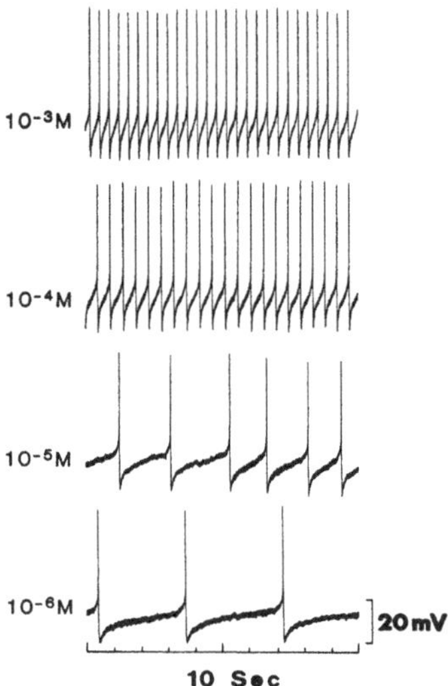

FIGURE 1. An example of the effects of serotonin on the spontaneous firing rate of the VV1 neuron in a *Limnea stagnalis* snail. As indicated, the traces are the cellular response to additions of 10^{-6} M, 10^{-5} M, 10^{-4} M, and 10^{-3} M serotonin.

using a Das-16F analog-to-digital (A/D) converter (Metrabyte Corp., Taunton, MA,) and an IBM-AT compatible microcomputer (Isotropic Computer Inc., Post Falls, ID). Frequencies were calculated between the previous AP and the most recent and then stored in the computer along with the time when the more recent AP occurred. The final analysis of the frequency versus time data was done off-line using in-house software.

4 RESULTS AND DISCUSSION

Of 15 VV1 and VV2 neurons exposed to serotonin it was found that all the cells showed similar increases in spontaneous firing frequency with increasing serotonin concentration. Figure 1 portrays an example of the graded increase in firing rate with serotonin concentration. As indicated in the figure, the traces correspond to the cellular responses to additions of 10^{-6} M, 10^{-5} M, 10^{-4} M, and 10^{-3} M serotonin. In addition to showing increased excitation with concentration, the figure also exemplifies the inherent digital nature of a neurotransducer which arises because the chemical information is encoded in the frequency at which the AP events occur. Thus, it is only necessary to monitor the time between events to determine concentration. This feature is important in sensor

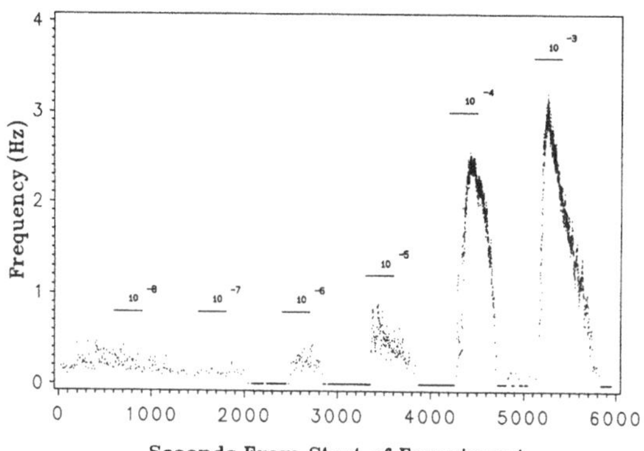

FIGURE 2. Firing frequency results from a one and a half hour experiment where the identified neuron VV1 was exposed to 5 minute applications of increasing levels of serotonin each followed by a 10 minute rinse. This is a typical example of the response obtained from both VV1 and VV2 neurons.

design because digital signals are less prone, than analog signals, to noise and interference. Also, since APs are very rapid, on the order of milliseconds, and have a uniform size and shape, they are easily recognized, making the sensing mechanism immune to baseline drift of the resting potential. In fact, wave shape recognition was used to generate all the firing frequency data presented in this paper and this technique was found to be insensitive to both electrical noise and baseline drift.

To analyze the concentration dependent response of the VV1 and VV2 neurons, several cells were exposed to 5 minute applications, each followed by a saline rinse, of increasing levels of serotonin between 10^{-8} M and 10^{-2} M. Figure 2 shows a typical example of results obtained from these experiments. For the cell represented in Figure 2, the addition of 10^{-8} M and 10^{-7} M serotonin during the first half hour of the experiment caused no discernible change in the baseline firing frequency. However, successive additions of 10^{-6} M, 10^{-5} M, 10^{-4} M, and 10^{-3} M serotonin resulted in a graded increase in firing rate. Application of 10^{-2} M serotonin, although not applied to the cell represented, resulted in a leveling off of the response perhaps indicating saturation of the serotonin receptors on the membrane surface.

Two other important considerations for sensor design result from analysis of Figure 2. First, response to serotonin is reversible, as indicated by the return to the baseline firing rate after the neuron was rinsed with fresh saline. This suggests that a neuron based sensor can be a reusable device. Second, it is clear from this figure, particularly at the higher concentrations of serotonin, that shortly after exposure, the firing frequency of the cell rapidly increases to

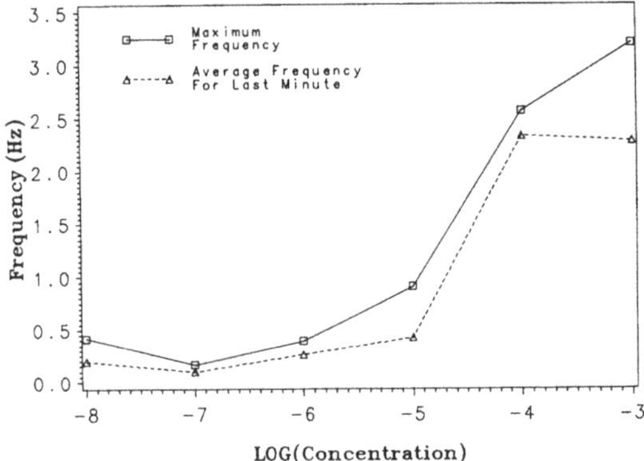

FIGURE 3. Maximum firing frequency and the average firing frequency for the last minute of each application, for the data shown in Figure 2, plotted against the logarithm of the serotonin concentration in the surrounding medium.

a maximum and then begins to diminish. This phenomenon is not desirable for sensing since it means the neuron is being desensitized with time. However, it has been shown with other neural preparations (5) that the maximum frequency response to a given concentration can be used as an indication of chemical concentration. This is also true for the *Limnea* preparation. The solid line on Figure 3 represents the maximum frequency for the data shown in Figure 2 as a function of the logarithm of the serotonin concentration in the surrounding medium. Also shown on Figure 3 by the dashed line is the average firing frequency for the last minute of serotonin exposure plotted against the logarithm of the serotonin concentration. Comparison of the two lines reveals that the desensitizing process causes a decrease in the response magnitude with time at all concentrations. This phenomena also leads to a reduction in the sensitivity at the 10^{-3} M level, where decay of the firing frequency occurs more rapidly. Therefore, use of neurons in a sensing device will require the measurement of maximum frequency values to obtain the broadest range of sensitivity.

5 CONCLUSIONS

Serotonin causes a reversible, concentration dependent increase in the spontaneous firing frequency of *Limnea stagnalis* giant ventral visceral neurons VV1 and VV2. The range of response is between 10^{-6} M to 10^{-3} M. Exposure to serotonin also causes the neurons to go through a desensitizing process causing the firing frequency to diminish shortly after the maximum response. It was found that the maximum firing frequency response gives the most sensitive indication of the chemical concentration. These results show that it is possible to use signals from VV1 and VV2 neurons in a neuron based serotonin sensor.

ACKNOWLEDGEMENTS

This project was supported under the Microsensor Technology Program of the Washington Technology Center. An equipment donation for the oscilloscope was received from Tektronix Corporation.

REFERENCES

1. Aizawa, A., Morioka, A., and Suzuki, S., (1980). An enzyme immunosensor for the electrochemical determination of the tumor antigen α-fetoprotein, Analytia Chemica Acta, 115: 61.
2. Tamiya, E., Seki, A., Karube, I., Gotoh, M., and Shimizu, I., (1988). Hypoxanthine sensor based on an amorphous silicon field-effect transistor, Analytia Chimica Acta, 215: 301.
3. Liang, B.S., Li, X., and Wang, H.Y., (1986). Cellular electrode for antitumor drug screening, Biotech. Progress, 2: 187.
4. Rechnitz, G.A., Kobos, R.K., Riechel, S.J., and Gebauer, C.R., (1977). A bio-selective membrane electrode prepared with living bacterial cells, Analytia Chimica, Acta, 94: 357.
5. Buch, R.M., and Rechnitz, G.A., (1989). Intact chemoreceptor-based biosensors: responses and analytical limits, Biosensors, 4: 215.
6. Belli, S.L., and Rechnitz, G.A., (1988). Biosensors based on native chemoreceptors, Fresenius Z Anal. Chem., 331: 439.
7. Middelhoek, S., French, P.J., Huijsing, J.H., and Lian, W.J., (1988). Sensors with digital or frequency output, Sensors and Actuators, 15: 119.
8. Brignell, J.E., (1986). Sensors in distributed instrumentation systems, Sensors and Actuators, 10: 249.
9. Koelman, W.A., and Regtien, P.L., (1984). Bus-organized data-acquisition systems, Sensors and Actuators, 5: 327.
10. Walker, R.J., (1986). Transmitters and modulators, The Mollusca, (A.O.D. Willows, ed.), 9, Academic Press, Florida, p. 279.
11. Curzon, G., (1978). Serotonin and neurological disease, Serotonin in Health and Disease, (W.B. Essman, ed.), 3, Spectrum Publications, New York, p. 407.
12. Coppen, A., (1972). Indoleamines and affective disorders, J. Psychiat. Res., 9: 163.
13. Winlow, W., and Benjamin, P.R., Neuronal mapping of the brain of the pond snail *Limnea stagnalis*, (1976). Neurobiology of Invertebrates (J. Salanki. ed.), Akademiai Kiado, Budapest Hungary, p. 41.

III

Modified Electrodes, Amperometric, and Potentiometric Sensors

6

Novel Sensing Membranes for Organic Guests Based on the Host Functionalities of Macrocyclic Polyamines and Related Compounds

KAZUNORI ODASHIMA and YOSHIO UMEZAWA

Department of Chemistry, Faculty of Science,
Hokkaido University, Sapporo 060, Japan

1. INTRODUCTION

Molecular recognition in biological systems consists of complicated processes that generally involve initial formation of highly structured complexes between macromolecular hosts and their specific guests, followed by expression of biologically significant functions such as discrimination of antigens by antibodies, chemical transformation of substrates by enzymes, translocation of metal ions by carriers, and transduction of signals by receptors. These biological molecular recognition processes are quite often displayed at membrane surfaces rather than in homogeneous solutions. Especially, signal transduction at membrane surface resulting in "transmembrane signalling" (Figure 1) is one of the most interesting biological processes in view of the development of novel sensing systems. The transmembrane signalling frequently involves transduction of a chemical signal to an electric signal at membrane surface, the general transduction mode being membrane potential change and permeation ion current [1].

In this chapter, our recent approaches of mimicking the biological signal transduction processes will be described. Some novel sensing membranes for potentiometric and voltammetric detection of organic guests (anionic and neutral) have been developed by the use of lipophilic derivatives of macrocyclic polyamine (**1**) and cyclodextrin polyamine (**2**) as membraneous receptor molecules [2-8]. The compounds used in this study are shown in Figure 2.

2. POTENTIOMETRIC SENSOR FOR ORGANIC ANIONS [2-4]

Synthetic host compounds with designed selectivities constitute a promising class of sensory elements for chemical sensors. This is best exemplified by the successful applications of acyclic carriers as well as crown ethers to potentiometric sensors for alkali and alkaline earth metal ions [9]. On the other hand, although the development of anion sensors using neutral, charged or associated charged carriers rather than ion-exchangers has been one of the current topics [10-13], it was not until recently that a relevant sensor for anions using a synthetic host compound was developed [2, 3].

A characteristic property distinguishing macrocyclic polyamines from the polyether counterparts (crown ethers) is their behavior of successive protonation, resulting in polycationic hosts capable of forming stable host-guest complexes with organic polyanions in acidic to neutral water. The complexation selectivities generally reflect electrostatic interaction between the host and guest [14, 15]. Accordingly, lipophilic derivatives of macrocyclic polyamines soluble in lipophilic solvents used for electrode membranes are expected to function as sensory elements of anion sensors.

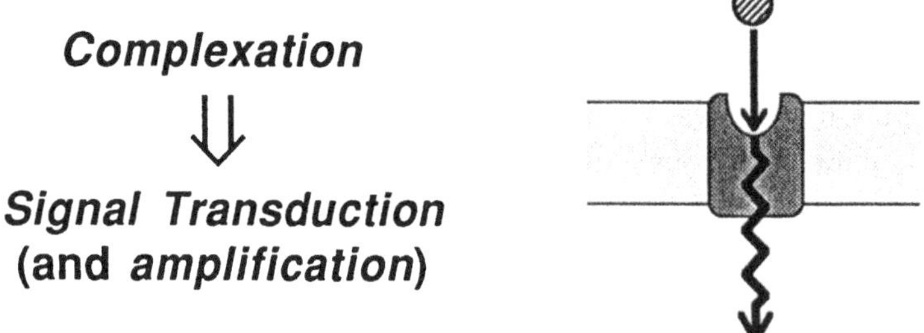

FIGURE 1. Molecular recognition at membrane surface involving host-guest complexation followed by signal transduction, resulting in "transmembrane signalling".

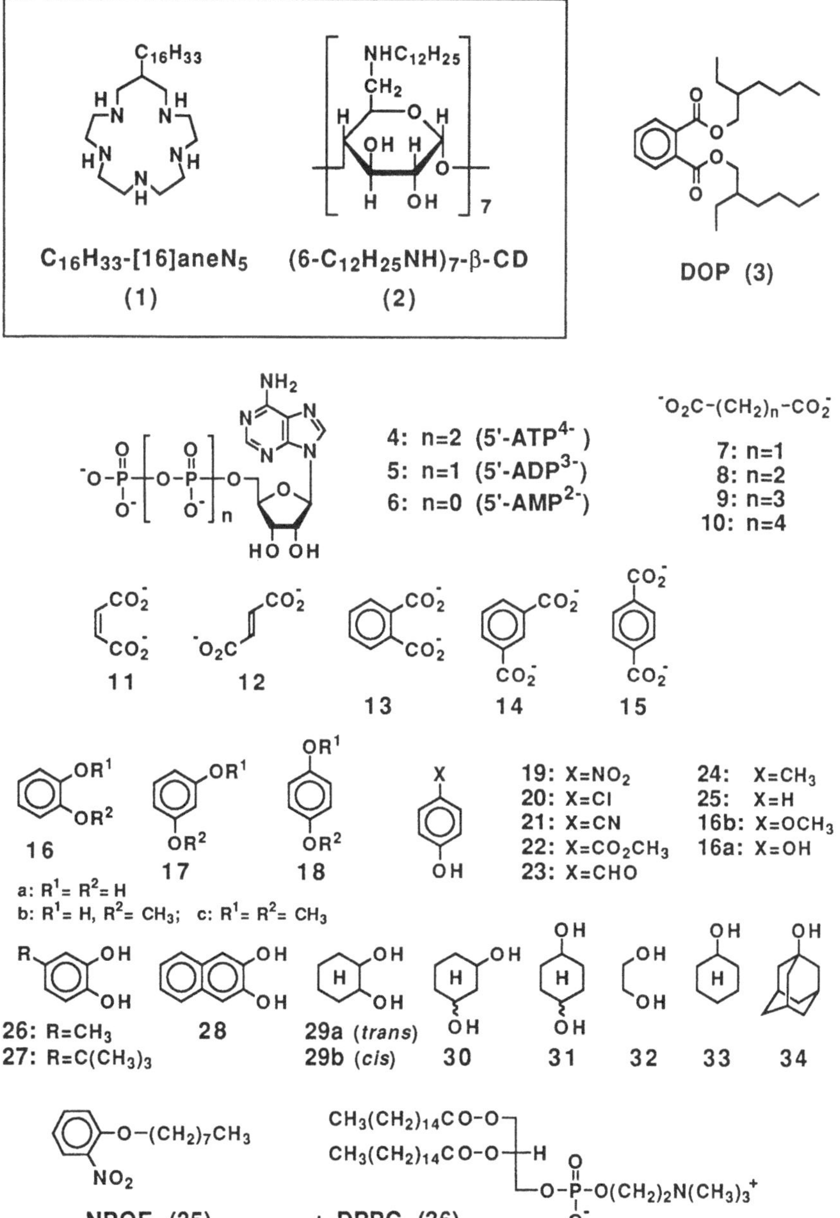

FIGURE 2. Structures of the receptors, anionic and neutral guests, electrode membrane solvent and lipid used in the present study.

2.1. Potentiometric sensor for ATP polyanion [2, 4]

A lipophilic 16-membered macrocyclic pentaamine, 15-hexadecyl-1,4,7,-10,13-pentaazacyclohexadecane ($C_{16}H_{33}$-[16]aneN_5, **1**), was synthesized and used as a sensory element for an impregnated liquid membrane electrode with dioctyl phthalate (DOP, **3**) as a membrane solvent and poly(vinyl chloride) (PVC) as a support [2].

A characteristic property of macrocyclic polyamine is successive protonation, resulting in a pH dependent magnitude of positive charge affecting the membrane potential of the electrode. Figure 3 shows pH-potential curves in the absence (curve 1) and presence (curve 2) of ATP^{4-} (**4**) as a polyanionic guest. The increase of the membrane potential with decreasing pH in the absence of the guest (curve 1) can be ascribed to the uptake of protons from the aqueous phase by macrocyclic polyamine **1** at the membrane surface. Upon addition of the anionic guest, the pH-potential curve (curve 2) deviated from curve 1 below pH 8.5, showing a

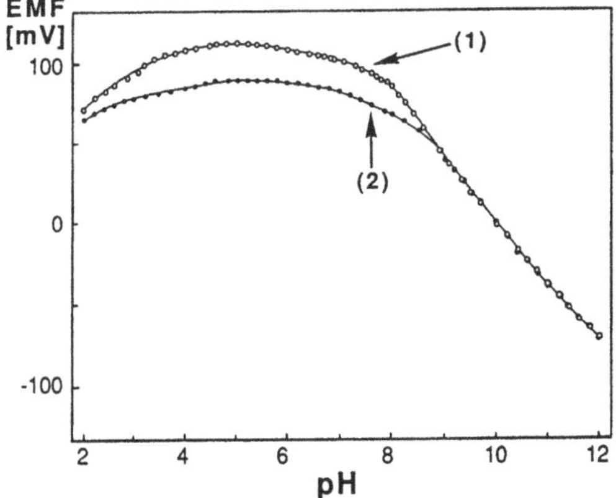

FIGURE 3. Effect of pH on the potentiometric response of the liquid membrane electrode containing macrocyclic polyamine **1** in the absence and presence of ATP (**4**). (1) 10^{-2} M H_2SO_4. The pH was adjusted by addition of NaOH containing 10^{-2} M Na_2SO_4. (2) 10^{-2} M H_2SO_4 + 10^{-3} M ATP. The pH was adjusted by addition of NaOH containing 10^{-2} M Na_2SO_4 and 10^{-3} M ATP.

negative potential shift. Such a pH profile was observed with many other anionic guests.

Figure 4 shows a possible mechanism leading to the potentiometric response. By the proton uptake, charge separation between the protonated polyamine and the hydrophilic counter anion is expected to occur at the membrane interface to generate a positive membrane potential. At the same time, protonated **1** becomes capable of binding with anionic guests (Figure 4a → 4b). Then, the host-guest complexation with an organic anion, which means an exchange of the hydrophilic counter anion to a more lipophilic one, would cause a decrease of charge separation, resulting in a negative potentiometric response (Figure 4c → 4d). The disappearance of potentiometric response in the higher pH region (Figure 3) may reflect the loss of host functionality of **1** due to decreased protonation.

Potentiometric response of the present sensor to a series of adenosine nucleotides, ATP (**4**), ADP (**5**) and AMP (**6**), was measured at pH 6.7, under which the guests mainly exist as ATP^{4-}, ADP^{3-} and AMP^{2-}, respectively. Figure 5 shows the concentration dependence of potentiometric response (log C vs E curve) for each of the adenosine nucleotides as well as for the inorganic phosphate (HPO_4^{2-}). A strong linear response was observed for ATP^{4-} in a concentration range of 10^{-3} to 10^{-7} M with a slope of -14.5 mV/decade (ca 20 °C) which is in good agreement with the theoretical Nernstian value for tetravalent anions. The response to ATP^{4-} was by far the strongest as compared with the other guests. The potentiometric selectivity coefficients (K^{Pot}), indicating relative magnitude of potentiometric response for each guest at a fixed guest concentration, were 1, 0.035, 0.030 and 0.0015 for ATP^{4-}, ADP^{3-}, AMP^{2-} and HPO_4^{2-}, respectively, as determined by the matched potential method [16]. This potentiometric selectivity correlates well with the complexation selectivity of [16]aneN_5 [17] and related hosts [18] in water as well as with the extraction selectivity of **1** in H_2O/CH_2Cl_2 system [2], both of which reflect the host-guest interaction based on the magnitude of electrostatic interaction between the protonated macrocyclic polyamine and the anionic guest.

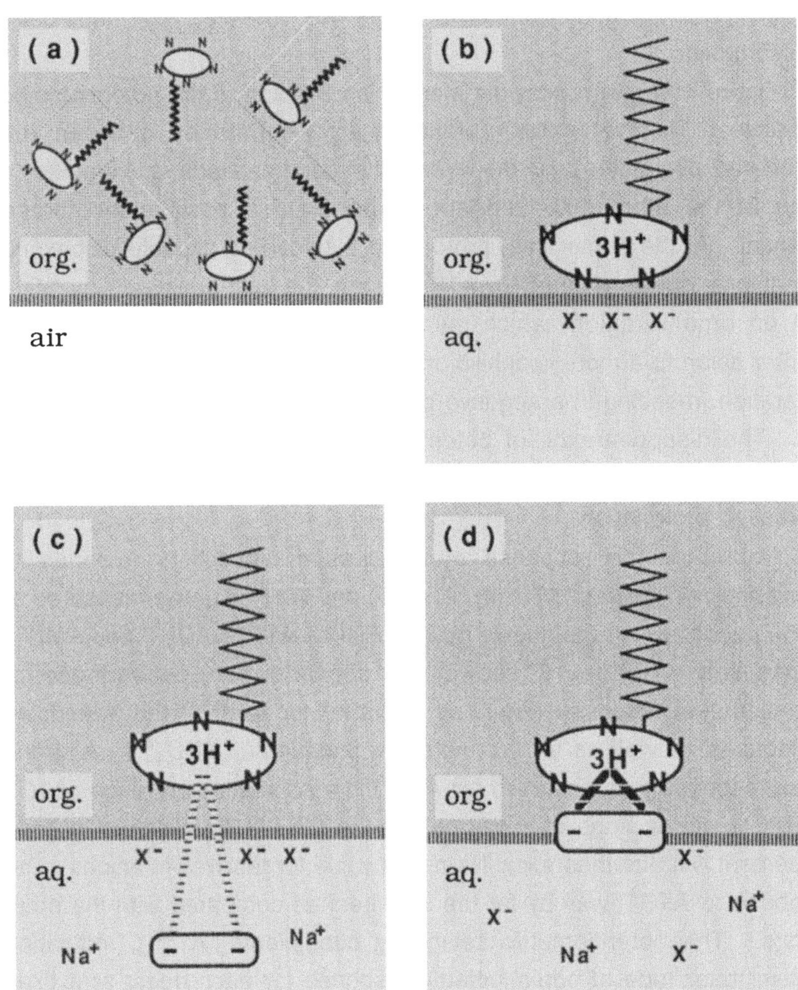

FIGURE 4. A possible mechanism of potentiometric response for anionic guest. (a) Before proton uptake. (b) Proton uptake by **1** at the membrane surface inducing charge separation, hence a positive membrane potential. (c) Host-guest interaction at the membrane surface. (d) Host-guest complex formation and decrease of charge separation, resulting in a negative potentiometric response. In the present figure, a triprotonated state is assumed for macrocyclic polyamine **1** at the membrane surface.

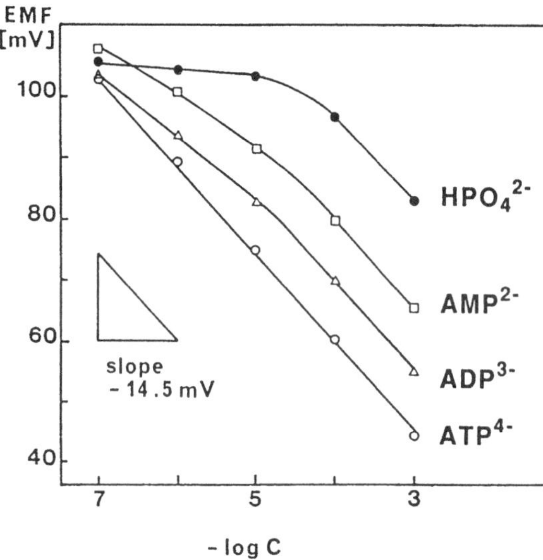

FIGURE 5. Potentiometric response of the liquid membrane electrode containing macrocyclic polyamine **1** toward adenosine nucleotides and inorganic phosphate at pH 6.7.

2.2. Potentiometric sensor for dicarboxylate guests [3, 4]

Discrimination of anionic guests with the same magnitude of charge but different positional relations of the anionic groups is a more sophisticated function displayed by protonated macrocyclic polyamines in water [19, 20]. In this context, potentiometric discrimination of series of dicarboxylate guests with different distances between the two negative charges was examined using the present electrode containing macrocyclic polyamine **1** [3]. To our knowledge, the only related example reported so far is potentiometric discrimination of maleic and phthalic acid isomers by the electrodes containing conventional ion-exchangers [21].

A systematic investigation was carried out with three series of dianionic guests, *i.e.*, linear homologs (**7**~**10**), geometrical isomers (**11**, **12**) and positional isomers (**13**~**15**) of dicarboxylates. The pH condition was carefully set for each series of guests to specifically observe potentiometric responses to the *dianionic* forms of the guests. This requirement is essential for the following two reasons. (i) The greatest discrimination of dicarboxylic acids based on electrostatic interaction with the host is expected when the guests exist in the dianionic forms. (ii) Since the magnitude of potentiometric response is different between monoanionic and dianionic species, it is ideal to set the pH condition at which the dicarboxylic acid almost exclusively exists in the dianionic form.

Table 1 shows the potentiometric selectivity coefficients determined by the separate solution method [22] for each of the three series of dianionic guests. For the linear homologs of terminal dicarboxylates (**7**~**10**), a small potentiometric discrimination was observed with a response order of **7** (n=1) > **8** (n=2) > **9** (n=3) > **10** (n=4), decreasing in the order of increasing distance between the two carboxylate groups. For the geometrical isomers of dicarboxylates, *i.e.*, maleate (**11**) and fumarate (**12**), much larger response was observed for **11** (*cis* isomer) than for **12** (*trans* isomer) (Figure 6, curves 1 and 2). Thus, the greater potentiometric response was obtained for the isomer with the shorter distance between the two negative charges. In addition, potentiometric discrimination of these rigid guests was much greater than that of the flexible linear homologs. For the positional isomers of dicarboxylates, *i.e.*,

TABLE 1. Potentiometric Selectivity Coefficients (K^{Pot}) for Linear Homologs, and Geometrical and Positional Isomers of Dicarboxylates [a)]

Guest	K^{Pot}	Guest	K^{Pot}
Linear homologs [b)]		**Geometrical isomers** [c)]	
7 (n=1)	1	**11** (*cis*)	1
8 (n=2)	0.78	**12** (*trans*)	0.08
9 (n=3)	0.74		0.55[d)]
10 (n=4)	0.68	**Positional isomers** [e)]	
		13 (*ortho*)	1
		14 (*meta*)	0.19
		15 (*para*)	0.04

a) Determined by the separate solution method [22]. b) pH 7.70 (HEPES buffer). c) pH 8.22 (HEPES buffer). d) Selectivity coefficient with the Capriquat® electrode. e) pH 7.41 (HEPES buffer).

phthalate (**13**), isophthalate (**14**) and terephthalate (**15**), potentiometric discrimination was observed with a response order of **13** (*ortho*) > **14** (*meta*) > **15** (*para*). Again, the magnitude of potentiometric response was in the order of decreasing distance between the two negative charges within the guest molecule. Potentiometric discrimination was the greatest for the positional isomers among the three series of dicarboxylate guests examined.

These potentiometric selectivities clearly reflects the general complexation selectivities displayed by protonated macrocyclic polyamines in water, which are based on electrostatic interaction between the host and guest [14, 15, 19, 20]. Potentiometric discrimination was proved to occur more efficiently with the rigid guests than with the flexible ones. Furthermore, although a classical ion-exchanger type electrode composed of Capriquat® (methyltrioctylammonium chloride, > 86%) also

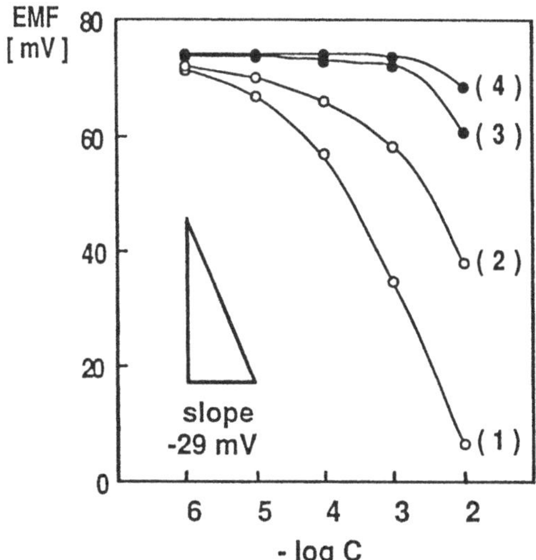

FIGURE 6. Potentiometric response of the liquid membrane electrode containing macrocyclic polyamine **1** (○) or Capriquat® (●) as a sensory element toward geometrical isomers of dicarboxylates (**11**, **12**) at pH 8.22. Curves 1 and 3, and 2 and 4 correspond to guests **11** (*cis*) and **12** (*trans*), respectively.

showed some discrimination for guests **11** and **12** (curves 3 and 4 in Figure 6, Table 1), the present macrocyclic polyamine sensor was superior in every important aspects of sensor, *i.e.*, selectivity, sensitivity, dynamic range, and response time.

The present sensor is characteristic in that the sensory element, initially existing as an uncharged, inactive form in the bulk membrane phase, changes to a charged, "active" form by multiple protonation at the membrane surface. This proton uptake is a prerequisite both for complexation with and potentiometric response to polyanionic guests. It is most likely that the protonated macrocyclic polyamines, charge-separated from the counter anions, exist only at the membrane surface and the electroneutrality in the bulk membrane still holds. Such aspect is not seen in classical ion-exchanger or neutral carrier type ion-selective electrodes. This is also supported by a rapid response time and the absence of hysteresis in the electrode behavior [2, 3].

3. POTENTIOMETRIC SENSOR FOR CATECHOL AND RELATED COMPOUNDS [4, 5]

The development of "potentiometric" sensors for neutral organic analytes is a puzzling problem, but involves a fundamental interesting problem concerning whether uncharged species can generate charge separation and, as a result, membrane potential. From this viewpoint, recent findings by Kimura *et al.* [23] are quite interesting because a protonated macrocyclic polyamine was found to form 1:1 complexes in neutral water with catechol and related compounds despite that these guests are in the uncharged, neutral forms under the experimental pH condition.

Based on these backgrounds, the availability of potentiometric response to catechol (**16a**) and related compounds (**16~34**) was examined using a PVC-supported membrane electrode containing macrocyclic polyamine **1** as a sensory element and *o*-nitrophenyl octyl ether (NPOE, **35**) as a membrane solvent [4, 5].

Figure 7 shows the log C vs E curves for catechol (**16a**), and its monomethoxy (**16b**) and dimethoxy (**16c**) derivatives at pH 6.1. Although guest **16a** (pK_1 = 9.5) almost exclusively exists in the uncharged form at this pH, a strong negative potentiometric response was unexpectedly observed. A negative potentiometric response, although much weaker, was also observed for guest **16b** having one OH group. However, the response to guest **16c** with no OH group was negligible.

In order to clarify the relation between the potentiometric response and the guest structure, potentiometric selectivity coefficients were determined by the matched potential method [16] for a series catechol related guests (**16~34**) (Table 2). This systematic investigation revealed the following tendencies. (i) A negative potentiometric response is generated by a wide range of guests having phenolic OH group(s) (**16a**,**b**, **17a**,**b**, **18a**,**b**, **19~28**) at the pH under which these guests exist almost exclusively in the neutral forms in the bulk aqueous phase. On the other hand, the response to the guests with no OH group (**16c**, **17c**, **18c**) was negligible. (ii) Comparing the three isomers of catechol, the magnitude of potentiometric response was in the order of **16a** (*ortho*) > **17a** (*meta*) >**18a** (*para*). In addition, among the aliphatic alcohols

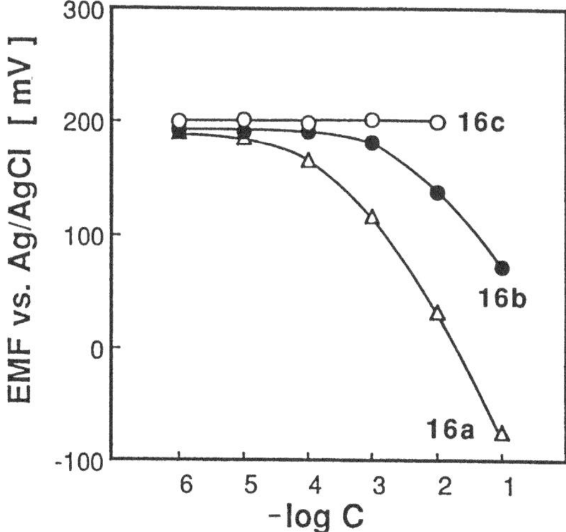

FIGURE 7. Potentiometric response of the liquid membrane electrode containing macrocyclic polyamine **1** toward catechol (**16a**) and its monomethoxy (**16b**) and dimethoxy (**16c**) derivatives at pH 6.1 (acetate buffer).

examined (**29**~**34**), *trans*-1,2-cyclohexanediol (**29a**) having a catechol-like steric structure exceptionally generated a potentiometric response. (iii) Comparing a series of catechol derivatives, the magnitude of potentiometric response was in the order of **28** > **27** > **26** > **16a**, the more hydrophobic guest generating the stronger response.

The fundamental condition for the generation of negative potentiometric response is that a positive species be transferred from the organic (membrane) to aqueous phase, or a negative species transferred from the aqueous to organic phase. The simplest mechanism consistent with this electrochemical requirement would be proton ejection from the organic to aqueous phase as shown in Figure 8. Thus, host-guest complexation between the protonated macrocyclic polyamine and the OH groups of catechol at the membrane surface might induce proton ejection, either by a decrease of basicity of the polyamine nitrogens or by a facilitated dissociation of the OH groups of catechol. An experimental result in homogeneous aqueous solution has been reported that might

TABLE 2. Potentiometric Selectivity Coefficients (K^{Pot}) and the first dissociation constants (pK_1) for Catechol and Related Compounds [a)]

Guest	K^{Pot}	pK_1	Guest	K^{Pot}	pK_1
16a (*ortho*)[b)]	1	9.5	**19**[c)]	25	7.2
17a (*meta*)[b)]	0.070	9.4	**20**[c)]	6.0	9.4
18a (*para*)[b)]	0.0077	10.0	**21**[c)]	3.9	8.0
			22[c)]	3.2	8.5
11b[b)]	0.052	10.0	**23**[c)]	1.4	7.6
12b[b)]	0.78	9.7	**24**[c)]	1.1	10.3
13b[b)]	0.25	10.2	**25**[c)]	0.58	10.0
			16b[c)]	0.49	10.2
26[b)]	2.0		**16a**[c)]	0.0089	10.0
27[b)]	18				
28[b)]	72		**29a**[b)]	0.0066	

a) Determined by the matched potential method [16].
b) pH 6.2 (acetate buffer). c) pH 4.2 (acetate buffer).

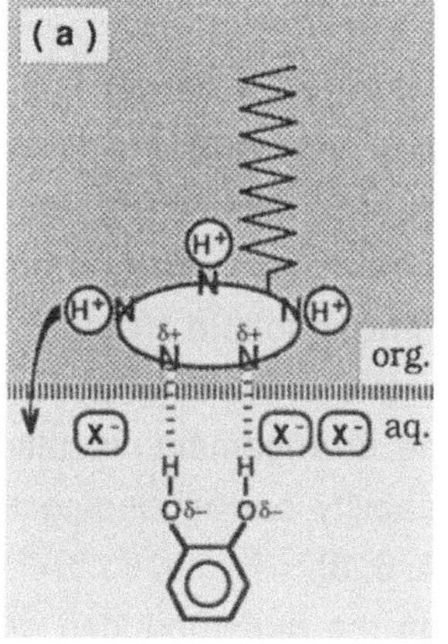

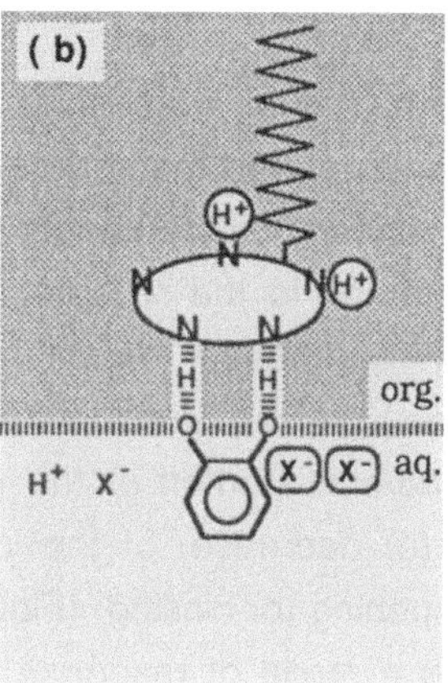

FIGURE 8. A possible mechanism of potentiometric response for catechol and related guests. (a) Proton uptake by **1** at the membrane surface inducing a positive membrane potential and host-guest interaction. (b) Host-guest complexation and a decrease of charge separation, resulting in a negative potentiometric response. In the present figure, a triprotonated state is assumed for macrocyclic polyamine **1** at the membrane surface.

indicate facilitated dissociation of proton as a result of host-guest complexation by macrocyclic polyamines [24].

4. ANION RESPONSIVE ION-CHANNEL MIMETIC SENSORS BASED ON LANGMUIR-BLODGETT (LB) MEMBRANE ASSEMBLIES [7, 8]

From the viewpoint of analytical chemistry, the most significant feature of receptor ion-channel proteins in biological membranes is intensive signal amplification based on controlled flux of a large amount of ions through the membrane by stimulant-triggered opening/closing of the channel [1]. Besides the approaches using real ion-channel proteins [25-29], those based on totally artificial systems are quite significant because of design versatility for a wide range of stimulants (analytes) as well as chemical stability of the systems, as clearly demonstrated in the development of ion-selective electrodes using synthetic ligands [9].

4.1. Principle of ion-channel mimetic function

Some prototypes of ion-channel mimetic sensors were developed using charged and ordered membrane assemblies deposited directly on glassy carbon electrodes by the Langmuir-Blodgett (LB) method [6]. Binding of a guest metal ion to the receptor site of a negatively charged membrane assembly composed of an anionic phospholipid (alone or with valinomycin) causes partial neutralization of the membraneous negative charge and/or distortion of the membrane arrangement, resulting in an increase (or decrease) of the ion permeability corresponding to model channel opening (or closing) (Figure 9a) [4, 6, 8].

Such a mode of response, based on the guest-induced change of ion permeability, can be detected at the underlying electrode by cyclic voltammetry (CV) using an appropriate marker ion such as $[Fe(CN)_6]^{4-}$ or $[Ru(bpy)_3]^{2+}$ (bpy: 2,2'-bipyridine). In this way, the concentration of guest as analyte in the sample solution can be quantitatively determined from the change of peak height (peak current) in the cyclic voltammogram. Because of the open/close switching of ion flux, the amount of the permeated marker ions thus detected is expected to be a markedly amplified measure of the guest (analyte) [4, 6, 8].

The generalization of the above principle to anion responsive sensors has been carried out by the use of polyamine hosts that function by multiprotonation as polycationic hosts capable of complexation with anionic guests [7]. Upon binding with an anionic guest, a decrease (increase) of the permeability for anionic (cationic) marker ion, corresponding to model channel closing (opening), is expected as a result of a decrease of the net positive charge and/or a change of the membrane arrangement (Figure 9b). The anion receptors used were macrocyclic polyamine **1** and cyclodextrin polyamine **2**. The latter host, heptakis(6-dodecylamino-6-deoxy)-β-cyclodextrin ($(6\text{-}C_{12}H_{25}NH)_7$-β-CD), was developed by Tagaki [30] as a new type of cyclodextrin derivative with an amphiphilic nature. This type of hosts [30, 31] are known to form stable LB membranes either with or without guest molecules [32-34]. Since host **2** has a cavity of 7~8 Å diameter capable of accommodating hydrophobic moieties of guests, the sensor containing host **2** is expected to show a different response selectivity compared with that containing simple macrocyclic polyamine **1**.

4.2. Response to anionic guests

Anion responsive ion-channel mimetic sensors were constructed with an LB membrane of macrocyclic polyamine **1** and lipid **36** (1:1 molar ratio, five layers) or that of cyclodextrin polyamine **2** alone (four to six layers), which were deposited directly on glassy carbon electrodes by the horizontal lifting method (Sensors 1 and 2, respectively). Differential scanning calorimetry showed that the LB membranes of the present sensors are most likely in a gel rather than liquid crystalline state under the CV measurement conditions.

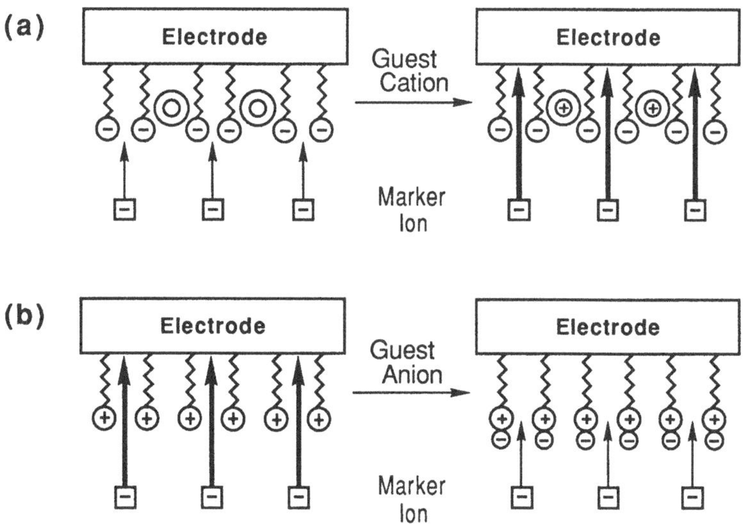

FIGURE 9. Schematic representations of the permeability change for anionic marker ion in the present "ion-channel" mimetic sensors, corresponding to model channel opening or closing behavior. (a) Cation responsive sensor with a composite LB membrane of valinomycin and phospholipid. (b) Anion responsive sensor with an LB membrane of protonated polyamine host.

In the present anion responsive sensors, proton uptake from the sample aqueous phase by the polyamine host at the membrane surface is a prerequisite for the membrane assembly to bear a positive charge. The acquired membraneous positive charge is, in turn, a prerequisite both for the binding with anionic guests and the control of ion permeation. This fundamental property is clearly reflected in the pH profile of the sensors.

For Sensor 1 containing macrocyclic polyamine **1** as a sensory element, the peak current in the cyclic voltammogram obtained by using $[Fe(CN)_6]^{4-}$ ($[Ru(bpy)_3]^{2+}$) as a marker ion increased (decreased) with decreasing pH. These cyclic voltammetric changes can be ascribed to an increasing electrostatic attraction (repulsion) between the anionic (cationic) marker ion and the protonated macrocyclic polyamine bearing a pH-dependent magnitude of positive charge. A similar pH-response profile was observed for Sensor 2 containing cyclodextrin polyamine **2**.

The response of the present sensors to anionic guests is represented in Figure 10 showing the cyclic voltammograms obtained at pH 6.0 for Sensor 1 in the absence and presence of anionic guest **11**. With the anionic marker ion ($[Fe(CN)_6]^{4-}$), the peak current decreased with an increasing concentration of the anionic guest (Figure 10a). On the other hand, when the cationic marker ion ($[Ru(bpy)_3]^{2+}$) was used, the peak current increased with an increasing guest concentration (Figure 10b). These observations can be explained by a decrease of the electrostatic attraction (repulsion) between the protonated macrocyclic polyamine and the anionic (cationic) marker ion due to partial neutralization by the anionic guest of the membraneous positive charge, resulting in a decrease (increase) of the permeability for the anionic (cationic) marker ion. Schematic representation is shown in Figure 9b for the guest-induced "channel closing" when an anionic marker ion is used. Similar CV changes were observed with Sensors 1 and 2 for a number of anionic guests including adenosine nucleotides, dicarboxylic acids, and inorganic anions.

4.3. Selectivity of response

Since the magnitude of response to guest anions by the present sensors will be most properly expressed, in a practical sense, by the change of the

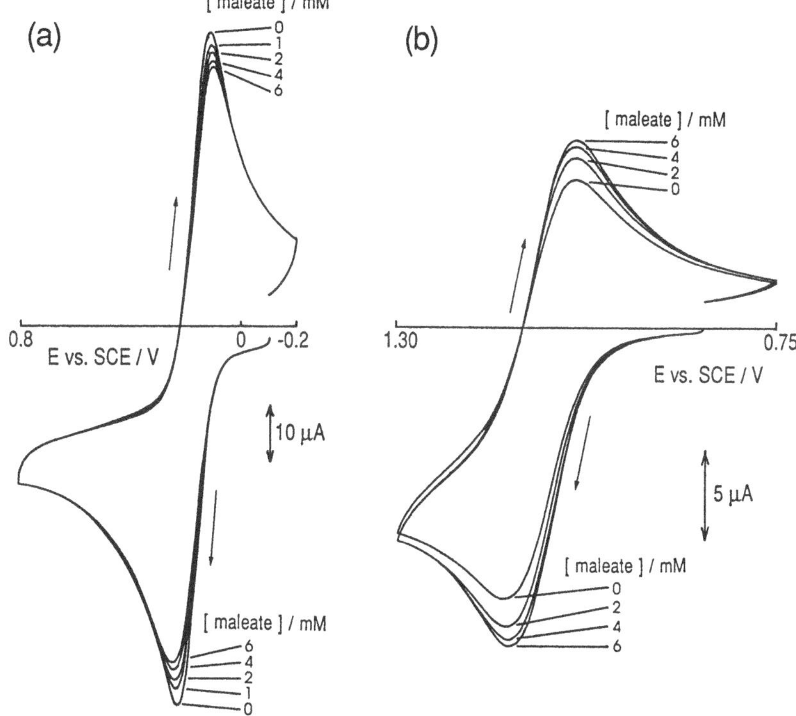

FIGURE 10. Cyclic voltammograms for the anion responsive sensor containing macrocyclic polyamine **1** in the absence and presence of maleate (**11**) as an anionic guest. The direction of potential scan is indicated with arrows. LB membrane composition: **1** + **3** (1:1 molar ratio, five layers). (a) pH = 6.0, $[[Fe(CN)_6]^{4-}]$ = 1.5 mM, and $[K_2SO_4]$ = 50 mM. (b) pH = 6.0, $[[Ru(bpy)_3]^{2+}]$ = 0.50 mM, and $[K_2SO_4]$ = 10 mM.

peak height (peak current) in the CV oxidation wave, the selectivity of response was calculated from the decrease percentage of the oxidation peak current for each guest (Table 3). The pH conditions for the CV measurements were set at pH 4.5~6.0 so that the polyamine hosts would be sufficiently protonated and at the same time the guests be sufficiently dissociated to be anionic forms.

Sensors 1 and 2 showed similar selectivities for the series of organic anions except for the phthalate series (**13~15**). The response orders of the adenosine nucleotides and the geometrical isomers of dicarboxylates were ATP^{4-} (**4**) > ADP^{3-} (**5**) > AMP^{2-} (**6**), and **11** (*cis*) > **12** (*trans*), respectively, for the both sensors (Table 3). For the adenosine nucleotides, the both sensors showed a greater response for the guest with a greater negative charge. On the other hand, for the *cis/trans* geometrical isomers of dicarboxylates, a greater response was observed for the guest with a shorter distance between the two anionic groups. For the inorganic anions, a response order similar to that for conventional ion-selective electrodes was observed with Sensor 1. However, the responses to bromide and chloride ions were negligible under the experimental conditions. The voltammetric selectivities displayed by Sensor 1 are qualitatively consistent with the complexation selectivities in water of macrocyclic polyamine hosts having related structures [17, 18, 19, 20]. Interestingly, the voltammetric selectivities are also consistent with the potentiometric selectivities of the liquid membrane ion-selective electrode containing host **1** [2, 3] (see Section 2).

For the positional isomers of phthalate, the response selectivities were different between Sensors 1 and 2 (Table 3). Sensor 1 showed a response order of **13** (*ortho*) > **14** (*meta*) > **15** (*para*), corresponding to an expected order of the magnitude of the host-guest interaction based on electrostatic interaction. On the other hand, Sensor 2 interestingly showed a different response order, *i.e.*, **14** (*meta*) > **15** (*para*) > **13** (*ortho*). This characteristic selectivity is possibly due to the host-guest interaction involving the β-cyclodextrin cavity capable of recognizing steric structures of guests.

4.4. Amplification

The important feature of the present ion-channel mimetic sensors is that they have a built-in ability of amplification, since binding of a single guest molecule to the membraneous receptor would trigger (or inhibit) the permeation of a large amount of ions. In the present study, the

TABLE 3. Selectivity and Amplification Factors of Anion Responsive Ion-Channel Mimetic Sensors Containing Lipophilic Macrocyclic Polyamine (**1**) and Cyclodextrin Polyamine (**2**)

	Sensor 1 a)		Sensor 2 b)	
Guest anion	Selectivity factor c,d)	Amplification factor e,f)	Selectivity factor c,g)	Amplification factor e,h)
Series 1				
ATP^{4-} (**4**)	1.00	5.4	1.00	18.8
ADP^{3-} (**5**)	0.78	4.5	0.44	17.0
AMP^{2-} (**6**)	0.19	4.1	0.15	12.1
Series 2				
11 (*cis*)	1.00	13.8	1.00	5.8
12 (*trans*)	0.03	7.3	0.41	4.3
Series 3				
13 (*ortho*)	1.00	3.3	0.55	11.7
14 (*meta*)	0.37	2.4	1.00	13.0
15 (*para*)	0.02	1.1	0.83	12.2
Series 4 i)				
ClO_4^-	1.00	4.0		
SCN^-	0.69	3.2		
I^-	0.40	1.2		
NO_3^-	0.06	0.13		

a) Membrane components: Macrocyclic polyamine **1** and lipid **35** (1:1 molar ratio; five layers). b) Membrane components: Cyclodextrin polyamine **2** (four to six layers). c) Relative value of the decrease percentage of the oxidation peak current in cyclic voltammogram for each series of guests (fixed guest concentration for each series; $[Fe(CN)_6]^{4-}$ (1.5 mM) as a marker ion). d) pH = 6.0 (acetate buffer). [Guest] = 1.0, 2.0, 2.0 and 4.0 mM for series 1, 2, 3 and 4, respectively. e) The changed molar amount of the oxidized marker ions relative to the total mole of the receptors embedded in the outmost layer of the LB membrane. f) pH = 5.7, 4.5, 6.0 and 6.0 (acetate buffer), and [guest] = 9.0, 7.0, 6.0 and 12.0 mM for series 1, 2, 3 and 4, respectively. g) pH = 6.0 (acetate buffer). [Guest] = 1.0, 2.0 and 2.0 mM for series 1, 2 and 3, respectively. h) pH = 6.0 (acetate buffer). [Guest] = 9.0, 7.0 and 6.0 mM for series 1, 2 and 3, respectively. i) The responses to bromide and chloride ions were negligible.

amplification factor was defined as the changed molar amount of the permeated marker ions relative to the total mole of the receptors embedded in the outmost layer of the LB membrane. The former was calculated from the guest-induced change of the peak area of the CV oxidation wave, and the latter from the A_0 value which indicates (average) molecular area of the membrane component(s) extrapolated at zero surface pressure. The A_0 values were determined from the π-A isotherm with a subphase corresponding to a typical condition of the present CV measurements .

The amplification factors for each guest are listed in Table 3. A value up to 19 was obtained with a scanning time of 9 s. Since saturation of the voltammetric response was not observed upon increasing the guest concentration, it can be presumed that the receptor molecules at the outmost layer are not fully occupied by the guest under the guest concentration range examined. Accordingly, the amplification factors calculated as above should be regarded as underestimated values.

5. CONCLUDING REMARKS

Two modes of signal transduction at membrane surface were studied by totally artificial systems using anion receptor molecules. The expected complexation selectivities in water are generally reflected, at least in a qualitative sense, to the potentiometric and voltammetric selectivities, which are based on different aspects of chemical phenomena in a sense that the latter selectivities involve complexation plus signal transduction at the membrane surface.

Potentiometric response by the electrode containing macrocyclic polyamine **1** described in Sections 2 and 3 are based on (i) charge separation by proton uptake, (ii) complexation with anionic or catecholic guests, and (iii) decrease of charge separation by a direct manner or proton ejection, resulting in a negative potentiometric response (Figures 4 and 8). All of these functions can be regarded as characteristic host functionalities displayed at membrane surface by protonated macrocyclic polyamines. The response mode of the ion-channel mimetic sensors described in Section 4 might be regarded as a simplest mimic of the channel opening/closing behavior of the biological ion-channel proteins, which would be a useful principle for signal transduction and amplification in the development of biomimetic sensors.

Considering the promising features of artificial host compounds as sensory elements, *i.e.*, designed selectivity as well as high chemical stability and synthetic versatility, systematic studies to elucidate quantitative relations between the host-guest complexation at membrane surface and the electrochemical signal transduction will certainly serve as reliable bases for rational design of biomimetic sensors.

ACKNOWLEDGMENTS

This work is supported by the Grant-in-Aids for Scientific Research from the Ministry of Education, Science and Culture, the Joint Studies Program (1988~1989) of the Institute for Molecular Science, and the Japan-U.S. Cooperative Science Program sponsored by Japan Society for the Promotion of Science and the U.S. National Science Foundation.

REFERENCES

1. B. Alberts, D. Bray, J. Lewis, M. Raff, K. Roberts, and J. D. Watson, *Molecular Biology of the Cell* (2nd ed.), Garland Publishing, New York, 1989; chapters 6 and 19.
2. Y. Umezawa, M. Kataoka, W. Takami, E. Kimura, T. Koike, and H. Nada, *Anal. Chem.*, **60**, 2392-2396 (1988).
3. M. Kataoka, R. Naganawa, K. Odashima, Y. Umezawa, E. Kimura, and T. Koike, *Anal. Lett.*, **22**, 1089-1105 (1989).
4. Y. Umezawa, M. Sugawara, M. Kataoka, and K. Odashima, in *Ion-Selective Electrodes, 5*, ed. by E. Pungor, Akadémiai Kiadó, Budapest, in press.
5. K. Odashima, H. Radecka, T. Kimura, R. Naganawa, M. Kataoka, Y. Umezawa, E. Kimura, and T. Koike, submitted for publication.
6. M. Sugawara, K. Kojima, H. Sazawa, and Y. Umezawa, *Anal. Chem.*, **59**, 2842-2846 (1987).
7. S. Nagase, M. Kataoka, R. Naganawa, R. Komatsu, K. Odashima, and Y. Umezawa, submitted for publication.
8. M. Sugawara, M. Kataoka, K. Odashima, and Y. Umezawa, *Thin Solid Films*, in press.
9. D. Ammann, W. E. Morf, P. Anker, P. C. Meier, E. Pretsch, and W. Simon, *Ion-Selective Electrode Rev.*, **5**, 3-92 (1983).
10. U. Wuthier, H. V. Pham, B. Rusterholz, and W. Simon, *Helv. Chim. Acta*, **69**, 1435-1441 (1986), and the references cited therein.
11. D. Ammann, M. Huser, B. Kräutler, B. Rusterholz, P. Schulthess, B. Lindemann, E. Halder, and W. Simon, *Helv. Chim. Acta*, **69**, 849-854 (1986), and the references cited therein.
12. N. A. Chaniotakis, A. M. Chasser, M. E. Meyerhoff, and J. T. Groves, *Anal. Chem.*, **60**, 185-188 (1988).
13. A. Hodinár and A. Jyo, *Chem. Lett.*, **1988**, 993-996; S. Daunert and L. G. Bachas, *Anal. Chem.*, **61**, 499-503 (1989).
14. E. Kimura, *Top. Curr. Chem.*, **128**, 113-141 (1985).
15. J. M. Lehn, *Science*, **227**, 849-856 (1985); *Angew. Chem., Int. Ed. Engl.*, **27**, 90-112 (1988).
16. V. P. Y. Gadzekpo and G. D. Christian, *Anal. Chim. Acta*, **164**, 279-282 (1984).
17. E. Kimura, A. Sakonaka, T. Yatsunami, and M. Kodama, *J. Am. Chem. Soc.*, **103**, 3041-3045 (1981).
18. B. Dietrich, M. W. Hosseini, J. M. Lehn, and R. B. Sessions, *J. Am. Chem. Soc.*, **103**, 1282-1283 (1981); M. W. Hosseini and J. M. Lehn, *Helv. Chim. Acta*, **70**, 1312-1319 (1987).

19. E. Kimura, M. Kodama, and T. Yatsunami, *J. Am. Chem. Soc.*, **104**, 3182-3187 (1982).
20. M. W. Hosseini and J. M. Lehn, *J. Am. Chem. Soc.*, **104**, 3525-3527 (1982); *Helv. Chim. Acta*, **69**, 587-603 (1986); *Helv. Chim. Acta*, **71**, 749-756 (1988).
21. N. Ishibashi, A. Jyo, and M. Yonemitsu, *Chem. Lett.*, **1973**, 483-484; N. Ishibashi, A. Jyo, and K. Matsumoto, *Chem. Lett.*, **1973**, 1297-1298; A. Jyo, M. Yonemitsu, and N. Ishibashi, *Bull. Chem. Soc. Jpn.*, **46**, 3734-3737 (1973).
22. K. Srinivasan and G. A. Rechnitz, *Anal. Chem.*, **41**, 1203-1208 (1969).
23. E. Kimura, A. Watanabe, and M. Kodama, *J. Am. Chem. Soc.*, **105**, 2063-2066 (1983).
24. E. Kimura, A. Sakonaka, and M. Kodama, *J. Am. Chem. Soc.*, **104**, 4984-4985 (1982).
25. P. Yager, *Biosensors*, **2**, 363-373 (1986).
26. M. Gotoh, E. Tamiya, M. Momoi, Y. Kagawa, and I. Karube, *Anal. Lett.*, **20**, 857-870 (1987).
27. M. E. Eldefrawi, S. M. Sherby, A. G. Andreou, N. A. Mansour, Z. Annau, N. A. Blum, and J. J. Valdes, *Anal. Lett.*, **21**, 1665-1680 (1988).
28. R. F. Taylor, I. G. Marenchic, and E. J. Cook, *Anal. Chim. Acta*, **213**, 131-138 (1988).
29. M. Uto, E. K. Michaelis, I. F. Hu, Y. Umezawa, and T. Kuwana, *Anal. Sci.*, submitted for publication.
30. H. Takahashi, Y. Irinatsu, S. Kozuka, and W. Tagaki, *Mem. Fac. Eng., Osaka City Univ.*, **26**, 93-99 (1985); H. Takahashi and W. Tagaki, *Yukagaku*, **37**, 1027-1031 (1988).
31. W. Tagaki, *Yukagaku*, **37**, 394-401 (1988), and the references cited therein.
32. M. Tanaka, Y. Ishizuka, M. Matsumoto, T. Nakamura, A. Yabe, H. Nakanishi, Y. Kawabata, H. Takahashi, S. Tamura, W. Tagaki, H. Nakahara, and K. Fukuda, *Chem. Lett.*, **1987**, 1307-1310.
33. Y. Kawabata, M. Matsumoto, T. Nakamura, M. Tanaka, E. Manda, H. Takahashi, S. Tamura, W. Tagaki, H. Nakahara, and K. Fukuda, *Thin Solid Films*, **159**, 353-358 (1988), and the references cited therein.
34. S. Taneva, K. Ariga, Y. Okahata, and W. Tagaki, *Langmuir*, **5**, 111-113 (1989).

7

Applications of Enzymes in Amperometric Sensors: Problems and Possibilities

PHILIP N. BARTLETT Department of Chemistry, University of Warwick, Coventry, CV4 7AL, UK

ABSTRACT

The combination of redox enzyme catalysts and amperometric electrochemistry is an attractive approach to chemical sensing. The successful development of devices using amperometric enzyme electrochemistry poses a number of problems; including those of the integration of the electrode and the biological components, stability, reproducibility, and interference. To overcome these problems, it is necessary to understand the interplay of mass transport and kinetics in amperometric enzyme electrodes and to develop strategies for the development of such electrodes.

In this paper we discuss some of the different approaches which exist to link the flow of electrons in biological electron transfer reactions to electrodes. These include the use of homogeneous mediators, modified electrodes, organic conducting salt electrodes, and covalent modificiation of the enzyme itself. We also discuss the application of conducting polymers to this problem.

INTRODUCTION

A brief consideration of undergraduate biochemistry texts

reveals that electron transfer reactions and electron transport play a key role in the processes of life.* In living cells electrons are transferred between redox partners in an orderly and ordered fashion in so called electron transport chains. At each link in these chains specific interactions between the redox partners ensure molecular recognition. Disruption of the sequential transfer of electrons along such chains, for example by the presence of low molecular weight indiscriminate electron transfer catalysts such as methyl-viologen (paraquat), is frequently fatal.

In developing amperometric biosensors the electrochemist seeks to exploit the high specificity of the biological electron transport chain to make sensors which can be used to detect particular components in complex mixtures. The very features which confer specificity also present a challenge. Frequently the biological molecules we wish to use show very poor electron transfer kinetics at metallic electrodes. With hindsight this is not surprising since a simple metallic electrode rarely presents a surface attuned to the particular requirements of the bio-molecule. In this article we shall examine some of the ways in which we may overcome this problem. We will concentrate on two classes of redox enzymes, dehydrogenases and flavoproteins.

DEHYDROGENASE BASED SYSTEMS

NADH (β-nicotinamide adenine dinucleotide) and the closely related NADPH (β-nicotinamide adenine dinucleotide phosphate) are two important coenzymes; over 250 NADH dependent, and over 150 NADPH dependent, dehydrogenases are known. Consequently there has been much interest in NAD(P)H electrochemistry and its application in biosensors. Table 1 lists a few NADH dependent hydrogenases and their potential applications.

---

* To quote H. A. O. Hill[1],
"Life is just one damned electron after another".[2]

TABLE 1 Some NADH dependent dehydrogenase enzymes

ENZYME	ANALYTE	APPLICATIONS
Alcohol Dehydrogenase	Ethanol	Fermantation Excise Food Industry
3α-Hydroxysteroid Dehydrogenase	Bile Acids	Clinical
Lactate Dehydrogenase	Lactate	Agriculture
Malate Dehydrogenase	Malate	Fermentation
Glutamate Dehydrogenase	Glutamate	Fermentation Food Industry
Glucose Dehydrogenase	Glucose	Fermentation Clinical
Amino Acid Dehydrogenase	Amino Acids	Clinical Food Industry
Tartrate Dehydrogenase	Tartrate	Food Industry
12α-Hydroxysteroid Dehydrogenase	Bile Acids	Clinical
Oestradiol 17α-Dehydrogenase	Oestradiol	Clinical
Aryl-alcohol Dehydrogenase	Aromatic Alcohols	Environmental
Testosterone 17β-Dehydrogenase	Testosterone	Clinical

In these systems the coenzyme undergoes oxidation or reduction in the course of the enzymatic reaction,

$$SH_2 + NAD^+ \xrightarrow{\text{dehydrogenase}} S + NADH + H^+$$

where SH_2 represents the substrate and S is the oxidised product. In nearly all cases which have been studied the enzyme catalyzed reaction proceeds by an ordered bisubstrate mechanism in which the

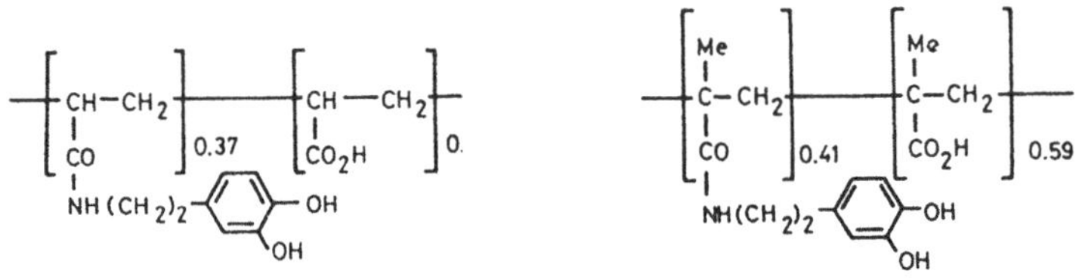

FIGURE 1 Structure of two ortho-quinone polymers used to prepare modified electrodes for the oxidation of NADH (from the work of Miller et al.[7,8]).

coenzyme must bind first (to give a complex called a haloenzyme) followed by binding of substrate. After reaction the product departs first, followed by the coenzyme.

The problem of utilising dehydrogenases in enzyme electrodes is essentially the problem of either oxidising or reducing the coenzyme at the electrode. Of these two processes the oxidation of NAD(P)H to biologically active $NAD(P)^+$ is by far the easier, although it is by no means trivial. This is because the reverse reaction, the reduction of NAD^+ to NADH, can lead to an enzymatically inactive isomer. In addition inactive dimers may also be produced.[3] Fortunately, for the majority of sensor applications, it is the oxidation of NAD(P)H to $NAD(P)^+$ which is of interest.

At clean metallic electrodes the oxidation of NADH only occurs at large overpotentials and proceeds through radical intermediates. This can cause problems with electrode fouling and/or

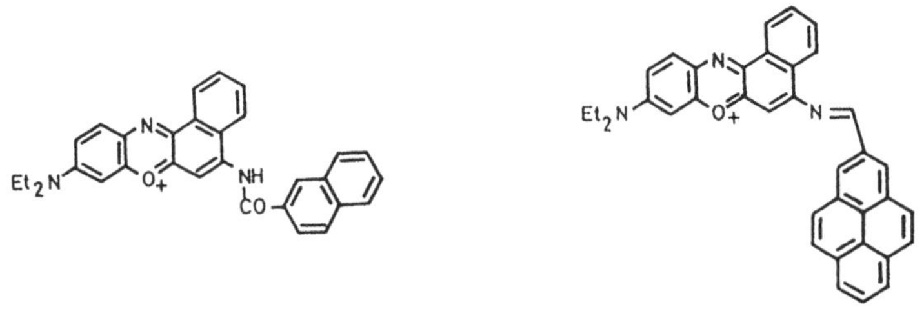

FIGURE 2 Redox dyes used to prepare modified carbon electrodes for NADH oxidation (from the work of Gorton et al.[4]).

interference when applied in electrochemical sensors. Hence there have been a number of attempts to produce a modified electrode surface at which the oxidation of NADH to enzymatically active NAD^+ can be achieved at more modest potentials. Much of this work has been discussed in an excellent review by Gorton.[4]

The general approach adopted towards this problem has been to try to identify species which react rapidly in homogeneous solution with NADH and then to immobilise these at the electrode surface using one or other of the techniques available to produce chemically modified electrodes.[5,6] For example Miller's group[7-10] have investigated the use polymers containing ortho-quinone groups, figure 1. They found that the electrodes initially catalyzed the oxidation of NADH to NAD^+ but that the effect rapidly decayed with use. They also found problems with the propagation of charge through the films; only those quinone groups close to the electrode were in electrical communication with the electrode. A more fruitful approach is to use redox dyes adsorbed on graphite, figure 2. In this way Gorton[11,12] and coworkers were able to get good stability and to achieve the oxidation of NADH at low potentials. This approach has now been applied in flow injection analysis using sensors based on NADH dependent dehydrogenases such as glucose dehydrogenase[13].

Conducting organic salts can also be used as electrode materials for these types of application. For example NMP.TCNQ (where NMP is N-methyl phenazine and TCNQ is tetracyanoquinodimethane, figure 3) is a good electrode material for the oxidation of NADH[14] and can be used with alcohol dehydrogenase or steroid dehydrogenases to make alcohol[15] or bile acid[16] sensors, figure 4. In this case the reaction is thought to proceed by adsorption of the NADH on the surface of the conducting salt followed by hydride transfer to the N-methylphenazinum present in the crystal lattice at the electrode surface. An advantage of this approach is that the material is sufficiently conducting that it can be formed into pressed pellets and used to make electrodes.[17] In this form a fresh electrode surface is then prepared simply by polishing and stability is not a problem.

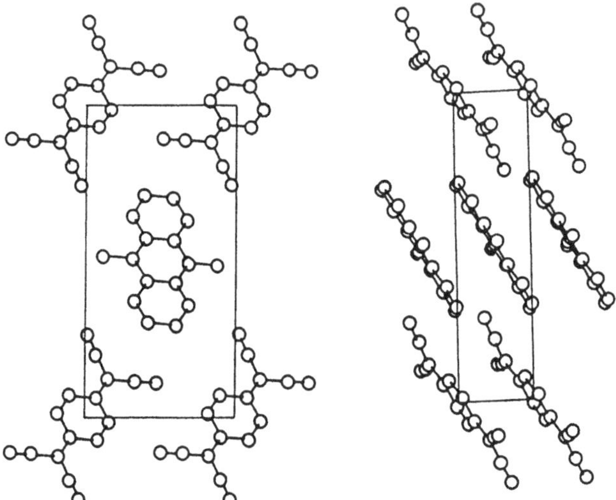

FIGURE 3 The crystal structure of NMP.TCNQ showing the segregated stack structure with TCNQ stacks at the corners of the unit cell. The central NMP stack is disordered with respect to the methyl group position. From Fritchie, C. J. Acta. Cryst. 1966,20,892.

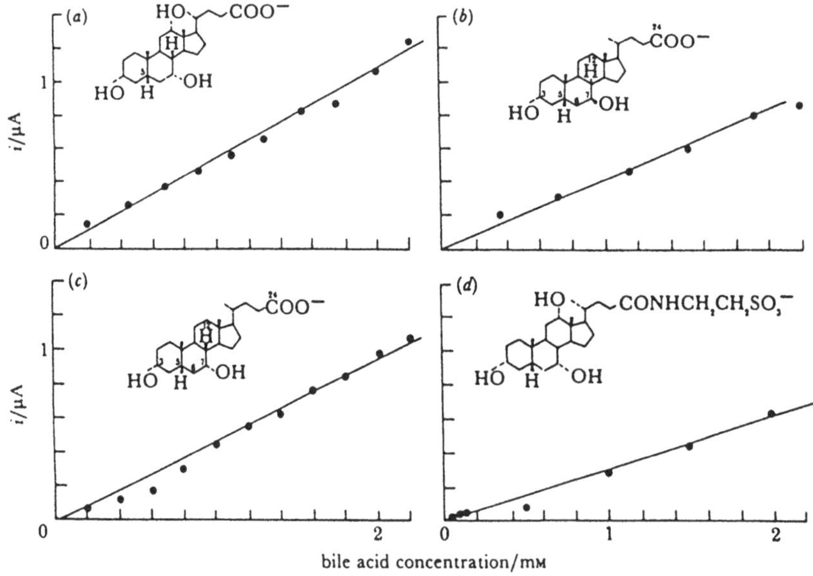

FIGURE 4 Results for the detection of four different bile acids using an NMP.TCNQ membrane electrode and 3-α-hydroxysteroid dehydrogenase: (a) cholic acid; (b) ursodeoxycholic acid; (c) chenodeoxycholic acid; (d) taurocholic acid (from Albery et al.[16]).

FLAVOPROTEIN ELECTROCHEMISTRY

In contrast to the dehydrogenases, the flavoproteins contain one or more flavin prosthetic groups which are reasonably tightly bound to the enzyme. Thus for this class of enzymes the enzyme itself exists in both oxidised and reduced forms depending upon the oxidation state of the flavin group. Table 2 lists some examples of flavoproteins along with possible areas for their application in biosensors. By far and away the most studied system is glucose oxidase. There are a number of reasons for this; most notably the enzyme is readily available, highly active, and very stable. Furthermore there is enormous interest in the development of diagnostic devices to monitor glucose for diabetics[18-21] and for fermentation control.[22]

Glucose oxidase catalyses the oxidation of glucose by oxygen to give gluconolactone and hydrogen peroxide as shown below:

$$\beta\text{-D-glucose} + \text{GOD(FAD)} \longrightarrow \text{gluconolactone} + \text{GOD(FADH}_2\text{)}$$
$$\text{GOD(FADH}_2\text{)} + O_2 \longrightarrow \text{GOD(FAD)} + H_2O_2$$

in this scheme GOD(FAD) represents the oxidised form of the enzyme and GOD($FADH_2$) the reduced form. The overriding problem for the development of amperometric enzyme electrodes using glucose oxidase, or any other flavoprotein, is to find a way to electrochemically reoxidise the enzyme and hence to avoid dependence on oxygen. This is not a trivial problem because the flavin group is buried within the protein and so may lie as much as 50 Å from the electrode surface. Experimental studies suggest that the probability of electron transfer falls exponentially as the distance between centres increases (see for example reviews by Marcus and Sutin[23] and McLendon[24]). Thus

$$k_{el} = k_{el,0} \exp(-\beta[r - r_o])$$

where k_{el} is the electronic transmission coefficient, $k_{el,0}$ its value when the separation is r_o, r is the distance between centres, and β is a constant. Values of β estimated from experimental measurements of long range electron transfer rates suggest that β

TABLE 2 Some flavoproteins and their applications

ENZYME	ANALYTE	APPLICATIONS
Glucose Oxidase	Glucose	Clinical Fermentation
Xanthine Oxidase	Purines	Food Industry
D-Amino Acid Oxidase	D-Amino Acids	Clinical
Cholesterol Oxidase	Cholesterol	Clinical
Mono Amine Oxidase	Mono Amines	Clinical Food Industry
Galactose Oxidase	Galactose	Food Industry

is about 12 nm^{-1}. This implies that the probability of electron transfer decreases by an order of magnitude for every 0.2 nm increase in distance between the two centres. Thus the conventional wisdom suggest that the rate of direct electron transfer between a clean metal electrode and a flavoprotein is likely to be very slow. A number of approaches have been used to tackle this problem. One of these is to employ a low molecular weight solution mediator.

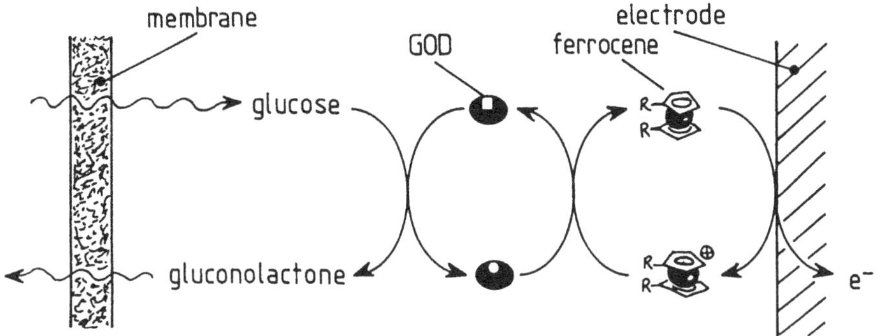

FIGURE 5 The operation of an amperometric enzyme electrode for glucose using a ferrocene mediator to shuttle electrons between the active site of the enzyme and the electrode.

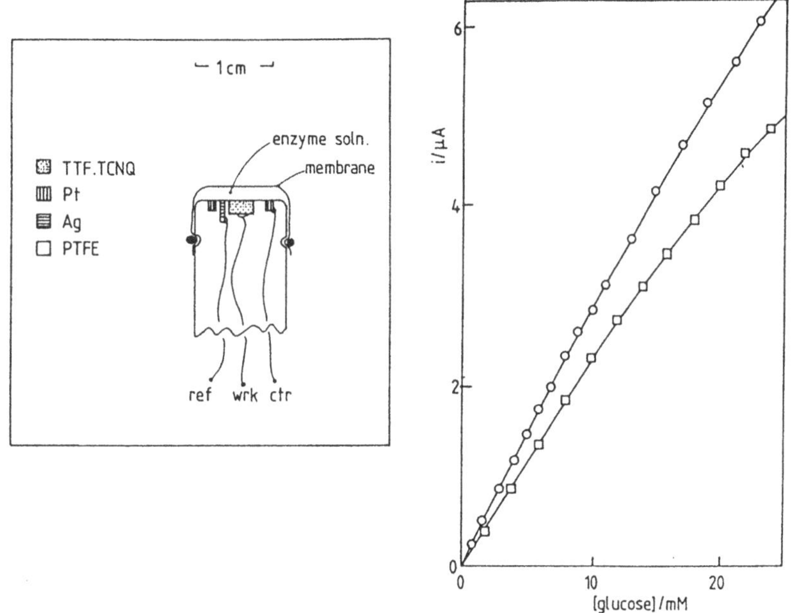

FIGURE 6 Construction of an amperometric membrane covered enzyme electrode using a TTF.TCNQ working electrode

FIGURE 7 Glucose calibration curves for a membrane electrode using glucose oxidase with TTF.TCNQ as the working electrode. The lower curve is the same electrode after 65 hours continuous operation in 30 mM glucose.

This species can then diffuse between the electrode surface and the active site of the enzyme transporting electrons back and forth and hence establish electrical contact between the two. Clearly there are a number of criteria which direct the choice of such a mediator. Firstly, it is essential that it have both rapid electrode kinetics and rapid homogeneous kinetics with the enzyme. Furthermore, it is desirable that the mediator be stable towards oxygen, non-toxic, and have a suitable redox potential. Finally, it would be very nice if we could use synthetic organic chemistry to tailor the properties of the mediator. All of these desirable properties are exhibited by ferrocenes, a fact which was first exploited by Cass et al.[25] to construct an amperometric sensor based on ferrocene mediated oxidation of glucose oxidase.

The ferrocene based glucose electrode is shown schematically in figure 5. The use of ferrocene as a mediator has proved a very successful strategy and one that has been commercialised to make disposable glucose sensors for diabetics.[26] The approach has also been successfully applied to a number of other flavoproteins[27,28] and to quinoproteins.[29]

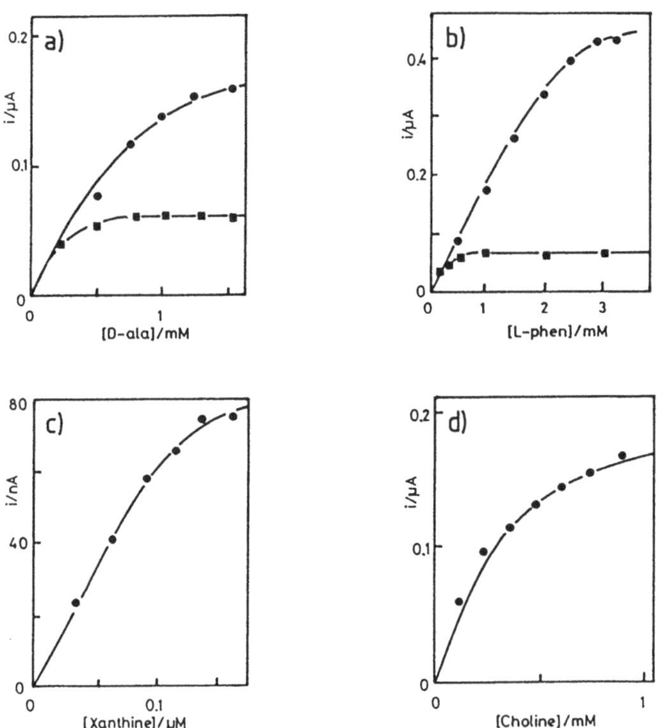

FIGURE 8 Results for four different flavoprotein amperometric enzyme electrodes based on a TTF-TCNQ working electrode: (a) D-amino acid oxidase; (b) L-amino-acid oxidase; (c) xanthine oxidase; (d) choline oxidase. The circles are for membrane electrode, the squares are results for adsorbed enzyme with no membrane.

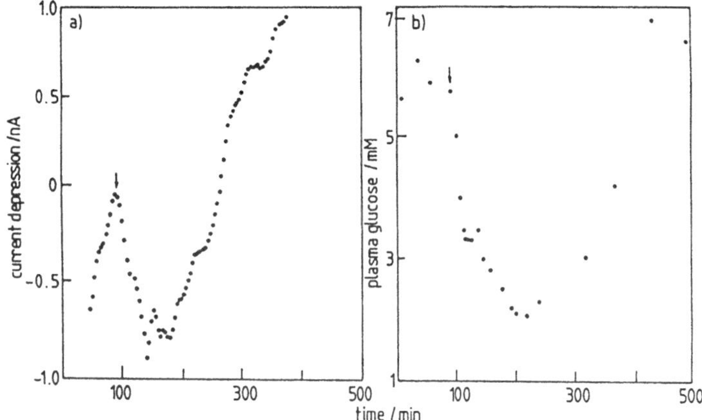

FIGURE 9 Results for in vivo glucose determination in the rat brain: (a) values from an implanted TTF.TCNQ glucose electrode; (b) blood glucose as determined by analysis of blood samples

An alternative approach which has also proved successful and applicable to a range of flavoproteins is the use of conducting organic salt electrodes for the oxidation of the reduced flavoprotein.[30-34] For this application TTF.TCNQ, where TTF is tetrathiafulvalene, appears to be the best choice.[30] TTF.TCNQ has been used with a range of flavoproteins including glucose oxidase, amino acid oxidases, xanthine oxidase and choline oxidase[31,35] Figure 6 shows a glucose membrane electrode based on TTF.TCNQ. Typical results for the detection of glucose are shown in Figure 7. Other flavoproteins can be used as shown by the results in Figure 8. Furthermore it is possible to dispense with the membrane and simply used enzyme directly adsorbed at the electrode surface. The response of these flavoprotein membrane electrodes can be analysed in terms of our published model[36] to establish the rate limiting processes for each electrode. Such analyses show that in all cases, with the exception of the choline electrode, the response is determined by diffusion of the substrate through the dialysis membrane. This is a very satisfactory situation for an enzyme electrode since it means that the response is independent of the enzyme activity. In the case of the choline electrode we fine that the response is determined by both enzyme kinetics and diffusion. At present the precise mechanism of the oxidation of the reduced flavoprotein is the subject of some debate.[16,33,37,38] Nevertheless electrodes of this type obviously work well and have been developed for in vivo applications,[39,40] Figure 9.

APPLICATIONS OF CONDUCTING POLYMERS

Another recent approach has been to immobilise glucose oxidase within conducting polymer films at electrode surfaces. This is attractive for several reasons; the process is simple, it is readily controlled, it is well suited to the immobilisation of enzymes on microelectronic substrates and microelectrodes, and multilayer structures can be developed. The immobilisation is achieved by adding the enzyme to the monomer solution before polymerisation. Typical polymerisation conditions are given in Table 3. The enzyme appears to be entrapped because of its high negative charge (-9 at neutral pH); in effect it is incorporated as a counter ion into the polycationic conducting polymer film. To date the immobilisation of glucose oxidase in polypyrrole,[41,42]

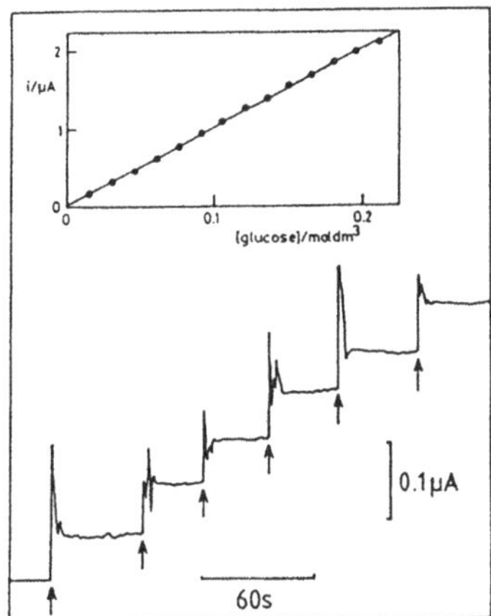

FIGURE 10 Measurement of glucose using glycose oxidase immobilised in poly-N-methylpyrrole film at a platinum electrode.

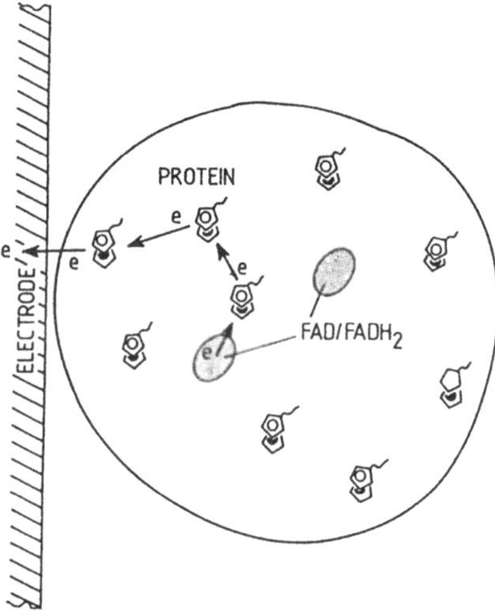

FIGURE 11 A cartoon showing the postulated electron transfer mechanism for modified glucose oxidase.

TABLE 3 Conditions for the electrochemical immobilisation of glucose oxidase

MONOMER	POLYMERISATION CONDITIONS[a]	COMMENTS
Pyrrole[b]	Potentiostatic 0.756 V. 0.2 M monomer.	Thick films. Fair stability. Saturation ca. 0.1 M glucose
N-Methylpyrrole	Potentiostatic 0.8 V 0.05 M monomer. pH 7.2 phosphate.	Thick films. Good stability. Saturation > 0.2 M glucose.
Aniline	Potentiostatic 1.5 V 0.02 M monomer. pH 7.2 phosphate.	Thin films. Poor stability. Saturation ca. 0.06 M glucose.

TABLE 3 (continued)

MONOMER	POLYMERISATION CONDITIONS[a]	COMMENTS
Phenol	Potentiostatic 1.4 V 0.05 M monomer. pH 7.0 phosphate	Very thin films. Good stability. Saturation ca. 0.1 M glucose.

[a]. All potentials vs. SCE, results refer to aqueous solutions and Pt electrodes. Typical enzyme concentrations 5-10 mg/ml.
[b]. From Foulds and Lowe.[41]

polyaniline,[43,44] polyindole,[45] poly-N-methylpyrrole,[46] and ferrocene substituted polypyrrole[47] films has been reported. Figure 10 shows results for the detection of glucose at a poly-N-methylpyrrole/glucose oxidase electrode. In nearly all cases there is little evidence of direct electron transfer between the flavin prosthetic group of the enzyme and the polymer although it is suggested that this may occur with the ferrocene derivatised polymer.[47] Direct, unmediated, electron transfer between redox proteins and conducting polymers remains a tantalising goal.

MODIFICATION OF ENZYMES

Finally an alternative approach which looks very promising is to modify the enzyme by the covalent attachment of redox centres to the protein.[48] In this case the suggestion is that the covalently attached redox centres act as 'stepping stones' allowing the electrons to get from the active site out to the electrode by a number of sequential, short steps, figure 11. Note that this is very similar to the mechanism of charge propagation through a redox polymer film discussed above.

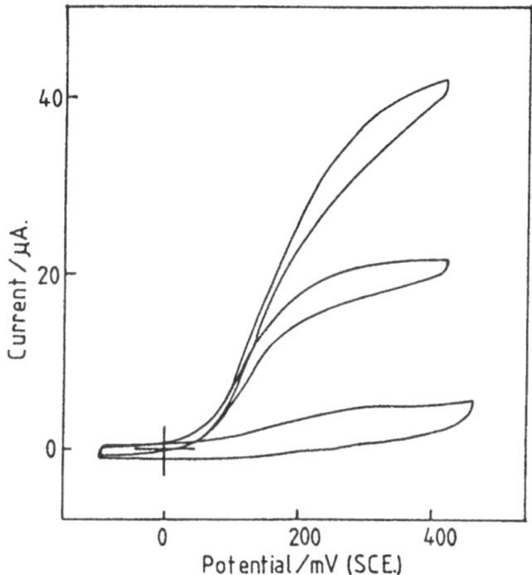

FIGURE 12 Cyclic voltammograms recorded at 10 mV s^{-1} at a glassy carbon electrode for ferrocene acetic acid modified glucose oxidase showing the effect of added (0, 2 and 44 mM) glucose.

Thus when glucose oxidase is modified by attachment of ferrocene carboxylic acid[49,50] or ferrocene acetic acid[51] direct electrochemical oxidation of the reduced flavoprotein at a clean metal electrode becomes possible, figure 12 and 13. This idea can be extended to other falvoproteins[50] and may prove to be generally useful.

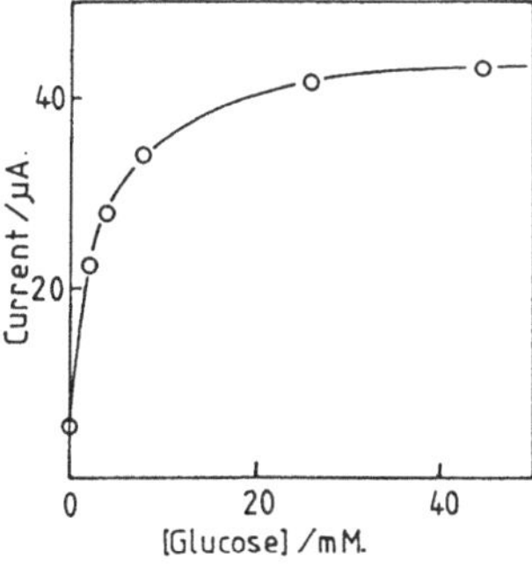

FIGURE 13 Plot of the limiting current for glucose oxidation using ferrocene acetic acid modified glucose oxidase as a function of the glucose concentration.

CONCLUSIONS

Interest in amperometric biosensors has stimulated considerable progress in the field of redox enzyme, redox protein, and coenzyme electrochemistry in the last few years. As our understanding of, and our ability to manipulate, biological electron transfer reactions increases we can expect to see further developments, not only in the biosensors field but also in bioelectronics. Central to much of this will be our ability to "interface" the biological system and the electrode.

ACKNOWLEDGEMENTS

We would like to thank the SERC and MediSense for financial support and Shani Ingram for her excellent typing.

REFERENCES

1. Hill, H. A. O. British Biophysical Society, Winter meeting, London, December 1988.
2. The original quotation, "Life is just one damned thing after another" is variously attributed to Elbert Hubbard (One thousand and One Epigrams) and Frank Ward O'Malley (Literary Digest 5 Nov. 1932).
3. Elving, P. J., Bresnahan, W.T., Moiroux, J., and Samec, Z. (1982). NAD/NADH as a Model Redox System: Mechanism, Mediation, Modification by the Environment, Bioelectrochem. Bioenerg. 9: 365.
4. Gorton, L. (1986). Chemically modified electrodes for the electrocatalytic oxidation of nicotinamide coenzymes, J. Chem. Soc., Faraday Trans. I, 82: 1245.
5. Murray, R. W. (1984). Chemically modified electrodes, Electroanalytical chemistry, vol. 13. (A. J. Bard, ed.), Marcel Dekker, New York, P. 191.

6. Hillman, A. R. (1987). Polymer modified electrodes: preparation and characterisation, Electrochemical science and technology of polymers, 1. (R. G. Linford, ed.), Elsevier, p. 103.
7. Degrand, C., and Miller, L. L, (1980). An electrode modified with polymer-bound dopamine which catalyses NADH oxidation, J. Amer. Chem. Soc., 102: 5728.
8. Fukui, M., Kitani, A., Degrand, C., and Miller, L. L. (1982). Propagation of a redox reaction through a quinoid polymer film electrode, J. Amer. Chem. Soc., 104: 28.
9. Lau, A. N. K., and Miller, L. L. (1983). Electrochemical behaviour of a dopamine polymer. Dopamine release as a primary analogue of a synapse, J. Amer. Chem. Soc., 105: 5271.
10. Carlson, B. W., and Miller, L. L. (1985). Mechanism of the oxidation of NADH by quinones. Energetics of one-electron and hydride routes, J. Amer. Chem. Soc., 107: 479.
11. Gorton, L., Torstensson, A., Jaegfeldt, H., and Johansson, G. (1984). Electrocatalytic oxidation of reduced nicotinamide coenzymes by graphite electrodes modified with an adsorbed phenoxazinium salt, meldola blue, J. Electroanal. Chem., 161: 103.
12. Gorton, L., Johansson, G., and Torstensson, A. (1985). A kinetic study of the reaction between dihydronicotinamide adenine dinucleotide (NADH) and an electrode modified by adsorption of 1,2-benzophenoxazine-7-one, J. Electroanal. Chem., 196: 81.
13. Appelqvist, R., Marko-Varga, G., Gorton, L., Torstensson, A., and Johansson, G. (1985). Enzymatic determination of glucose in a flow system by catalytic oxidation of the nicotinamide coenzyme at a modified electrode, Anal. Chim. Acta. 169: 237.
14. Albery, W. J., and Bartlett, P. N. (1984). An organic conductor electrode for the oxidation of NADH, J. Chem. Soc., Chem. Commun.: 234.
15. Albery, W. J., Bartlett, P. N., Cass, A. E. G., and Sim, K. W. (1987). Amperometric enzyme electrodes. Part IV. An enzyme electrode for ethanol, J. Electroanal. Chem., 218: 127.
16. Albery, W. J., Bartlett, P. N., and Cass, A. E. G. (1987).

Amperometric enzyme electrodes, Phil. Trans. R. Soc. Lond., B316: 107.

17. Bartlett, P. N. (1989). Conducting organic salt electrodes, Biosensors: a practical approach. (A. E. G. Cass ed.), IRL Press, in press.
18. Tatershall, R. B. (1979). Home Blood Glucose Monitoring, Diabetologia 16: 71.
19. Free, H. M., and Free, A. H. (1984). Analytical Chemistry in the Conquest of Diabetes, Anal. Chem. 56: 664A.
20. Turner, A.P.F., and Pickup, J. C. (1985). Diabetes Mellitus: Biosensors for Research and Management, Biosensors 1: 85.
21. Velho, G.D., Reach, G., and Thevenot, D.R. (1987). The Design and Development of in vivo Glucose Sensors for an Artificial Pancreas, Biosensors. Fundamentals and Applications. (A. P. F. Turner, I. Karube and G.S. Wilson, eds.), Oxford University Press, Oxford, p.390.
22. Enfors, S.-O. (1987). Compensated enzyme-electrodes for in situ process control, Biosensors. Fundamentals and Applications. (A. P. F. Turner, I. Karube and G. S. Wilson, eds.), Oxford University Press, Oxford, p. 347.
23. Marcus, R. A., and Sutin, N. (1985). Electron transfers in Chemistry and biology, Biochim. Biophys. Acta., 811: 265.
24. McLendon, G. (1988). Long-distance electron transfer in proteins and model systems, Acc. Che,. Res., 21: 160.
25. Cass, A. E. G., Francis, D. G., Hill, H. A. O., Aston, W. J., Higgins, I. J., Plotkin, E. V., Scott, L. D. L., and Turner, A. P. F. (1984). Ferrocene-mediated Enzyme Electrode for Amperometric Determination of Glucose, Anal. Chem. 56: 667.
26. Matthews, D. R., Holman, R. R., Bown, E., Steemson, J., Watson, A., Hughes, S., and Scott, D. (1987). Pen-sized Digital 30-Second Blood Glucose Meter, Lancet April 4: 778.
27. Cass, A. E. G., Davis, G., Green, M. J.., and Hill, H. A. O. (1985). Ferricinium Ion as an Electron Acceptor for Oxidoreductases, J. Electroanal. Chem. 190: 117.

28. Dicks, J., Aston, W. J., Davis, G., Turner, A. P. F. (1986). Mediated Amperometric Biosensors for D-galactose, Glycolate, and L-amino acids based on a Ferrocene-modified Carbon Electrode, Anal. Chim. Acta 182: 103.

29. D'Costa, E. J., Higgins, I. J., and Turner, A. P. F. (1986). Quinoprotein Glucose Dehydrogenase and its Application in an Amperometric Glucose Sensor, Biosensors 2: 71.

30. Albery, W. J., Bartlett, P. N., and Craston, D. H. (1985). Amperometric enzyme electrodes, part II. Conducting organic salts as electrode materials for the oxidation of glucose oxidase. J. Electroanal. Chem., 194: 223.

31. Albery, W.J., Bartlett, P. N., Bycroft, M., Craston, D. H., and Driscoll, B. J. (1987). Amperometric enzyme electrodes, part III. A conducting organic salt electrode for the oxidation of four different flavoenzymes, J. Electroanal. Chem., 218: 119.

32. Albery, W. J., and Craston, D. H. (1987). Amperometric enzyme electrodes: theory and experiment, Biosensors; fundamentals and applications. (A. P. F. Turner, I. Karube, and G. S. Wilson, eds.), Oxford University Press, Oxford, p. 180.

33. Kulys, J. J. (1986). Enzyme electrodes based on organic metals, Biosensors, 2: 3.

34. Kulys, J. J., Samalius, A. S., and Svirmickas, G.-J. S. (1980). Electron exchange between the enzyme active centre and organic metal, FEBS Lett., 144: 7.

35. McKenna, K., and Brajter-Toth, A. (1987). Tetrathiafulvalene tetracyanoquinodimethane xanthine oxidase amperometric electrode for the determination of biological purines, Anal. Chem., 59: 954.

36. Albery, W. J., and Bartlett, P. N. (1985). Amperometric Enzyme Electrodes. Part I. Theory, J. Electroanal. Chem. 194: 211.

37. Cenas, N. K., and Kulys, J. J. (1981). Biolytic oxidation of glucose on conductive charge transfer complexes, Bioelectrochem. Bioenerg., 8: 103.

38. Hill, B. S., Scolari, C. A., and Wilson, G.S. (1988). Enzyme

electrocatalysis at organic salt electrodes, J. Electroanal. Chem., 252: 125.

39. Boutelle, M. G., Stanford, C., Filenz, M., Albery, W. J., and Bartlett, P. N. (1986). An amperometric enzyme electrode for monitoring brain glucose in the freely moving rat, Neurosci. Lett., 72: 283.

40. Hale, P. D., and Wightman, R. M. (1988). Enzyme-modified tetrathiafulvalene tetracyanoquinodimethane microelectrodes: direct amperometric detection of acetylcholine and choline, Mol. Cryst. Lig. Crys., 160: 269.

41. Foulds, C. N., and Lowe, C. R. (1986). Enzyme entrapment in electricially conducting polymers. Immobilisation of glucose oxidase in polypyrrole and its application in amperometric glucose sensors, J. Chem. Soc., Faraday Trans. I, 82: 1259.

42. Umana, M., and Waller, J. (1986). Protein-modified electrodes. The glucose oxidase/polypyrrole system, Anal. Chem., 58: 2979.

43. Bartlett, P.N., and Whitaker, R. G. (1987/1988). Strategies for the development of amperometric enzyme electrodes, Biosensors, 3: 359.

44. Shinohara, H., Chiba, T., and Aizawa, M. (1988). Enzyme microsensor for glucose with an electrochemically synthesised enzyme polyaniline film, Sensors and Actuators, 13: 79.

45. Pandey, P. C. (1988). A new conducting polymer-coated glucose sensor, J. Chem. Soc., Faraday Trans. I, 84: 2259.

46. Bartlett, P. N., and Whitaker, R. G. (1987). Electrochemical immobilisation of enzymes. Part II. Glucose oxidase immobilised in poly-N-methylpyrrole, J. Electroanal. Chem., 224: 37.

47. Foulds, C. N., and Lowe, C. R. (1988). Immobilization of glucose oxidase in ferrocene-modified pyrrole polymers, Anal. Chem., 60: 2473.

48. Hill, H. A. O. (1984). Assay Techniques utilising specific binding agents, European Patent Application No. 84303090.9.

49. Degani, Y., and Heller, A. (1987). Direct electrical communication between chemically modified enzymes and metal electrodes.

1. Electron transfer from glucose oxidase to metal electrodes via electron relays, bound covalently to the enzyme, J. Phys. Chem., 91: 1285.

50. Degani, Y., and Heller, A. (1988). Direct electrical communication between chemically modified enzymes and electrodes. 2. Methods of bonding electron-transfer relays to glucose oxidase and D-amino-acid oxidase, J. Amer. Chem. Soc., 110: 2615.

51. Bartlett, P. N., Whitaker, R. G., Green, M. J., and Frew, J. (1987). Covalent binding of electron relays to glucose oxidase, J. Chem. Soc., Chem. Commun.: 1603.

8

Electrochemical Reactions, Enzyme Electrocatalysis, and Immunoassay Reactions in Hydrogels

B. N. Oliver, Louis A. Coury, J. O. Egekeze, C. S. Sosnoff, Yining Zhang and Royce W. Murray* *Kenan Laboratories of Chemistry, University of North Carolina, Chapel Hill, NC 27599-3290.*

C. Keller and Mirtha X. Umaña*,[a] *Research Triangle Institute, Research Triangle Park, NC 27709.*

1 ABSTRACT

Hydrogels of poly(acrylamide) and poly(ethylene oxide) are convenient and biocompatible media for use as physically rigid, solid state voltammetry solvents. Thin gel slices containing supporting electrolyte, buffer components and other reagents can be laid atop in-plane patterns of working, reference and auxiliary electrodes, dried in place and then reswelled with microdroplets containing electroactive species, enzyme substrates, or haptens to observe, respectively, conventional electrochemical voltammetry of the electroactive probe, electrocatalytic currents resulting from electron-transfer mediated turnover of an enzyme in the presence of the added substrate, or enhanced electrocatalytic currents resulting from displacement of redox-labelled hapten from an antibody by the added hapten. Examples of such reactions in hydrogels are given, including the mediated oxidation of sulfite by sulfite oxidase, of glucose by glucose oxidase, and enzyme-enhanced immunoassay of phenytoin. The hydrogel films are potentially useful packaging strategies for electrochemical assays employing microlithographically-defined, disposable electrochemical microcells.

2 INTRODUCTION

In keeping with the current general importance of solid state chemistry within the chemical sciences, we have initiated a number of projects aimed at developing electrochemical methods and investigating chemical and electrochemical phenomena in physically rigid solvents. In contrast to numerous previous studies (1) where electrodes coated with films of polymeric materials are contacted with fluid electrolyte solutions, the present experiments include no fluid media; the electroactive ingredients and electrolyte are dissolved in a rigid matrix (or are part of it) to which the electrodes are contacted. Our studies (2-9) in "solid state voltammetry" have included organic polymer electrolytes in amorphous, partly crystalline, and plasticized forms, gelling alkoxysilanes (10), and hydrogels of poly(ethylene oxide), and poly(acrylamide) (11). The polymer electrolytes are more nearly true solids, having correspondingly meager ionic conductivities, thus our voltammetric methodologies rely heavily on microdimensioned electrodes. The gelling alkoxysilanes and hydrogels, while physically rigid, have a large internal aqueous solvent content (low microviscosity), exhibit large ionic conductivities, and allow use of conventional sized electrodes as well as microelectrodes.

It is the object of this paper to illustrate quantitative voltammetry and bioanalytically interesting electrochemical reactions in physically rigid, hydrogel solvents. The electroanalytical utility of hydrogels includes their biocompatibility (12) and the potentialities for packaging of reagents and design of disposable electrochemical cells for routine electroanalysis. To this end, it is necessary to understand effects of the hydrogel environment on transport, and chemical and heterogeneous charge transfer processes, as well as practical matters like how to add chemical reagents and samples to physically rigid solvents.

3 VOLTAMMETRY IN A GELLING ALKOXYSILANE

A hydrogel consists of a large fraction of water with thinly interspersed, but cross-linked, organic or inorganic polymer chains.

The nature and density of the polymer cross-link connections strongly controls how the gel swells, or collapses. Transport rates in gels, and thereby electrochemical diffusion currents, are thus sensitive to hydrogel cross-linking. This point is readily illustrated by the example (11) in Fig. 1 in which voltammetry of a redox solute is measured at a working electrode immersed in a gelling mixture of the monomer $(EtO)_4Si$, water and a catalyst. The main

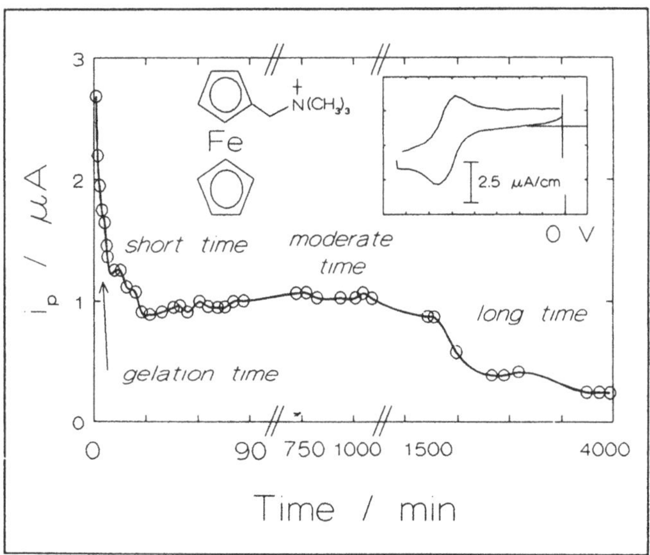

Figure 1. Time dependence of cyclic voltammetric peak currents for 1 mM $[CpFeCpCH_2N(CH_3)_3]^+$ at 2 mm diameter GC disk in a gelling mixture of 8 x 10^{-2} mol H_2O, 4 x 10^{-2} mol EtOH, 1 x 10^{-2} mol $(EtO)_4Si$, 1.5 x 10^{-4} mol HCl, and 1.3 x 10-3 mol HF. At indicated gelation time, the mixture had become a rigid solid. At long time, the rigid gel began to collapse and to extrudes wolvent (*viz.*, EtOH and H_2O). **Inset:** CV of 1 mM $[CpFeCpCH_2N(CH_3)_3]^+$ PF_6^- at GC disk during gelation.

voltammetric effect observed is a decrease in the diffusion current for a ferrocene-derivative redox species, reflecting an alteration of its diffusion coefficient as polymerization proceeds.

We see that the time course of the process shows a gradual early decrease in the diffusion rate as gelation takes place, followed by a long period of a relatively steady transport rate in the now-rigid gel, and eventually a further decrease in current as the silicate gel collapses and exudes water solvent. The main points of Fig. 1 are: (*i*) that it is straightforward to observe voltammetry in a gelling and in a gelled solvent medium, (*ii*) that gels are capable of supporting stable voltammetry for extended periods of time, and (*iii*) that diffusion rates in gels are lowered, but only modestly, from those in fluid solutions.

4 VOLTAMMETRY IN POLY(ACRYLAMIDE) HYDROGELS

Poly(acrylamide), PAM, is a well-known hydrogel material whose preparation is straightforward (16) and which has been widely used as a solvent medium in chemical procedures, in particular gel electrophoretic methods. We have found PAM to be readily adaptable as a solvent for electrochemical voltammetry, applicable both to large metalloproteins such as cytochromes as well as to smaller redox probes (12).

In designing experiments with rigid solvents, including gels, the physical shape of the solvent becomes a significant experimental choice and can even influence the diffusion geometry operative at the working electrode (3). While not the only possible choice, we have found (12) convenient a format in which the electrodes of the electrochemical cell are designed to lie in a plane with a thin slice of PAM gel placed over them. The electrodes may be macrosized disks, metal foil edges or wire tips, as illustrated schematically in Panel A of Fig 2., or may be microsized and microlithographically defined (15). The slice of gel, if dry, can be wetted after which it conforms to the cell surface and becomes reasonably adherent thereto. We have previously employed PAM at a low cross-linking composition (12), thinking to promote mobility of large redox

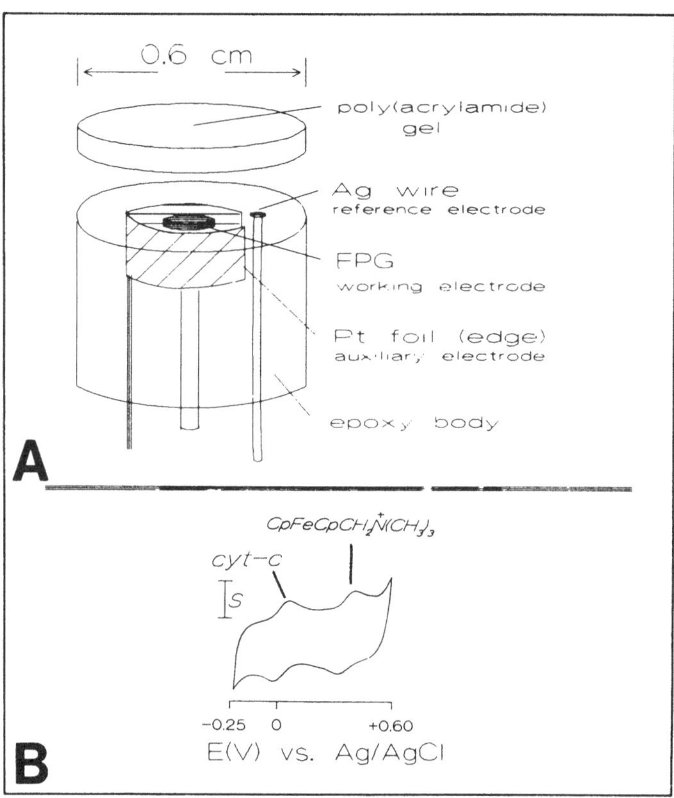

Figure 2. *Panel A*: Schematic of electrochemical gel-cell. *Panel B*: Voltammogram in dry gel slice to which is added 10 μL of 0.15 m<u>M</u> cytochrome-<u>c</u>, 0.025 m<u>M</u> $[CpFeCpCH_2N(CH_3)_3]^+$ PF_6^-, dissolved in 0.1 <u>M</u> KCl, via method *ii*. S = 1 μA.

proteins. Higher cross-linking compositions, however, have not been tested and may perform equally well. Poly(ethylene oxide), PEO, similarly of good biocompatibility, was also investigated as a hydrogel material, but we have not found it to be as attractive as PAM for voltammetric studies. A detailed study of voltammetry in PAM and in PEO will be presented in a separate publication (17).

A significant factor of practical concern in gel voltammetry is deciding how to add chemical reagents to the rigid polymer. When the gel polymer is cross-linked, as is the case with PAM, it cannot be co-dissolved with the reagents, thus the latter must be imbibed into the gel. The three tactics for reagent addition are: (*i*) soaking the gel slice in the reagent solution, (*ii*) absorbing a microdroplet of reagent solution into a slice of dried gel, and (*iii*) hydrating a dried gel slice after (*i*) or (*ii*) in a stream of humidified gas. The degree of swelling of the gel with these procedures is typically (*i*) >> (*ii*) > (*iii*). For example, a reagent loaded into a gel by (*i*), followed by drying and reswelling by (*ii*) or (*iii*), is in a more concentrated form after the latter reswelling.

All three methods can be employed either before or after mounting the gel slice on the electrode; usually the latter is more convenient. Generally, we have found it convenient to load supporting electrolytes and buffer components, whose concentrations need not be precisely known, into gels using procedure (*i*), blotting off excess liquid and drying the gel in preparation for subsequent steps.

When it is important to know the concentration of components of the solution in which voltammetry is to be performed (such as that of the electroactive species), method (*ii*) is an effective approach. A microdroplet (say 5-30 μL) of the solution is added to a dry, electrode-mounted gel slice, and the voltammetry is performed before significant evaporation of the droplet has taken place. It is easy to use gel slices thin enough that the volume fraction of the organic polymer is a small percentage of the swollen gel; *i.e.*, the reagent concentration in the swollen gel is nearly the same as that in the applied droplet of solution. An example of the voltammetry obtained in a PAM gel in such an experiment is illustrated in Panel B of Fig. 2 for a microdroplet of a mixture of the redox protein cytochrome-*c* and a water-soluble ferrocene derivative, the ferrocenyl methyltrimethylammonium cation ($[CpFeCpCH_2N(CH_3)_3]^+$). The solution was added to a dry gel slice which had been previously soaked in 0.1 M KCl, blotted and then dried. Note that the S/N in this example is quite reasonable, even though very low concentrations were employed (*viz.*, 150 and 25 μM for the cytochrome and ferrocene, respectively). In fact, gel voltammetry is generally as well (or better) defined as that obtained in an aqueous buffer solution. In the voltammogram shown, the Ag/AgCl reference electrode potential is shifted from that observed in 0.1 M KCl because the droplet-swollen gel (method (*ii*)) is less swollen than the original, solution-soaked gel (method (*i*)), enhancing C_{KCl}. The $[CpFeCpCH_2N(CH_3)_3]^+$ in this example serves as an internal redox standard for re-calibration of the potential scale, allowing the observation to be made that the formal potential of the cytochrome-*c* couple is unchanged in the PAM gel, as compared to water (12).

When gel solutions are prepared in this way, various redox couples have been observed to give voltammetric peak currents that follow the expected linear diffusion laws, *i.e.*, currents proportional to (potential sweep rate)$^{1/2}$ and to concentration (Fig. 3). From the slopes of plots like these, gel diffusion coefficients for cytochrome-*c* and $[CpFeCpCH_2N(CH_3)_3]^+$ of 2.1×10^{-7} and 3.6×10^{-6} cm^2/s, respectively, were measured (12) and were found to be 4.1 and 1.4 times slower, respectively, than those measured in fluid aqueous solutions of the same electrolyte. Diffusion of the large redox protein is slowed the most, as would be expected.

We have also measured the heterogeneous electron transfer rate constant for the cytochrome-*c* reaction from the voltammetric peak potential separations. The result in the gel solution, 2.7×10^{-3} cm/s, at an edge-plane pyrolytic graphite electrode, was indistinguishable from that measured at the same electrode in aqueous solution but not coated with a gel slice, 3.5×10^{-3} cm/s. In this example, the presence of polymer strands in the interfacial environment had no detectable effect on the electron transfer process. Heterogeneous electron transfer rates have been observed to decrease in other viscous media (18, 19). The absence of a kinetic effect in PAM gels, which are macroscopically quite viscous, points out the important difference between the physically observable polymer

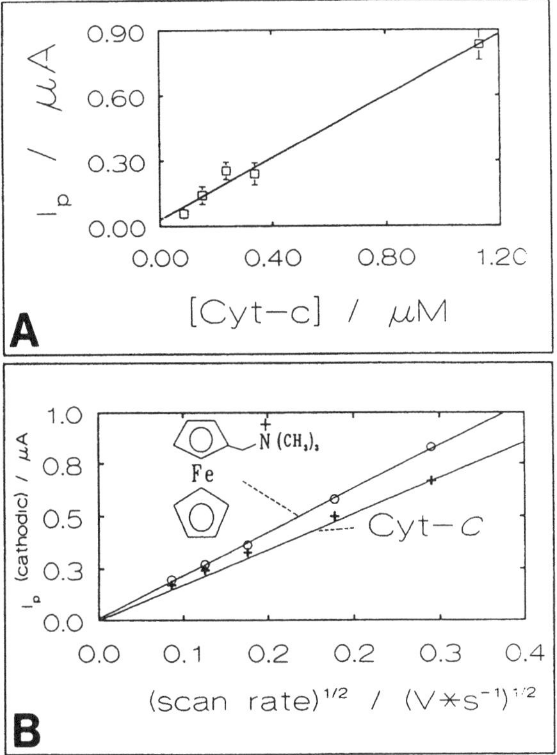

Figure 3. *Panel A:* Voltammetric peak currents monitored for addition to dry gel slices (method *ii*) 20 μL droplets with varying concentrations of cytochrome-c. *Panel B:* Voltammetric peak currents for dry gel slices to which was added (method *ii*) 20 μL 0.12 mM $[CpFeCpCH_2N(CH_3)_3]^+ PF_6^-$, or 20 μL of 0.34 mM cytochrome-c at varying scan rates.

solvent macroviscosity and its less-readily observable microviscosity, the latter of which is the more relevant parameter for molecular reactions and electron transfer dynamics (20).

5 ENZYME SYSTEMS IN PAM

Sulfite Oxidase. The enzyme sulfite oxidase, (SO), is a two-redox site, molybdo-heme protein which, in its reduced form, is known (21) to undergo an *in vivo* reaction sequence with ferricytochrome-*c* in which the SO heme center is oxidized, followed by an internal electron transfer from the Mo to Fe centers of the enzyme. Sulfite is oxidized to sulfate at the Mo site, thus re-reducing SO. While activity assays of this enzyme based on reduction of simple electron acceptors such as ferricyanide have been employed for some time (22), coupling of SO to an electrochemically driven electron-transfer mediated electrocatalytic scheme was only recently demonstrated by studies in this laboratory (23-25).

In fluid electrolyte solution experiments, we have found (25) that a number of electrogenerated oxidants will drive the SO enzyme system. Because of lack of prior work, our investigation began in, and has largely been limited to, conventional aqueous electrolyte solutions in pH 7.5 TRIS buffer. We find that a large number of simple redox couples with $E^{o'}$ values ranging from 0 to +0.4 V *versus* NHE may serve as electron acceptors for the enzyme. Enzymic re-reduction of electrogenerated oxidants such as ferricyanide, $[Co(phen)_3]^{3+}$, ferricytochrome-*c*, $[Ru(NH_3)_6]^{3+}$, and the radical cation of N,N,N',N'-tetramethyl-*p*-phenylenediamine ($TMPD^+$) leads to electrocatalytic currents, according to the (simplified) scheme:

$$TMPD \xrightarrow[\text{electrode}]{} TMPD^+ \qquad [1]$$

$$(SO)_{red} + 2\ TMPD^+ \xrightarrow[k1]{} (SO)_{ox} + 2\ TMPD \qquad [2]$$

$$(SO)_{ox} + SO_3^{2-} \xrightarrow[k2]{} (SO)_{red} + SO_4^{2-} \qquad [3]$$

where TMPD is used as the example mediator and no distinction is made in the reactions of SO as to whether its Fe or Mo site is involved. An example of this kind of mediation is shown in Panel A of Fig. 4. The current for the $TMPD^{o/+}$ couple itself is the same whether sulfite or enzyme, taken singly, are present or not, but is considerably enhanced, as shown, in the presence of mixtures of sulfite and its oxidase enzyme, SO.

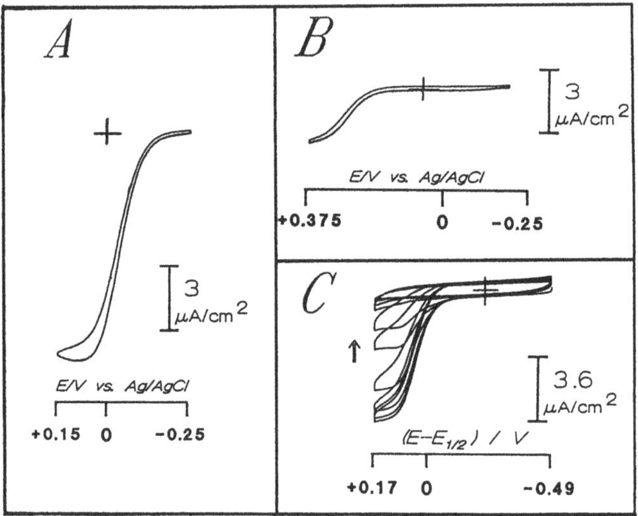

Figure 4. Electrocatalytic oxidation of sulfite via mediation of sulfite oxidase with N,N,N',N'-tetramethyl-*p*-phenylenediamine (TMPD). *Panel A:* Aqueous solution wave; [TMPD] = 35 μM, [enzyme] = 0.68 μM, [SO_3^{2-}] = 0.36 mM, v = 2mV/s. *Panel B:* PAM gel wave; 1.7 nmol TMPD, 0.2 nmol enzyme and 144 nmol SO_3 sorbed into dry gel. Gel volume *circa* 65 μL. v = 2 mV/s. *Panel C:* PAM gel waves during drying in Ar stream; 2.1 nmol TMPD, 0.2 nmol enzyme and 129 nmol SO_3^{2-} sorbed into initially dry gel. v = 10 mV/s.

The solution in Panel A of Fig. 4 contains a small concentration of enzyme and a large concentration of sulfite ion, relative to that of the mediator, which for this and other mediator couples often produces the sigmoidal, steady-state current-potential curve shape observed. The limiting current on the voltammogram is proportional to the concentration of TMPD mediator, but is essentially independent of sulfite ion concentration (above about $C_{sulfite}$ = 0.3 mM, under these solution conditions). Analogous results are found using Co phenanthroline complexes, where we have also established (25) that the limiting current is proportional to the square-root of the enzyme concentration. These are electrochemical criteria (26) for the current being controlled by the rate of Rxn. (2) in the above scheme, and serving as a measure of the rate constant k_1. That is, the electrocatalytic rate is controlled by the enzyme-mediator reaction rate, the rate of the enzyme-sulfite reaction being much larger. We calculate that $k_1 = 2 \times 10^6$ $\underline{M}^{-1}s^{-1}$ in Rxn. (2).

As expected, use of smaller sulfite ion concentrations and larger enzyme concentrations shifts control of the electrocatalytic currents toward Rxn. (3) and makes the currents both non-steady-state as well as more responsive to sulfite concentration. This circumstance, of course, is the more interesting one from the chemical sensor point of view, whereas the situation observed in Panel A of Fig. 4 is interesting from the enzyme electron-transfer dynamics point of view.

The Rxn. scheme (1-3) functions in the PAM gel solution in an analogous manner, as shown in Panel B of Fig. 4, where the gel was prepared by sequential sorption of solutions of the various components as in method *(ii)*. Again, large sulfite and small enzyme concentrations produce a sigmoidally-shaped, steady-state current-potential curve with a sulfite concentration-independent limiting current. Evaluation of k_1 from this experiment, using a separately determined value for the diffusion coefficient of TMPD in the gel of 6×10^{-7} cm^2/s, yields a value of 5×10^5 $\underline{M}^{-1}s^{-1}$. This value, slightly less than the solution result, must be regarded as a preliminary result, since the proper dependencies of the current on mediator and enzyme concentrations have not yet been experimentally tested in the gel.

The decrease in the value of the bimolecular rate constant for the gel reaction compared to the aqueous solution data may be indicative of any one of several effects. Decreased mobility of the enzyme might result in such an effect, although covalent immobilization of other oxidase enzymes often leads to *enhanced* activity. Equally plausible are ionic strength influences on the homogeneous electron transfer rates or inhibition of the enzyme due to altered pH or chloride activity in the gel. Further experiments are underway to elucidate the cause of the apparent decreased catalytic rate in the gel.

Panel C of Fig. 4 demonstrates the results of allowing the swollen gel to dry out in a stream of Ar. The currents reproducibly decrease during drying, then abruptly vanish at a later point in drying, in contrast to the increasing behavior of currents for small redox probes alone (*vide infra*). The response is observed to reappear if the dried gel is then rehydrated by sorption of a droplet of buffer solution. This result demonstrates that, at least over a brief period, the enzyme sulfite oxidase tolerates a dry PAM environment.

Glucose Oxidase. That the above approach to eliciting electron transfer-mediated electrocatalysis of redox enzyme reactions has some generality was demonstrated using the glucose/ glucose oxidase reaction system. Mediated electron transfer to glucose oxidase in the presence of glucose, previously known (27-29) in fluid electrolyte solutions, is demonstrated in a PAM gel solvent by the results in Fig. 5. The reaction scheme operative is:

$$\mathrm{Fer} \xrightarrow[\text{electrode}]{} \mathrm{Fer}^{+} \quad [4]$$

$$(\mathrm{GO})_{red} + 2\ \mathrm{Fer}^{+} \xrightarrow[k1]{} (\mathrm{GO})_{ox} + 2\ \mathrm{Fer} \quad [5]$$

$$(\mathrm{GO})_{ox} + \mathrm{Glu} \xrightarrow[k2]{} (\mathrm{GO})_{red} + (\mathrm{Glu})_{ox} \quad [6]$$

where the mediator is ferrocene (Fer), which was loaded into the gel by a droplet of acetonitrile solution. Interestingly, ferrocene functions quite well in this capacity, although it is nominally of limited solubility in the subsequently aqueous enzyme and glucose solutions added to the gel by a sequence of method (*ii*) steps. Panel A of Fig. 5 shows the enhancement of the ferrocene oxidation current upon addition of glucose to the enzyme containing gel, and Panel B shows the linear relationship between electrocatalytic

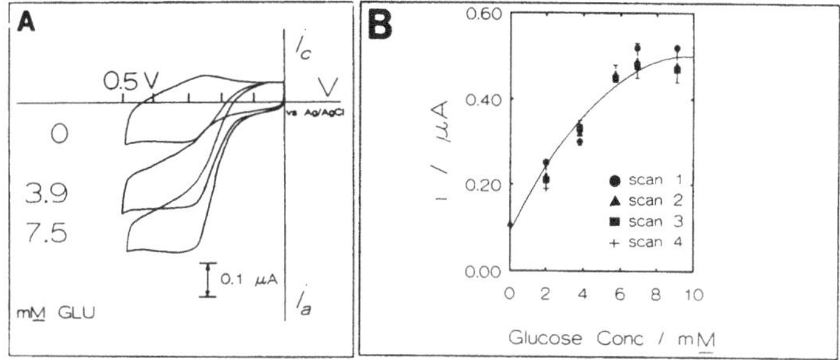

Figure 5. Electrocatalytic oxidation of glucose in PAM gel via mediation of glucose oxidase with ferrocene. *Panel A:* Upper curve-gel contains 60 nmol ferrocene, applied in 20 μL CH_3CN solution, dried, and then hydrated with 60 μL 0.1 M aqueous phosphate, 0.5 M KCl buffer. Lower curves- gel contains 20 μL glucose oxidase (Sigma, 400 units/mL) and 2 or 4 μL 1.2 M glucose in addition to ferrocene mediator. *Panel B:* Catalytic limiting currents (as in Panel A, lowest curve) as a function of glucose concentration in gel.

current and glucose concentration in the gel. The latter result shows that the electrocatalysis is responsive to the rate of Rxn. (6), although at high glucose concentrations the reaction is becoming saturated in glucose and the current-glucose concentration linearity is lost. This result is consistent with the fluid solution reaction results (30).

A more ambitious scheme is presented in Fig. 6, where we seek to employ the glucose/glucose oxidase reaction as an amplifier to detect binding of a tagged ferrocene mediator to an antibody. In this case, a large glucose concentration is employed to drive control of the electrocatalysis toward Rxn. (5). The design of the scheme in Fig. 6 is to detect displacement of the ferrocene mediator, tagged with a hapten (*viz.*, phenytoin) so as to become bound as an antigen by antibody. Upon addition of unlabelled hapten-

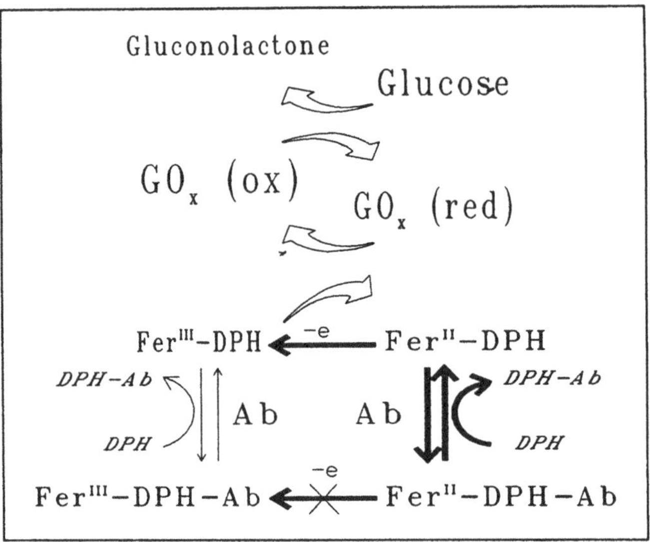

Figure 6. Reaction scheme for glucose-oxidase enzyme amplified detection of competitive binding of phenytoin and phenytoin-labelled ferrocene (28).

analyte (*i.e.*, the drug phenytoin) to the gel solution, the ferrocene-labelled hapten is released from the antibody binding site and detected as it functions as a mediator in the electrocatalytic scheme, Rxns. (4-6).

The scheme in Fig. 6 has been previously demonstrated (31) in fluid electrolyte solution, and its preliminary success in a gel solution is demonstrated in Fig. 7. The initial electrocatalytic current produced by Rxns. (4-6), shown by voltammogram *b* in Fig. 7, is essentially completely quenched by adding phenytoin anti-serum to the gel (voltammogram *c*), and is partly restored by adding a sample of unlabelled phenytoin to the gel (voltammogram *d*). The additions of solutions to the gel were made by method (*ii*). While the currents observed were small, the manner in which they changed by the above sequence of reagent additions provides reasonable support for the scheme proposed in Fig. 6.

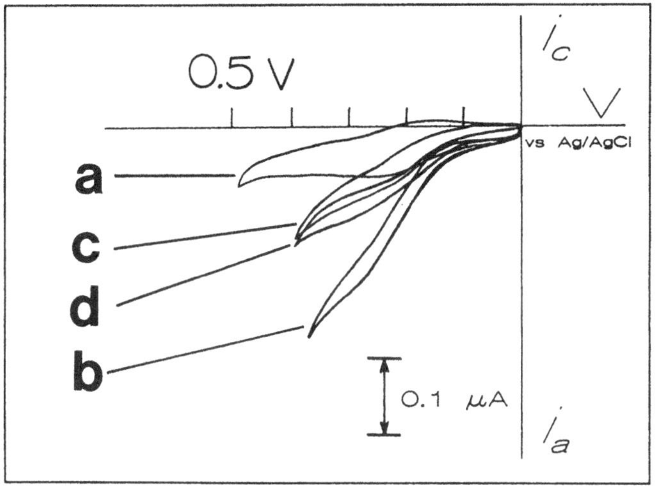

Figure 7. Voltammetry in PAM gel slice. *Curve a:* gel contains 30 μL 0.1 M K_2HPO_4, 0.5 M KCl; 2 μL 1.0 M glucose; and 5 μL 1.2 mM Fer-DPH (*viz.*, ferrocene carboxylic acid amide - coupled to phenytoin; applied as CH_3CN solution). *Curve b:* after subsequent addition of 4 μL glucose oxidase (400 units/mL). *Curve c:* after subsequent addition of 10 μL serum solution containing polyclonal anti-DPH antibodies (31,32). *Curve d:* after subsequent addition of 0.5 μL 15 mM phenytoin in CH_3CN; total concentration of CH_3CN in gel approximately 10% by volume.

Figures 4, 5 and 7 present results for electrochemically driven bioredox systems which support the reaction schemes represented by Rxns. (1-3), (4-6), and Fig. 6. We have limited quantitative characterization of the gel bioredox reactions at present, but are greatly encouraged by the fact that these reactions could be designed fairly explicitly from information about their behavior in fluid electrolyte. To a first approximation, from these and from the quantitative voltammetry results, it appears that PAM gels should be generally applicable to all forms of aqueous solution voltammetry that do not involve chemically aggressive reagents that could react with the gel itself.

6 DRYING EFFECTS IN GELS

Finally, we return to the matter of the behavior of voltammetry of gels containing electroactive species as they are dried and rehydrated. Figure 8 presents peak current data measured following the application of a droplet of the soluble redox probe $[CpFeCpCH_2N(CH_3)_3]^+$ as in Fig. 2, but over a time span during which the droplet gradually evaporates. The voltammetric currents remain

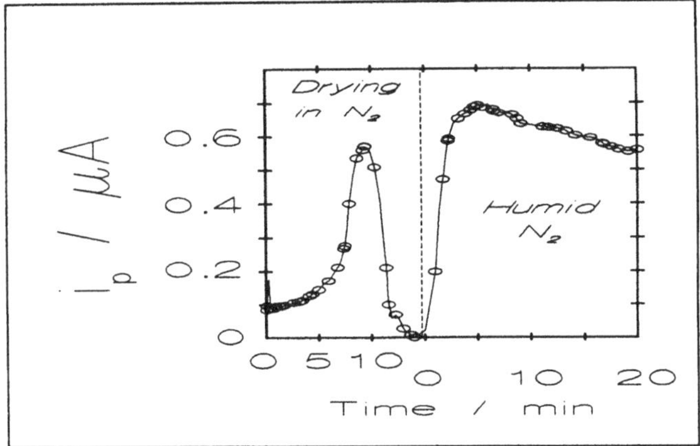

Figure 8. Time course of magnitude of voltammetric peak currents during drying in N_2 stream (left panel) and rehydration in humid N_2 (right panel) of gel slice containing 20 μL 0.025 mM $[CpFeCpCH_2N(CH_3)_3]^+$.

relatively constant for a period of time (*circa* 5 minutes), during which the outer portions of the gel may undergo considerable drying without affecting the water content of the gel solution immediately adjacent to the electrode surface. Later, the drying process concentrates the solution next to the electrode with the redox probe, *i.e.*, a drying-induced transport process moves redox material toward the working electrode, which enhances the diffusion current. Eventually, however, the gel water content becomes insufficient to support voltammetric performance, and the current (rather abruptly) falls to zero and remains there (time > 10 min.).

Rehydration of the gel by placing the electrode in a stream of humidified gas reveals, crudely, a general reversal of the drying events (right side of Fig. 8). The initial currents continue to reflect the redistributed concentrations (*i.e.*, enriched concentration of redox probe near the electrode), and are initially larger than the maximum current monitored during drying, but gradually fall at longer times (time = 10-20 min after rehumidification).

The essential message of these results, which will be elaborated upon in another publication (17), is that drying and rehydration events can drive spatial movement of gel solutes so that the chemical reagents in a gel can become spatially redistributed in a drying process. Quantitative electrochemical (and spectroscopic) procedures which involve drying of gel solutions must accordingly take possible concentration inhomogeneities into consideration.

ACKNOWLEDGEMENT. This research was supported in part by grants from the National Science Foundation and the Office of Naval Research (RWM, at UNC) and from the Army Office of Research (MU, at RTI, glucose experiments). The authors thank E. Cook of RTI for the anti-DPH serum employed in Fig. 7.

REFERENCES

a. Present address: Consultant, 6823 Falconbridge Rd., Chapel Hill, NC 27514.

1. R. W. Murray, Annu. Rev. Mater. Sci. **1984**, 14, 145.
2. R. A. Reed, L. Geng, and R. W. Murray, J. Electroanal. Chem. **1986**, 185, 208.
3. R. A. Reed, L. Geng, M. Longmire, and R. W. Murray, J. Phys. Chem. **1987**, 91, 2908.
4. L. Geng, M. Longmire, R. A. Reed, J. F. Parcher, C. J. Barbour, and R. W. Murray, Chem. Mat. **1989**, 1, 58.
5. A. Bettelheim, R. A. Reed, N. H. Hendricks, J. P. Collman, and R. W. Murray, J. Electroanal. Chem. **1988**, 238, 259.

6. L. Geng, R. A. Reed, M.-H. Kim, T. Wooster, B. N. Oliver, J. O. Egekeze, R. Kennedy, J. W. Jorgenson, J. F. Parcher, and R. W. Murray, J. Am. Chem. Soc. **1989**, 111, 1614.
7. J. F. Parcher, C. J. Barbour, and R. W. Murray, Anal. Chem. **1989**, 61, 584.
8. M. Watanabe, M. L. Longmire, and R. W. Murray, J. Phys. Chem., submitted.
9. M. L. Longmire, M. Watanabe, H. Zhang, T. T. Wooster, and R. W. Murray, Anal. Chem., submitted.
10. R. A. Reed, T. T. Wooster, R. W. Murray, J. S. Tonge, D. R. Yaniv, and D. F. Shriver, J. Electrochem. Soc. **1989**, 136, 2565.
11. Y. Zhang, University of North Carolina at Chapel Hill, unpublished results, 1989.
12. B. N. Oliver, J. O. Egekeze, and R. W. Murray, J. Am. Chem. Soc. **1988**, 110, 2321.
13. M. S. Hershfield, R. H. Buckley, M. L. Greenberg, A. L. Melton, R. Schiff, C. Hatem, J. Kurtzberg, M. L. Markett, R. H. Kobayashi, A. L. Kobayashi, A. Abuchowski, New Engl. J. Med. **1987**, 316, 589.
14. F. F. Davis, A. Abuchowski, T. van Ea, N. C. Palezuk, K. Savoca, R.H-L. Chen, P. Pyatak, in "Biomedical Polymers: Polymeric Materials and Pharmaceuticals for Biomedical Use", E. P. Goldberg, A. Nakajima, Eds., Academic Press, N.Y. 1980, p. 441.
15. M. Morita, M. L. Longmire, and R. W. Murray, Anal. Chem. **1988**, 60, 2770.
16. O. Gaal, G. A. Medgyesi, and L. Vereczkey, "Electrophoresis in the Separation of Biological Molecules;" John Wiley: New York, 1980.
17. B. N. Oliver, J. O. Egekeze, L. A. Coury and R. W. Murray, manuscript in preparation.
18. X. Zhang, H. Yang, and A. J. Bard, J. Am. Chem. Soc. **1987**, 109, 1916.

19. X. Zhang, J. Leddy, and A. J. Bard, J. Am. Chem. Soc. **1985**, 107, 3719.

20. D. A. Zichi, G. Ciccotti, J. T. Hynes, M. Ferrario, J. Phys. Chem. **1989**, 93, 6261, and references cited.

21. K. V. Rajagopalan, in "Molybdenum and Molybdenum-Containing Enzymes, " M. Coughlan, Ed., Pergammon Press: Oxford, UK, 1980.

22. H. J. Cohen and I. Fridovich, J. Biol. Chem. **1971**, 246, 359.

23. L. Geng, J. Jernigan, R. A. Reed, M. Longmire, M. Morita, B. N. Oliver, C. J. Barbour, J. F. Parcher, and R. W. Murray; 1988 C. N. Reilley Award Address, 1988 Pittsburgh Conference, New Orleans, LA, 2/24/1988; abstract number 804.

24. L. A. Coury, Jr., B. N. Oliver, J. P. Egekeze, C. Sosnoff, and R. W. Murray, 175th Nat. Meeting Electrochem. Soc., Los Angeles, CA, May 1989, Extended Abstract 448.

25. L. A. Coury, B. N. Oliver, J. O. Egekeze, C. S. Sosnoff, J. C. Brumfield, and R. W. Murray, Anal. Chem., submitted.

26. A. J. Bard and L. R. Faulkner, "Electrochemical Methods: Fundamentals and Applications," John Wiley: New York, 1980.

27. A. E. G. Cass, G. Davis, G. D. Francis, H. A. O. Hill, W. J. Aston, I. J. Higgins, E. V. Plotkin, L. D. L. Scott, and A. P. F. Turner, Anal. Chem. **1984**, 56, 667.

28. A. L. Crumbliss, H. A. O. Hill, and D. J. Page, J. Electroanal. Chem. **1986**, 206, 327.

29. W. J. Albery, P. M. Bartlett, D. H. Cransten, J. Electroanal. Chem. **1985**, 194, 223.

30. M. Umaña, and J. Waller, Anal. Chem. **1986**, 58, 2979.

31. M. Umaña, J. Waller, M. Wani, C. Whisnant, and E. Cook, J. Res. Nat. Inst. Stds. and Technol. **1988**, 93, 1.

32. C. E. Cook, J. A. Kepler, and H. D. Christensen, Res. Commun. Chem. Pathol. Pharmacol. **1973**, 5, 769.

9
Amplification Possibilities with Neuroreceptor-Based Biosensors

LEMUEL B. WINGARD JR. Department of Pharmacology, School of Medicine, University of Pittsburgh, Pittsburgh, Pennsylvania

1 BIOCHEMICAL COMPONENT OF BIOSENSORS

The functional components of a biosensor can be divided into those that provide molecular level recognition and those that provide transduction. The selectivity of the biosensor for one or more analytes is based on the ability of the recognition element to carry out some physical or chemical process with the analyte while rejecting similar processes with potentially interfering compounds. The transduction component is needed to convert the recognition process into a discernable readout signal.

In many biosensor designs, a biochemical compound such as an enzyme or an antibody provides the recognition function, while a non-biochemical material is used to generate the transduction function. Some enzymes and immunocompounds show highly selective catalytic acitvities and binding affinities for specific analytes; in addition they are stable at room temperature and available in relatively large (milligram to gram) quantities. Thus, such proteins have found wide applicability as recognition elements for the development of numerous biosensor designs.

A class of proteins known as neuroreceptors also possesses high affinity binding sites and therefore constitutes another source of molecular recognition components for biosensors (1,2). However, the highly complex structures of neuroreceptors, their general labile nature at room temperature, and the difficulty in obtaining sufficient quantities of receptor protein for biosensor studies have restricted attempted biosensor applications of these proteins until recently. One of the enticing attributes of neuroreceptors is the possibility for signal amplification by several orders of magnitude (3). Thus, in spite of the significant technical difficulties to be overcome for the development of neuroreceptor-based biosensors, the possibility for signal amplification makes this route worth exploring.

2 DESCRIPTION OF NEURORECEPTORS

Mammalian cells utilize neuroreceptors for the transmission of signals across the lipid membrane that separates the extracellular from the intracellular regions. Neuroreceptor proteins are embedded in the membrane and extend into the adjoining regions,

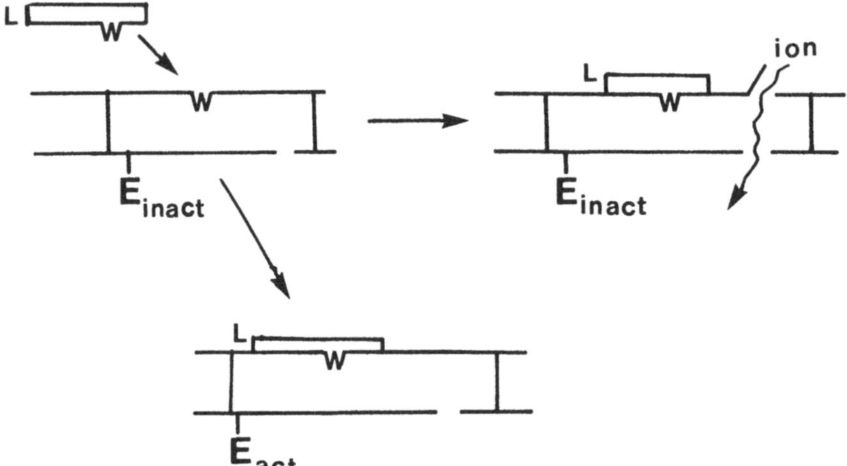

FIGURE 1. Neuroreceptor functioning, showing ligand L binding to receptor to open ion channel or activate enzyme E.

with the specific binding sites for molecular recognition of certain ligands on the extracellular side and signal generators extending into the intracellular region. The general scheme for functioning of neuroreceptors is shown in Fig. 1, with the main elements consisting of an extracellular ligand binding site and an intracellular signal generator based on either a transmembrane ion channel that opens as a result of ligand binding or a membrane enzyme that undergoes activation or inhibition as a result of ligand binding. The ion channel generated change in concentration of specific ions within the cell can lead to activation or inhibition of intracellular processes; and the change in activity of the membrane enzyme activates secondary messenger systems that in turn govern the activities of selective intracellular processes.

The more common neuroreceptors are listed in Table 1. The receptor names are based largely on the first experimental compounds or types of compounds that were observed to bind and activate these receptors. The present nomenclature system makes wide use of the concept of receptor "subtypes" to acknowledge a common endogenous ligand, termed a neurotransmitter, but to acknowledge that different pharmacological results are observed

TABLE 1. Types and Subtypes of Common Neuroreceptors.

Receptor Type	Subtypes
cholinergic	nicotinic, muscarinic (M_1, M_2)
adrenergic	$alpha_1$, $alpha_2$, $beta_1$, $beta_2$
GABA	A, B
acidic amino acids	NMDA, quis, kainate
calcium	L, N, T
opioid	mu, delta, kappa, sigma, epsilon
serotonin	$5\text{-}HT_1$, $5\text{-}HT_2$, $5\text{-}HT_3$
dopamine	D_1, D_2
adenosine	A_1, A_2
glycine	--

with different groups of ligands (1). It is not clear whether all of the subtypes of a particular receptor type belong together or whether one or more subtypes may actually represent another type of receptor. The relationships between receptor types and subtypes should become more evident as the amino acid sequences and the resulting three-dimensional structures of the different receptor protein types and subtypes become known and can be compared.

The three dimensional structure has not been determined yet for any of the neuroreceptors by x-ray crystallography because of the small amounts of available receptor protein and the great difficulty in forming suitable crystals. However, some structural information is available, primarily for the nicotinic cholinergic receptor for which acetylcholine is the endogenous neurotransmitter ligand.

The nicotinic acetylcholine receptor is made up of five subunits arranged in a circle with a Na^+/K^+ channel in the center of the circle and with each subunit consisting of a sequence of roughly 500 amino acids (subunit molecular weight about 50,000 daltons) (4,5). Four different subunits are present, with the alpha subunit appearing twice in the circle of five subunits that makes up the intact ion channel-binding site receptor complex. The assembled five-subunit complex is thought to have a cylindrical shape about 80 A in diameter by 140 A long, thus spanning the entire 40 A thick bilayer cell membrane and extending well into the extracellular space and also slightly into the intracellular region. The amino acid sequence of each subunit passes through the membrane more than once, with the nicotinic alpha subunit passing five times through the membrane lipid, as shown schematically in Fig. 2. The ion channel normally is closed and opens for a few milliseconds only when acetylcholine or other agonist molecules are bound to each of the two alpha subunits. When open, the channel diameter of approximately 7 A is sufficient for a hydrated Na^+ ion to pass through (4,5).

The GABA Type A neuroreceptor constitutes another interesting candidate for exploration as a biosensor component. The major

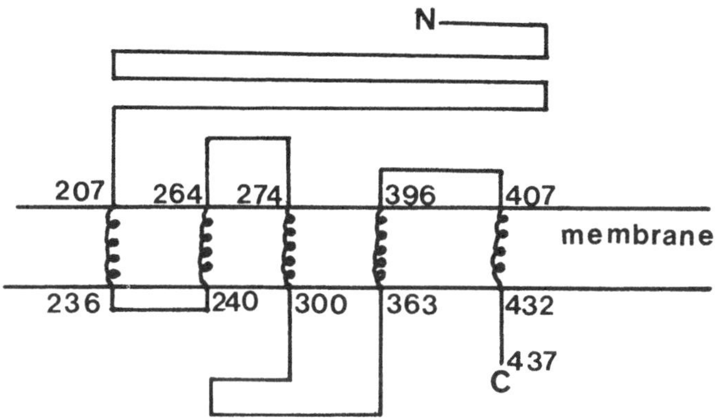

FIGURE 2. Proposed membrane crossings by amino acid chain of alpha subunit of acetylcholine nicotinic receptor. (from data in Ref. 4)

features of this receptor system are shown in Fig. 3 and consist of a chloride ion channel and separate binding sites for GABA (and agonists), benzodiazepines, barbiturates, and toxins such as picrotoxin (6). Only binding of GABA can open the chloride channel; but binding of benzodiazepines or barbiturates at the same time as

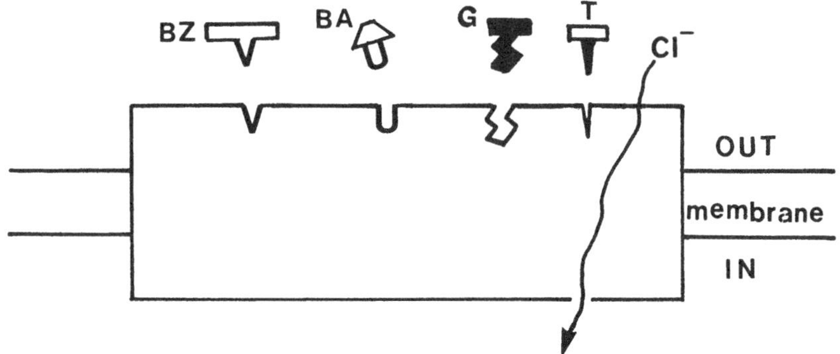

FIGURE 3. GABA Type A neuroreceptor, showing GABA (G), benzodiazepine (BZ), barbiturate (BA), and toxin (T) binding sites and chloride channel.

GABA binding occurs can prolong the duration or frequency of channel opening. Benzodiazepine and barbiturate compounds appear to act in an allosteric manner as their binding serves to augment the channel opening capabilities observed with GABA binding alone. Toxins act by apparent binding at the channel opening and thus act to block transport thru the channel. The GABA Type A receptor is composed of at least two types of subunits of approximately 50,000 daltons each with each type subunit precent in duplicate in the assembled ion channel system (7).

3 SOURCES OF NEURORECEPTORS

Neuroreceptors extracted from mammalian tissues can be obtained roughly in amounts of 50 to 100 ng per 100 g of tissue. This low production level is the result of the very small concentrations of receptor protein in the tissue and also because of the generally labile nature of isolated neuroreceptor proteins. Efforts are underway in many laboratories to develop cultured cell lines for production of receptor protein, and some success has been achieved, for example for opioid delta receptors with a hybrid mouse neuroblastoma crossed with a rat glioma NG 108-15 cell line (8) or a human neuroblastoma SK-N-SH cell line (9) that expresses the mu opioid receptor. Other routes involve expression of the cDNAs for the receptor subunits in foreign cell lines, as a method for the production of large amounts of receptor protein. A particularly attractive expression system involves a baculovirus-based insect cell line (10). The baculovirus system has been used successfully for the expression of numerous mammalian proteins and has the advantage of carrying out post translational receptor glycosylation and possibly receptor assembly processes. This laboratory has a collaborative project underway to express the DNA for the GABA Type A subunits in the baculovirus-insect cell system.

The nicotinic acetylcholine receptor is the only neuroreceptor for which an alternative natural source exists. The electric organ of the _Torpedo californica_ electric eel shows high amino acid sequence homology between the nicotinic acetylcholine receptor subunits from the electric eel and those from mammalian skeletal muscle (4,5). Therefore, the nicotinic acetylcholine receptor has become a model for studies of receptor characterization as well as receptor applications, as in biosensors. However, the presence of five subunits makes the acetylcholine receptor more complex than many others, such as the glycine and GABA Type A receptors. With the availability of the Torpedo electric organ, the acetylcholine receptor protein can be obtained in quantities of 10 to 100 milligram or greater.

In general isolated, purified neuroreceptors are labile and need to be stabilized in some manner for use in biosensors. Placing the receptors in an appropriate lipid bilayer, such as a liposome or even a synaptosome may be one route for partial stabilization (11). Some investigators have elected not to isolate the receptors but to use them in their native environment in tissue slices or in isolated whole cells (12); however, the presence of protein degrading enzymes and of signal artifacts and the difficulty in sterilizing such tissue slices to prevent added tissue destruction and the generation of additional aritfacts from microbial growth makes this approach much less attractive for practical applications.

4 NEURORECEPTORS IN BIOSENSORS

In principle, neuroreceptors ahould be usable in biosensors as follows:

1) to detect binding without amplification.
2) to detect binding with ion channel amplification.
3) to detect binding with enzyme amplification.

The first category is the only one that appears practical at present because techniques for receptor immobilization and stabilization with retention of ion channel or enzyme functionality still need to be developed. A short review of the literature on receptor biosensors to detect binding is included prior to further discussion of receptor amplification in biosensors.

4.1 Receptor Biosensors Based on Detecting Binding

Several reports have appeared in which isolated acetylcholine receptors have been utilized with a transducer in attempted demonstrations to recognize selective ligand binding to the receptor. In one test, a fixed amount of phencyclidine-labeled enzyme was added to lipid vesicles containing reconstituted acetylcholine receptors (13). Phencyclidine binds strongly to acetylcholine receptors; however the enzyme label was inactivated when the phencyclidine-enzyme moeity bound to the receptor but became active when displaced by free phencyclidine added in an unknown sample. The activity of the enzyme could be calibrated to indicate the concentration of free phencyclidine in the sample. Although this was an innovative method and incorporated an amplication step, the amplication was not carried out through the receptor but through the enzyme label.

In another report acetylcholine receptors were immobilized on the gate of an ion selective field effect transistor (ISFET) (14) by means of 1) a glutaraldehyde-coupled diamine matrix or 2) adsorption in a lecithin (lipid) film. Potentials were measured with respect to a reference ISFET that did not contain the receptor protein. Although a number of interesting results were obtained, it is difficult to rule out artifacts , since acetylcholine is a quaternary ammonium compound and thus carries a charge and since no independent test was devised to show that the specific binding capability of the receptor was functioning, although the signal caused by acetylcholine disappeared after the immobilized receptor was held at 60° C for 30 minutes. It is extremely difficult to devise tests to determine the functional integrity of a receptor preparation immobilized on some type of transducer, so this report represents some progress in the evaluation of receptor-based biosensors.

Two other reports are available in which acetylcholine receptors were immobilized by adsorption onto an electrical capacitor (15) and by entrappment or crosslinking in a polymer matrix (16). The occurrence of selective binding was tested by noting a change in electrical capacitance or electrical impedance, respectively. In both cases it is doubtful that the reported electrical changes could be attributed only to binding of acetylcholine or toxin to the immobilized receptors.

The acetylcholine receptor optical biosensor results presented elsewhere in this volume (17) show more convincing results for signal generation related to specific binding to the immobilized receptors.

Several additional transduction methods should be applicable to use with neuroreceptors for the determination of specific binding. Piezoelectric crystals, surface acoustic wave devices, and evanescent wave optical techniques are several approaches that need to be investigated.

The change in oscillation frequency of a quartz piezoelectric crystal has been shown to result from binding of ligands to antibody immobilized on the crystal surface, with the ligands either in the gas (18) or liquid (19) phase. Similar piezoelectric determination of mass changes caused by selective binding of ligands to immobilized neuroreceptors also may be possible; although the sensitivity of the method may not be sufficient to detect ligands of only a few hundred daltons in molecular weight. This estimate is based on the liquid phase sensitivity of 1.0 Hz change in frequency for 10 ng of ligand added to a 0.22 cm^2 area of immobilized antibody (19); for a receptor surface size of 100 A by 100 A and a ligand molecular weight of 100, a maximum of 0.2×10^{12} receptor molecules could fit on the 0.22 cm^2 area but 10^{13} molecules of ligand would be required for 10 ng.

Surface acoustic wave devices utilize an electrically generated wave that travels between two points on a quartz crystal with immobilized antibody placed between the same two points. The change in propagation velocity that results when mass is added to the immobilized antibody, as through binding of ligands, can be used to quantify the degree of ligand binding with gas and more recently liquid samples (20,21). With a large molecular weight protein, such as IgG, the limit of detection is 1-2 pg of ligand/mm^2 of surface area (at a signal to noise ratio of 3); and the sensitivity is about 600 ppm/ng/mm^2, with the relative velocity change expressed as parts per million and the ng refering to the amount of immobilized material. The feasibility of using this technique with immobilized neuroreceptors and liquid samples remains to be demonstrated.

The use of evanescent optical techniques is especially attractive because the light energy inside the fiber optic waveguide is modulated by those external (to the optical fiber) factors that are within a few nanometers of the fiber surface. Thus materials immobilized on the external fiber surface can modulate the signal but not those materials in the bulk of the solution surrounding the fiber. This has the advantages of not requiring a separation step in the procedure and of not requiring the addition of a label (22). The methodology is discussed elsewhere (23).

An alternative method is to introduce spectroscopic probes into receptor binding sites so that fluorescence, for example, is quenched when ligand binding occurs, as demonstrated for a model antibody system (24). However, such a transduction process likely will require more knowledge than currently is available about the structure of specific receptors.

4.2 Amplification Schemes

If methodology can be developed for immobilization of receptors such that either the ion channel or enzyme activation-inhibition activity remains functional, then signal amplification should be achievable. The discussion here is limited to the ion channel case since more is known about that system at present. One to two molecules of ligand bind to the extracellular side of the receptor, thereby opening the channel and allowing an unknown number of ions to pass through the membrane. Individual channels are either open or closed, there are no intermediate stages. In native tissue the degree of channel opening can be modulated by changing the total number of channels that are open at any time.

If the number of ions that pass through the membrane while the channel is open can be determined, then the amplification ratio can be calculated. Patch clamp techniques are available for recording the ion current that flows through individual ion channels and for determining how long a channel stays open (25,26). A plot of the distribution of channel open times for GABA Type A receptors from mouse spinal cord neurons (Fig. 4 I) shows a mean value of 4 milliseconds, and a typical recording of channel current versus time (Fig. 4 II) gives a value of 2 picoamperes for the conditions used (27).

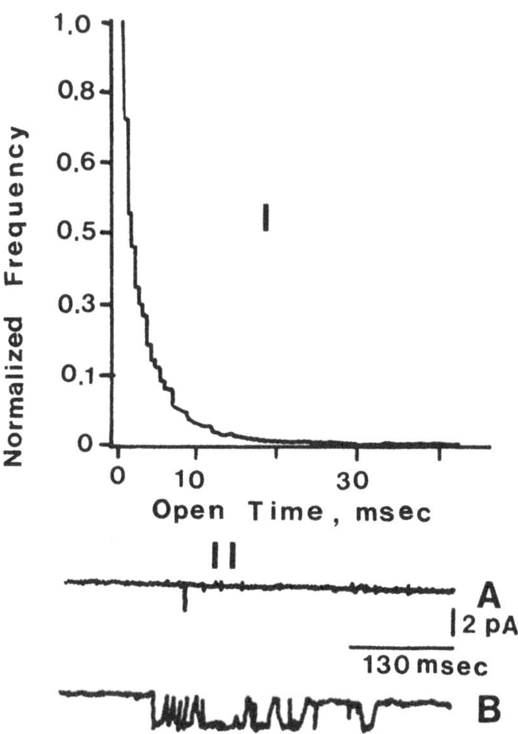

FIGURE 4. Single channel open time and ion currents. I: distribution of open time divided into segments of 0.5 msec each in presence of 2 uM GABA. II: single channel ion current in absence (control) (A) and presence (B) of 2 uM GABA. (From Ref. 27 with permission)

Since an ampere is a coulomb/sec, 2 picoampere (2×10^{-12} coulombs/sec) for 4 milliseconds would allow 8×10^{-15} coulombs to pass through the channel. Using the Faraday constant of 96,000 coulombs/equivalent gives a value of 8.3×10^{-20} equivalents or 50,000 ions. Thus, the amplication factor would be 50,000/2 or 25,000 for this set of conditions. With revised conditions, the channel may stay open considerably longer and therefore result in an amplification factor of 50,000 to 100,000 or more.

4.3 Potential Difficulties

In addition to the need to demonstrate methodology for reconstitution and immobilization of receptors with retention of ion channel or enzymatic activity and overall binding and structural stability, two other problems must be addressed. These are 1) non-specific binding and 2) possible shifts in receptor conformation to give different degrees of binding affinity with apparent conformations where binding does not lead to channel opening.

A typical plot of specific, non-specific, and total ligand bound to a receptor preparation (in natural intact, isolated and purified, or reconstituted forms) as a function of increasing concentration of free ligand is shown in Fig. 5. Specific binding is characterized by a fixed number of sites and therefore the concentration of bound ligand reaches saturation as the free ligand concentration is increased; while non-specific binding continues to increase linearly with greater concentrations of unbound ligand. Biosensor designs in which binding to a neuroreceptor, antibody, or other protein or similar material is an integral part of the recognition process need to incorporate a procedure to correct the output in some way for non-specific binding.

The nicotinic acetylcholine receptor exists in at least three conformations: 1) conformation 1 with two molecules of acetylcholine bound to the alpha subunits (channel does not open), 2) conformation 2 with the same molecules bound (channel opens), and 3) conformation 3 with one or two molecules of acetylcholine

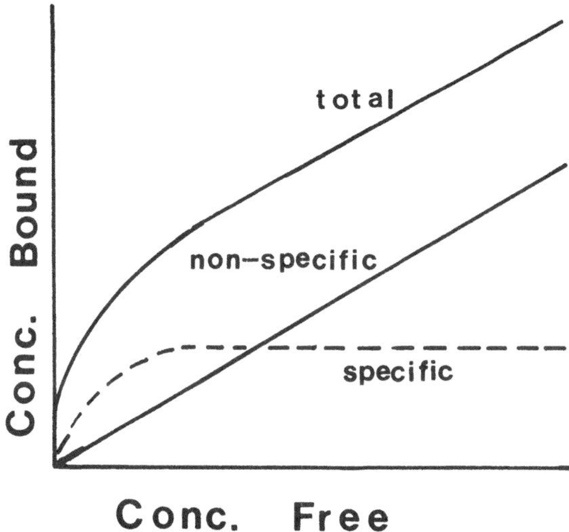

FIGURE 5. Variation of specific and non-specific bound ligand with concentration of free ligand.

bound but with different binding affinities than in 1 or 2 (channel does not open) (28). Whether such conformational changes will occur or be a problem with this receptor as part of a biosensor and whether such conformational changes occur with other types of neuroreceptors remains to be tested experimentally.

ACKNOWLEDGMENTS

This work was supported by a grant from The Upjohn Company.

REFERENCES

1. S. H. Snyder, Science, 224, 22 (1984).
2. L. B. Wingard Jr., Possibilities for Biosensors Based on Neuroreceptors, in Biosensors International Workshop 1987

(R. D. Schmid, ed.), VCH Publishers, Weinheim, 1987, pp. 133-137.

3. L. B. Wingard Jr., Biosensors from Neuroreceptors: What Can We Expect to Detect, in Biotechnology Research and Applications (J. Gavora, D. F. Gerson, J. Luong, A. Storer, and J. H. Woodley, eds.), Elsevier Applied Science, London, 1988, pp. 230-239.
4. F. Hucho, Eur. J. Biochem., 158, 211 (1986).
5. M. P. McCarthy, J. P. Earnest, E. F. Young, S. Choe, and R. M. Stroud, Ann. Rev. Neurosci., 9, 383 (1986).
6. R. W. Olsen, J. Yang, R. G. King, A. Dilber, G. B. Stauber, and R. W. Ransom, Life Sci., 39, 1969 (1986).
7. P. R. Schofield, M. G. Darlison, N. Fujita, D. R. Burt, F. A. Stephenson, H. Rodriguez, L. M. Rhee, J. Ramachandran, V. Reale, T. A. Glencorse, P. H. Seeburg, and E. A. Barnard, Nature, 328, 221 (1987).
8. W. F. Simonds, T. R. Burke Jr., K. C. Rice, A. E. Jacobson, and W. A. Klee, Proc. Nat. Acad. Sci. USA, 82, 4974 (1985).
9. V. C. Yu, M. L. Richards, and A. Sadee, J. Biol. Chem., 261, 1065 (1986).
10. I. R. Cameron, R. D. Possee, and D. H. L. Bishop, Trends Biotechnol., 7, 66 (1989).
11. M. Montal, R. Anholt, and P. Labarca, The Reconstituted Acetylcholine Receptor, in Ion Channel Reconstitution (C. Miller, ed.), Plenum Press, New York, 1986, pp. 157-204.
12. R. M. Buch and G. A. Rechnitz, Anal. Chem., 61, 533A (1989).
13. S. F. Hallowell and G. A. Rechnitz, Anal. Lett., 20, 1929 (1987).
14. M. Gotoh, E. Tamiya, M. Momoi, Y. Kagawa, and I. Karube, Anal. Lett., 20, 857 (1987).
15. M. E. Eldefrawi, S. M. Sherby, A. G. Andreou, N. A. Mansour, Z. Annau, N. A. Blum, and J. J. Valdes, Anal. Lett., 21, 1665 (1988).
16. R. F. Taylor, I. G. Marenchic, and E. J. Cook, Anal. Chim. Acta, 213, 131 (1988).
17. K. Rogers, D. Richman, and M. Eldefrawi, this volume.

18. J. Ngeh-Ngwainbi, P. H. Foley, S. S. Kuan, and G. G. Guilbault, J. Am. Chem. Soc., 108, 5444 (1986).
19. K. A. Davis and T. R. Leary, Anal. Chem., 61, 1227 (1989).
20. S. L. Rose-Pehrsson, J. W. Grate, D. S. Ballantine Jr., and P. C. Jurs, Anal. Chem., 60, 2801 (1988).
21. G. J. Bastiaans, Proc. Biosensors "89, Cambridge, UK, Sept. 1989.
22. J. F. Place, R. M. Sutherland, and C. Dahne, Biosensors, 1, 321 (1985).
23. L. B. Wingard Jr. and D. Wise (editors), Biosensors with Fiber Optics, Humana Press, Clifton, (in press).
24. S. J. Pollack, G. R. Nakayama, and P. G. Schultz, Science, 242, 1038 (1988).
25. E. Moczydlowski, Single-Channel Enzymology, in Ion Channel Reconstitution (C. Miller, ed.), Plenum Press, New York, 1986, pp. 75-113.
26. F. Franciolini and A. Petris, Experientia, 44, 183 (1988).
27. R. L. Macdonald, R. E. Twyman, C. J. Rogers, and M. G. Weddle, Pentobarbital Regulation of the Kinetic Properties of GABA Receptor Chloride Channels, in Chloride Channels and Their Modulation by Neurotransmitters and Drugs (G. Biggio and E. Costa, eds.), Raven Press, New York, 1988, pp. 61-71.
28. J. B. Udgaonkar and G. P. Hess, Proc. Nat. Acad. Sci. USA, 84, 8758 (1987).

10

Enzyme-Analyte Conjugates as Signal Generators for Amperometric Immunosensors: Immunochemical Phenomena Related to the Detection of Hapten Molecules

WILLFRIED SCHRAMM, SE-HWAN PAEK, and TONY YANG University of Michigan, Reproductive Sciences Program and Bioengineering Program, Ann Arbor, Michigan

1 INTRODUCTION

The majority of immunoassays that use enzymes as signal generators are designed for the colorimetric, i.e., spectrophotometric detection of products generated by the enzymatic biocatalyst in response to varying analyte concentrations in the sample. Spectrophotometric detection has a long tradition in analytical chemistry and it is therefore not surprising that enzyme immunoassays from their early inception were adapted to the measurement of colored reaction products. Furthermore, the immobilization of antibodies to solid matrices, the utilization of this technology in microplates for which multiple pipettors were already available, and the subsequent development of the microplate reader, a spectrophotometer that can measure the color intensity of 96 wells in about 1.5 minutes, established the colorimetric immunoassay as a standard technique in the analytical laboratory. Other techniques for signal generation using microplates followed suit: luminescent, fluorescent, and γ-radiation detection. In principle, an enzyme immunoassay can be as easily quantified by amperometric detection of products generated by enzymatic reactions. Although research groups began to explore this technology in the early seventies, there was no strong commercial incentive for the development of other detection methods such as electrochemical detection in immunoassays.

It appears that this situation is changing. Analytical chemists are being challenged to provide methods for the quantitative detection of analytes outside the laboratory. This requires simple, reliable, inexpensive procedures that do not confuse the user with techniques familiar only to the clinical chemist. If these methods are based on immunoglobulins as bioreceptors, electrochemical detection of products generated by enzymes in response to varying analyte concentrations in biological samples has unique advantages. No other instrumentation can successfully compete with an amperometric or potentiometric electrode with regard to size, accuracy, sensitivity, reliability, and price.

The prerequisites for further progress in the development of commercially available electrochemical detection methods combined with immunochemistry are available. One is the technique of ELISA (enzyme-linked immunosorbent assay) in its many variations. Another is the Clark electrode, an enzyme electrode developed for the quantitative detection of glucose [1]. Although the Clark electrode has been used in the past in research laboratories in combination with immunoglobulins, commercial products combining the two technologies have not yet entered the market.

Electrochemical detection of substrates, particularly amperometric measurement of products generated by enzyme reactions, can be highly sensitive and specific. However, when this method of signal generation is combined with immunochemical detection, the antibody-antigen interaction might impose certain limitation on the analytical system.

In this communication, we will focus on potential limitations of the immunochemical component in amperometric immunosensors. However, the problems outlined are of equal importance for other methods of signal generation in enzyme immunoassays. We will consider a competitive solid-phase immunoassay with the immunoglobulin immobilized on a flat surface, preferably directly on the electrode surface or in it's close vicinity. In addition, we will outline potential problems that might be encountered for the immunochemical detection of small analytes, also referred to as "haptens," with enzymes as signal generators for electrochemical detection. Conclusions can be projected to other model systems.

2 THE MODEL SYSTEM: COMPETETIVE IMMUNOASSAY

Amperometric immunosensors can make use of the technique of the competitive immunoassay. There are three major components in this type of immunoassay (Figure 1): An antibody that specifically recognizes the analyte (or antigen) to be measured in a sample (Fig. 1A). This event, the formation of an antibody-antigen complex, can usually not be measured directly, i.e., it does not generate a detectable signal. Therefore, the third component, the analyte-enzyme conjugate, is introduced

(Fig. 1B). This conjugate should bind to the antibody in a similar fashion as the native antigen.

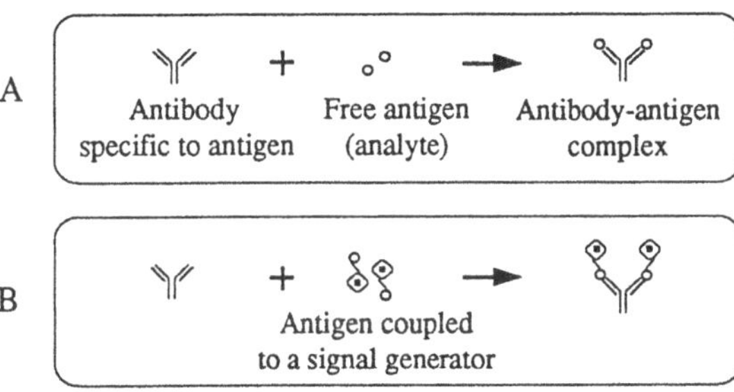

Figure 1. Components of an immunoassay. The antibody-antigen complex (A) cannot be measured with conventional detectors. If the antigen is coupled to a signal generator (B), the resulting antibody-antigen complex can be monitored.

Provided the analyte plus analyte-enzyme conjugate are in excess with respect to the antibody, these two species compete for limiting binding sites (Figure 2).

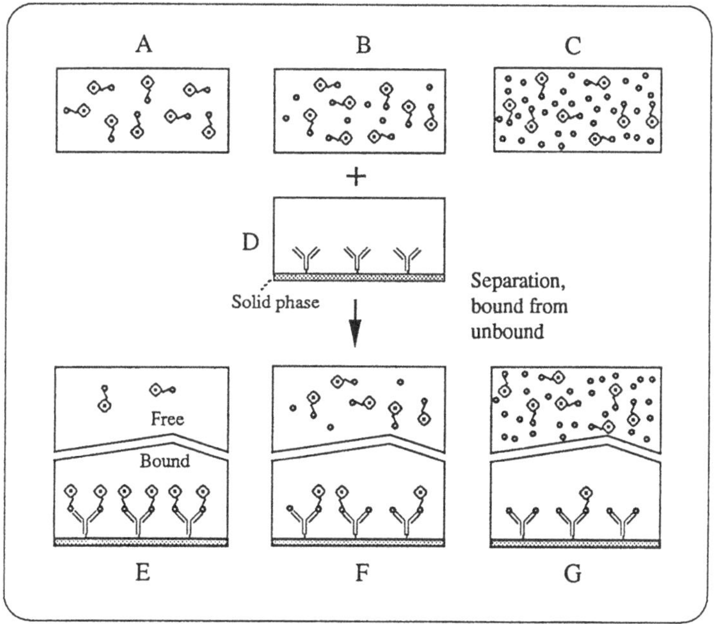

Figure 2. Principle of the competitive immunoassay. Either labeled antigen (A) or a mixture of labeled antigen and native antigen (e.g. analyte from the sample, B and C) are incubated with an antibody (D). After a period of incubation, the bound and free components are separated (A+D=E, B+D=F, C+D=G) and a signal proportional to the concentration of the free analyte is measured.

Competitive immunoassays usually require separation of the free from the bound signal generator. This is often done by immobilizing the antibody on a solid surface and washing off the components that are not bound to the antibody.

For example, in an amperometric immunosensor, the antibody can be immobilized on or in close proximity to the electrode and an analyte-glucose oxidase conjugate can serve as a signal generator. After immersing the electrode in a sample containing the conjugate, the separation can be achieved by a quick rinse to remove the free conjugate. Thereafter, the electrode is exposed to glucose and the generated electroactive species (either a mediator or hydrogen peroxide) is measured. This immunosensor is, in principle, a modified Clark electrode [1] with the difference that an antibody is immobilized that captures glucose oxidase proportional to analyte concentration in samples.

In the examples in Figures 1 and 2, the signal generator, bound to the antigen, is only twice the size of the antigen proper. For immunoassays with electrochemical detection, the label is usually an enzyme that generates the electrochemically active species. The size of the enzyme (e.g. glucose oxidase) can exceed the size of the antigen up to 500-fold, particularly if the analytes are small molecules (haptens) such as drugs of abuse, steroid hormones, many therapeutic drugs, or other physiological markers. We will now focus on some unique features that require special attention in the detection of hapten molecules in immunoassays utilizing enzymes as signal generators.

3 STEREOCHEMICALLY CONTROLLED IMMOBILIZATION OF ANTIBODIES

The shape of an immunoglobulin (IgG) molecule can be portrayed as the letter Y, with the stem representing the Fc fragment and the two branches representing the Fab fragments that contain idiotypic, or antigen-binding, sites. Physical immobilization of IgG molecules to solid surfaces can lead either to multilayers (Figure 3, top) or to monolayers (Figure 3, middle). The formation of monolayers seems to be thermodynamically favored if the concentration of IgG exposed to the surface is sufficiently low. In these first two examples, the immunoglobulins are shown to be immobilized in the "ends-on" configuration [2], i.e., by means of the Fc fragment (Figure 3, bottom). The "ends-on" configuration is the optimal orientation for immobilization in that both idiotypic sites on the antibody are accessible to the analyte. The least favorable case is a "top-on" configuration in which both idiotypic sites are bound to the surface, thereby preventing any interaction between that antibody molecule and the analyte. The physical binding of this protein to a solid surface might also be expected to occur in a less ordered fashion than described by these two limiting cases with the antibody binding to the surface in a "side-on" position in which only one of the two idiotypic sites are available for binding the analyte.

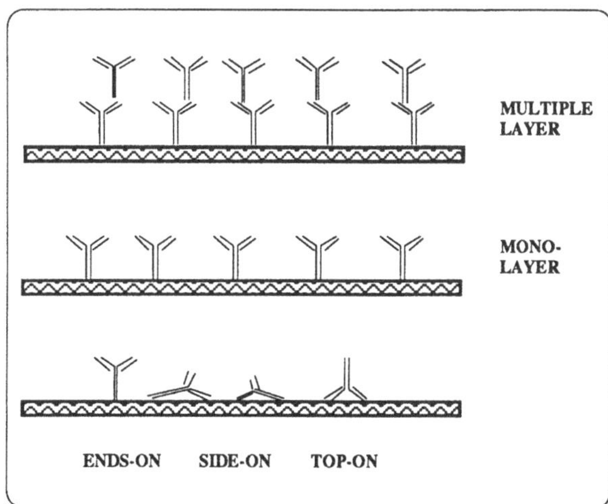

Figure 3. Immobilization of antibody in a multi-layer (top) and a monolayer (middle) in the "ends-on" position. Although binding of the antibody "ends-on" is desirable for optimal assays, most molecules are likely to be bound "side-on" (bottom). The "top-on" position constitutes another border case (bottom).

To keep the antibody from collapsing onto the surface of the solid matrix with the result that the idiotypic site might not be accessible for antigen binding, the surface can be coated first with an excess of Protein A [3]. This protein binds specifically to the Fc region of immunoglobulins, thus exposing the idiotypic, antigen binding site (Figure 4). Likewise, Fab fragments that specifically recognize the Fc region of a primary antibody to the analyte have been used to achieve the same effect [4].

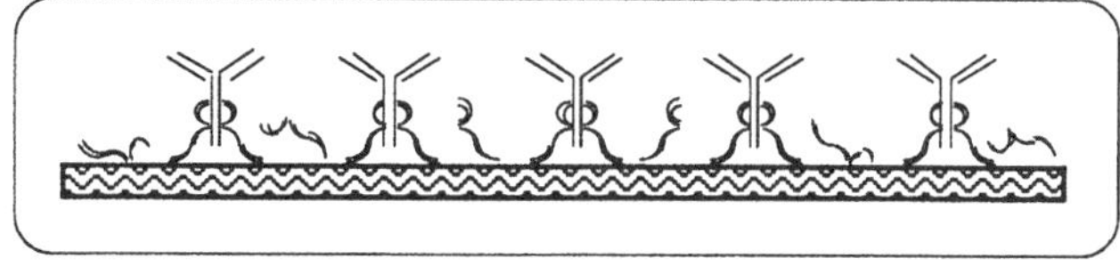

Figure 4. Immobilization of immunoglobulins via Protein A. The antibodies are prevented from collapsing to the "side-on" position and, therefore, the idiotypic site is exposed for unimpaired antigen binding.

The effect of the method by which immunoglobulins are bound to surfaces is striking. Antibody immobilized directly by physical adsorption on polystyrene microwells binds antigen with a substantial variability in sequential wells, especially if the antibody concentration is low (Figure 5, top panel). For the experiment shown in Figure 5, an average of 2.6 fmol of a monoclonal antibody was physically adsorbed per well [5]. The variation in binding was overcome when the immunoglobulin was bound via Protein A (Figure 5, bottom panel).

The physical structure of the solid matrix at the molecular level can have a pronounced effect on binding of proteins. Investigators have demonstrated temperature variations in microplates during incubation due to differences in evaporation between the inner wells and the wells located around the periphery of plates [6]. Likewise, the surface structure of polymers differs as a result of the manufacturing process: after the molten plastic is extruded into molds, cooling creates a temperature gradient that changes the surface characteristics of the polymer. This can cause subtle differences such as the orientation of ligands in the polymer (e.g. the degree of atactic, syntactic, or isotactic orientation) which subsequently has an amplified effect on the lipophilic interaction with absorbed proteins.

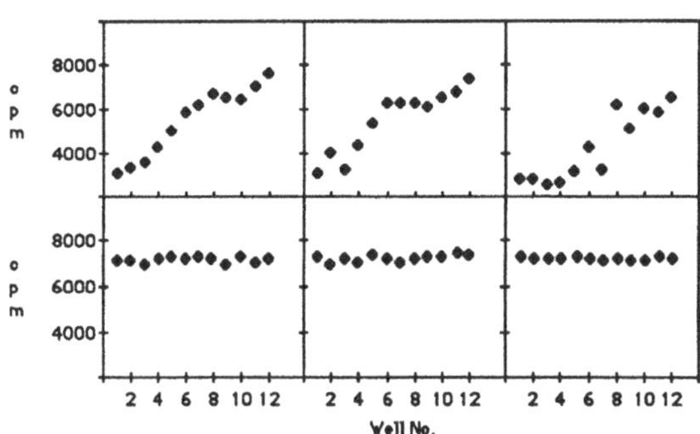

Figure 5. Variation of immunoglobulin binding by physical absorption (upper panel) and binding via Protein A (lower panel). Each square represents the data obtained from 12 sequential wells. The monoclonal antibody to progesterone was quantitated with a radiolabeled progesterone derivative. (From Ref. [5])

Immobilization via another binding protein has two advantages: 1) the first protein can be applied in excess so that variations in binding to the surface are buffered; and 2) the combination of first binding protein plus immunoglobulin can form a complex that provides more than one attachment point to the polymer surface (Figure 4). For example, Protein A has four potential binding sites for the Fc region of immunoglobulins, at least two of them are able to bind simultaneously to a single IgG molecule thus forming complexes in the liquid-phase [7].

If microwells with a monoclonal antibody immobilized via Protein A were incubated for extended periods of time with buffer, only a small percentage dissociated [3]. Therefore, we conclude that IgG molecules are bound by more than one binding site to Protein A. Furthermore, additional interaction between the solid surface and the IgG molecule may account for the strong adherence of the immunoglobulin. Scatchard plots [8] indicate that the idiotypic sites are freely available for antigen binding. We obtained dissociation constants for the antibody that were similar for the immobilized antibody and in the liquid phase ($K_d = 1.1 \times 10^{-10}$ mol/L, [3]). If the immunoglobulin is absorbed by electrostatic interaction, however, it is impossible to construct a meaningful Scatchard plot (Figure 6, right). In this case, binding sites of the antibody are obscured and not fully accessible to the antigen, and immunoglobulin can be desorbed during the incubation process [9].

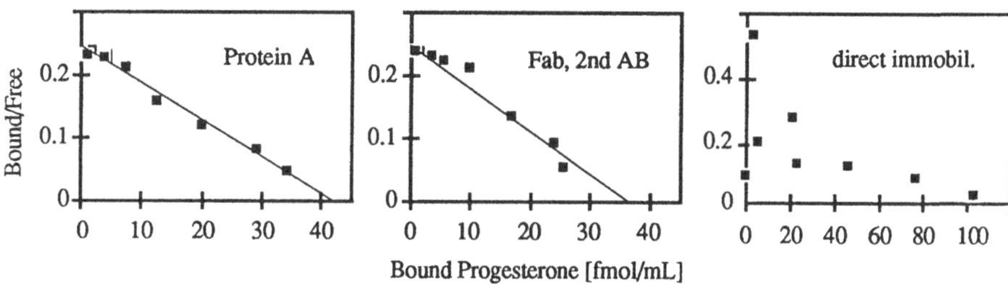

Figure 6. Scatchard plots with monoclonal antibody immobilized via Protein A (left); via the Fab fragment of an antibody binding to the Fc segment of the primary monoclonal antibody (middle); and via direct, physical immobilization by absorption (right).

4 ACCESSIBILITY OF LIGANDS IN ANALYTE-ENZYME CONJUGATES

While the accessibility of the binding site of immunoglobulins in immunosensors is one concern for sterically unimpaired antibody-antigen interaction, free access of the analyte in the analyte-enzyme conjugate is another. In the following analysis, we will concentrate on issues related to enzyme-analyte conjugates where the analyte is small (about 100-400 times smaller) compared with the enzyme. The analyte may not be accessible to the antibody binding site due to the short bridging sequence between the enzyme and the analyte ligand (Figure 7A). Only by extending the chemical link between the analyte and the enzyme may the attached analyte become available for binding to the immunoglobulin.

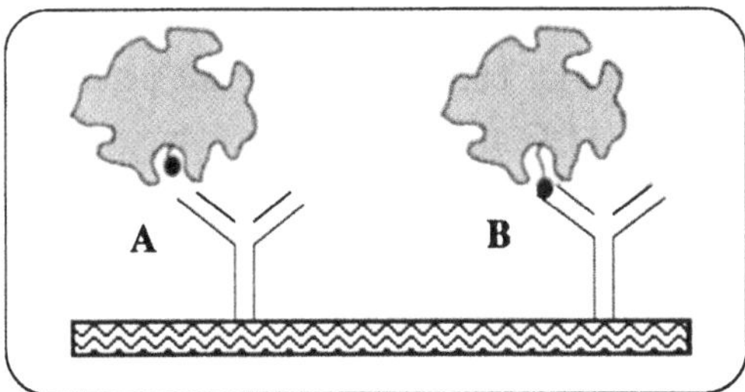

Figure 7. In conjugates between small analytes and enzymes, the analyte ligand might not be accessible to the idiotypic binding site of an antibody due to steric hindrance.

Antigens with the molecular mass of up to about 700 dalton can be "site-filling," i.e., they may be completely immersed in the three dimensional amino acid structure of the idiotypic site of the immunoglobulin. Therefore, impaired accessibility can severely effect antibody binding. In practice, the situation is more complicated than shown in Figure 7. If the analyte in the enzyme conjugate is completely masked by the protein, this product is not suitable as a signal generator in immunosensors. Accessibility as shown in Figure 7B, however, is usually not an all-or-none issue.

Table 1. Three tracers of progesterone and their immunochemical properties in binding to a monoclonal antibody: 1) radiolabeled derivative, 2) and 3) enzyme-labeled derivatives with a different bridge group.

	Tracer	Spacer Distance [nm]	Binding Constant K_a [L/mol]	50% inhib. [pg/well]
1		0.4	1.1×10^{11}	101
2		0.4	5.0×10^{9}	33
3		0.9	7.6×10^{10}	87

We have tested three different progesterone derivatives for their immunochemical properties as signal generators in immunoassays with an immobilized monoclonal antibody (Table 1). A tyrosine methyl ester suitable for labeling with ^{125}I was bound to progesterone with a spacer molecule of about 0.4 nm length (1 in Table 1). Using the same chemical linkage, a horseradish peroxidase conjugate was prepared (2, Table 1). With a different chemical reaction and using a different position in the enzyme for conjugation (i.e., a carbohydrate moiety), a steroid-enzyme conjugate with a longer bridge was obtained (3, Table 1).

The association constant, K_a, for the radiolabeled derivative was the highest among the three tracers. Although the same chemical linkage was used for one of the enzyme tracers, the dissociation constant was lower (2, Table 1). It appears that the large enzyme molecule interferes with antibody binding to some degree. By applying a larger bridge between the analyte and the enzyme, the binding constant increases, although not to the value of the small radiolabeled tracer (3, Table 1).

The tracer with the highest binding constant, the radiolabeled derivative, has the lowest sensitivity in immunoassays (1 in Figure 8 and 1 in Table 1) whereas the highest sensitivity was found for the enzyme tracer that has the lowest binding constant (2 in Figure 8 and 2 in Table 1). This is not surprising, since it is easier for the native antigen in the sample to compete with a tracer of low binding constant. Hence, smaller amounts of analyte can be detected. This phenomenon can be exploited only to a certain point in an analytical system. The lower the binding constant of the tracer, the smaller the number of molecules that are available for signal generation. Therefore, the greater sensitivity obtained with a weakly binding tracer must be balanced against the need for a minimal amount of bound enzyme conjugate necessary to obtain a measurable signal.

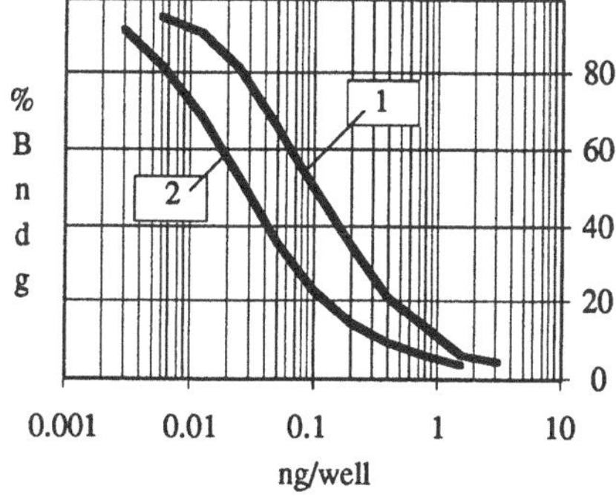

Figure 8. Standard curves in binding assays with immobilized antibody and a radiolabeled derivative as tracer (1, see also Table 1), and an enzyme-labeled tracer (2). The amount of immobilized antibody (2.6 fmol/well) and the amount of tracer (10 fmol/well) was the same for both systems.

5 NUMBER OF LIGANDS IN ANALYTE-ENZYME CONJUGATES

Radiolabeled derivatives of small analyte molecules are usually much easier to obtain in defined quality than their enzyme-labeled counterparts. Because of the high quantum yield of the radioactive decay of ^{125}I, the majority of tracers are derivatives of the analyte that can be iodinated, i.e., tyrosine methyl esters, histamines, or tyramines [10, 11]. As these can be easily purified by HPLC, well defined reagents with one signal generator per analyte molecule are obtained. The synthesis of analyte-enzyme conjugates, on the other hand, is more challenging. Enzymes typically have more than one functional group that can react with the activated analyte, and conjugates may be obtained with more than one ligand attached to the protein. Such species can bind very strongly to antibodies in immunoassays. As outlined above, the higher the binding constant of the signal generator, the less sensitive is the analytical system. Thus, enzymes with multiple ligands can substantially decrease the assay sensitivity. This is exemplified in Figure 9, in which a single enzyme molecule containing two analyte molecules simultaneously binds to two different, immobilized antibody molecules. For a free analyte to displace this conjugate, two analyte molecules would have to compete simultaneously and *at the same time,* an event of low probability.

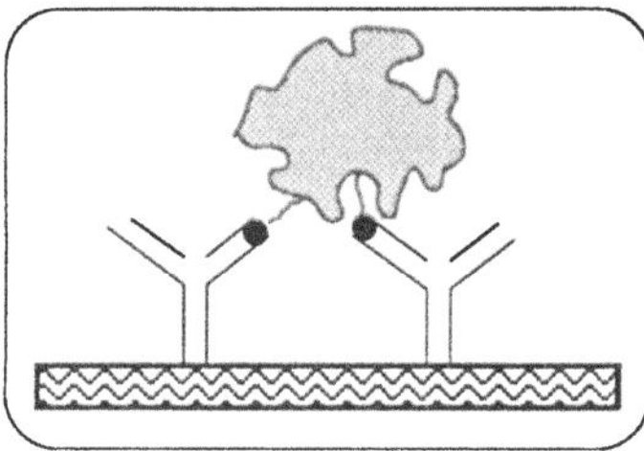

Figure 9. An analyte-enzyme conjugate with two ligands of analyte bound to the enzyme. Such a conjugate can bind simultaneously to two binding sites either of different (as shown) or to the same antibody resulting in lower sensitivity in immunoassays.

Standard curves using an enzyme-analyte conjugates with multiple ligands usually have a flat slope (B in Figure 10) extending over a wide range of analyte concentrations. For some applications this can be advantageous. However, most applications require the determination of small changes in analyte concentration and, therefore, standard curves with a steep negative slope are preferred (e.g. A in Figure 10).

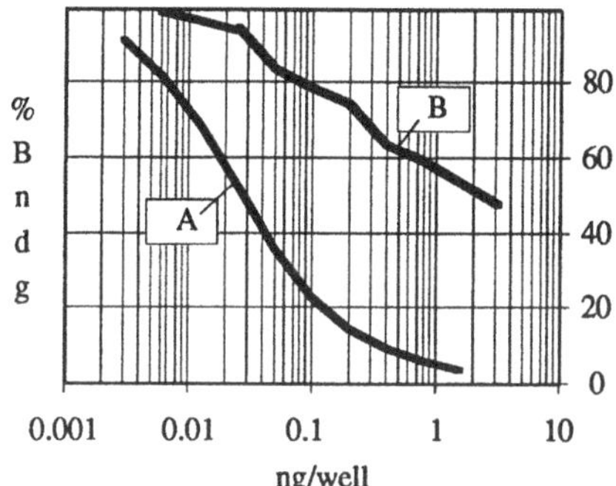

Figure 10. Standard curves with analyte-enzyme conjugates. The conjugate either contains predominantly one analyte ligand per enzyme (A) or multiple ligands (B).

High-quality conjugates between analytes and enzymes for immunochemical sensors should meet the following criteria:

- Chemical modification of the analyte molecule for subsequent conjugation occurs at a known and defined position of the analyte.
- The effect of chemical modification of the analyte molecule on its binding affinity to the immunoglobulin is known.
- The activated analyte reacts with the enzyme without impairing its biocatalytic activity.
- The activated analyte is attached to defined epitopes at the enzyme.
- The analyte ligand in the conjugate binds to the antibody with a binding constant that is within a certain range.
- Methods are available to control the number of analyte ligands that react with the enzyme, or to separate conjugates with different numbers of analyte ligands.

Other criteria might apply such as shelf life of the conjugate, ease of electrochemical detection of the enzyme product, low non-specific binding, contribution to fouling of electrodes, and effect on diffusion kinetics which we will analyze in the following section.

Electrochemical immunosensors that use analyte-enzyme conjugates for amperometrical detection of signals are much more demanding with regard to a well defined signal generator than are traditional immunoassays using radiolabeled tracers. The reproducible synthesis of analyte-enzyme conjugates with a known ratio of analyte to enzyme per molecule of conjugate may turn out to be a substantial challenge. For the studies shown above we used horseradish peroxidase as enzyme.

Similar experiments have been carried out with conjugates between small analytes and glucose oxidase for the utilization in systems with electrochemical detection. The molecular weight of glucose oxidase is about four times higher and, therefore, the synthesis of a well-defined conjugate is more complex since more potentially reactive groups (e.g. amino groups from lysine residues) are available for chemical binding.

6 DIFFUSION OF ANALYTE-ENZYME CONJUGATES

Enzyme electrodes usually use an immobilized enzyme on or in close vicinity of the electrode proper. The integrity of the enzyme is, within limits, of secondary concern. A large excess of enzyme can compensate for loss of some activity during immobilization. In immunochemical enzyme electrodes, on the other hand, the enzyme-analyte conjugate is applied in a well-defined amount in concentrations that can be 1000 times lower than in enzyme electrodes. The integrity of the enzyme molecules is crucial for the performance of the analytical system. Loss of activity results in inaccurate quantitation of analytes. Finally, the analyte enzyme conjugate is in solution and migrates by diffusion to the immobilized antibody. We have analyzed some of the potential limitations that molecular diffusion of the analyte and the analyte-enzyme conjugate may impose on the system.

Immunosensors based on electrochemical detection of signals frequently use membranes on top of the electrodes to protect these from fouling by components from the sample solutions. A typical example is the Clark electrode covered by a thin film of acetyl acetate or other polymers. Hydrogen peroxide, the electroactive species generated by the enzyme, is sufficiently small to penetrate the membrane while other components remain excluded. Diffusion through the protective polymer can slow down the response time of the electrode. Although disposable electrodes may not require the membrane, another problem arises with the utilization of an antibody-antigen reaction in electrochemical sensors: diffusion of analyte and analyte-enzyme conjugate from the bulk solution to the surface of the electrode where the antibody is immobilized might affect the reaction kinetics of the sensor. For the construction of an immunosensor, it is of consequence if the kinetics of antibody-antigen binding are determined by diffusion or if they are reaction controlled, i.e., by the on- and off-rate of antibody-antigen complex formation.

The model system that we will consider in the following assumes a well of a microplate filled with 200 μL of aqueous medium containing the sample and the enzyme-analyte conjugate. On the bottom of the well, for example, an electrode may be attached. Three different diffusion processes occur involving the enzyme-analyte conjugate and the analyte from the sample (not taking into consideration the diffusion of the electroactive species to the electrode surface): 1) three dimensional diffusion (Figure 11, A) from the bulk solution to the surface of the electrode; 2) lateral or two-dimensional diffusion along the surface of the system (Figure 11, B); and C) orientational diffusion that directs the ligand on the conjugate towards the idiotypic site of the immunoglobulin for proper binding. (Figure 11, C).

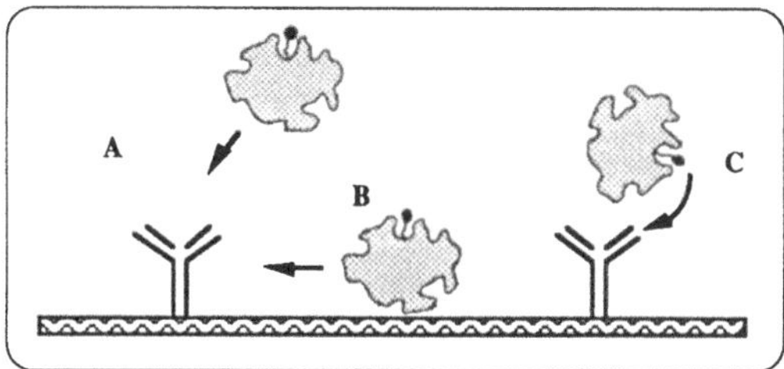

Figure 11. Diffusion of analyte-enzyme conjugate to antibody molecules immobilized on the surface of an electrode. A: three dimensional, B: lateral (two dimensional), and C: orientational diffusion

Three-dimensional diffusion can be accelerated by agitating the solution (e.g. by stirring or shaking which we will summarily refer to as "stirring conditions"). Under stirring conditions, a layer forms on the surface that is organized by the electrostatic properties of the electrode and polymer surface, the immunoglobulins immobilized, and by oriented water and medium molecules. Although the thickness of this layer becomes infinitesimally small with increasingly optimal stirring, it never reaches zero in practical terms. This layer, sometimes referred to as the "film layer" or "penetration layer," constitutes the volume for molecular diffusion under stirring conditions. We have experimentally determined the thickness of this penetration layer for the microwells mentioned above as 85 μm [12] using 0.01 mol/L phosphate buffer containing 1 g/L of gelatin and with moderate agitation on an orbital shaker. This compares to 30 μm reported for phosphate buffer without gelatin and vigorous stirring by other investigators [13]. For comparison, an immunoglobulin, immobilized in the "ends-on" configuration (i.e., via the Fc fragment, Figure 3), extends about 23.5 nm in the end-on adsorption [14, 2] from the surface. Hence, the penetration layer under stirring conditions is still more than 1000 times thicker than the extension of an immobilized IgG.

Mathematical modeling by taking into consideration only three dimensional molecular diffusion (A in Figure 11) results in kinetic curves that coincide with experimental results (Figure 12). Since the experiment provides the sum of all three types of diffusion, we conclude that lateral and orientational diffusion are substantially faster and contribute, therefore, very little to the kinetics of antibody-antigen binding.

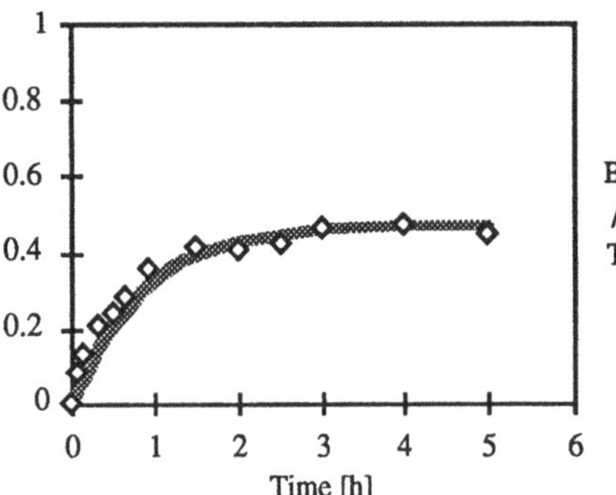

Figure 12. A mathematical model for the diffusion rate of an enzyme-analyte conjugate under stirring conditions (solid line) explains experimental results satisfactorily (dots). The ratio of conjugate bound to antibody immobilized to microwells vs. total amount incubated (B/T) over time is shown. The incubation volume was 200 µL per well.

The size of the molecule determines the time when equilibrium between the on- and off-rate of antibody-antigen complex formation has been reached. As expected, the larger the size of the molecule, the longer it takes until the binding with the antibody is in equilibrium (Figure 13). We have experimentally determined that binding of the molecule with the mass of 740 dalton is reaction controlled while the other two species are diffusion controlled.

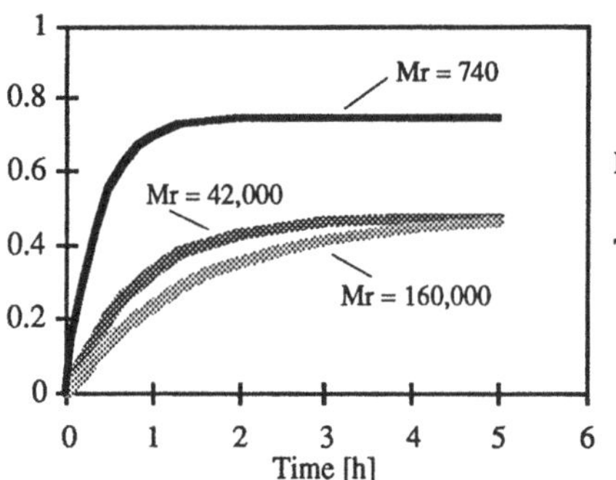

Figure 13. Kinetics of antibody-antigen binding with three tracers of different molecular mass, M_r. The top curve is related to a radiolabeled tracer, the second curve to a horseradish peroxidase conjugate, and the third curve to a glucose oxidase conjugate.

The fraction of the total antigen that is bound to the antibody at equilibrium (B/T) is determined by the binding constant to that antigen (Figure 14, ordinate). However, the time when equilibrium is reached is either reaction controlled or diffusion controlled (Figure 14, abscissa). For the radiolabeled signal generator with the molecular mass of $M_r = 740$ (an iodinated tyrosine methyl ester of progesterone), we have experimentally determined that attaining equilibrium is reaction controlled and, under the applied conditions, diffusion can be neglected. That is not so with the enzyme-antigen complexes with the molecular masses of $M_r = 42{,}000$ and $M_r = 160{,}000$.

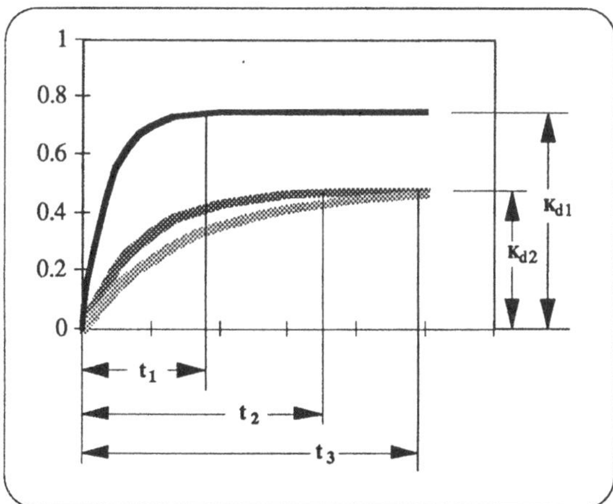

Figure 14. The time when equilibrium for antigen-antibody binding is reached (t_1 to t_3) is either reaction controlled (e.g. for the species determined by t_1) or diffusion controlled (t_2 and t_3). The binding constant (K_{d1} and K_{d2}) determines the amount of antigen bound. The binding constant for the two enzyme-analyte species (lower curves) is the same but the time of equilibrium differs due to their variation in size.

In practical terms, this means that in an amperometric immunosensor for the detection of a small analyte and with an enzyme as signal generator, the analyte will reach the antibody first and can bind. Therefore, competition with the enzyme-labeled tracer can be established only at a later time. Competitive immunoassays do not require equilibrium conditions for the formation of the antigen-antibody complex. In fact, it is not even necessary that the two species competing for binding sites, the antigen and the enzyme-antigen conjugate, reach the surface at an equal rate. However, dose-response curves generated under these conditions will be time-dependent. Therefore, if the sensor has been calibrated for a certain time of incubation, it is essential for the user to observe this incubation period for accurate results. The advantage of electrochemical detection is that circuits can be included into the recording device that initiate a count down for taking a measurement after a predetermined time interval.

CONCLUSIONS

Amperometric immunosensors combine two basic technologies: the methodologies of immunoassay with special emphasis on enzyme-linked immunoassays, and the techniques of detection of enzyme-generated electroactive molecules, most advanced to date in amperometric enzyme electrodes [15]. However, the enzyme in enzyme electrodes is used in a different setting than in immunosensors. An excess of enzyme is immobilized in enzyme electrodes. The enzyme in immunoassays is a mobile species, available in limited amount, and used as an enzyme-analyte conjugate to participate in an immunochemical reaction.

This communication analyzes issues related to the utilization of the full potential of immunoassays with enzymes as signal generators. The quantitative detection of small molecules (haptens) by means of a large enzyme-hapten as signal generator is subject to special considerations. We have shown that the availability of the idiotypic site of immobilized immunoglobulins can substantially affect the performance of the analytical system. Methods for stereospecific binding of immunoglobulins and uniform distribution on solid surfaces have been reviewed. Furthermore, the effect of the structure of enzyme-hapten (enzyme-analyte) conjugates as signal generators on the performance of immunoassays has been described: 1) the immunochemical availability of the analyte ligand in the conjugate; 2) the effect of the binding constant of the conjugate; and 3) the effect of multiple analyte ligands in the conjugate. Since the structure of this conjugate can profoundly affect quantitative analysis, special emphasis has to be put on the reproducible synthesis, purification, and characterization of the enzyme-analyte conjugates. Finally, kinetic considerations related to the quantitative determination of small molecules by means of large enzyme-analyte signal generators have been outlined. Different diffusion and binding kinetics of the two species binding to an immunoglobulin require well-controlled timing of the immunochemical reaction.

ACKNOWLEDGEMENTS

This work was supported in part by the Army Research Office (246655-LS). We are indebted to Drs. Paul A. Craig and Richard H. Smith for critical discussions.

REFERENCES

1. L.C. Clark, L.D. Bowers. Electrode system for continuous monitoring in cardiovascular surgery. *Ann. N.Y. Acad. Sci.* 102:29-45, 1962.

2. I. Oreskes, J.M. Singer. The mechanism of particulate carrier reactions. I. Adsorption of human γ-globulin to polystyrene latex particles. *J. Immunol.* 86:338-344, 1961.

3. W. Schramm, T. Yang, A.R. Midgley. Surface modification with Protein A for uniform binding of monoclonal antibodies. *Clin. Chem.* 33:1338-1342, 1987.

4. G.M. Sankolli, R.A. Stott, L.J. Kricka. Improvement in the antibody binding characteristics of microtitre wells by pretreatment with anti-IgG Fc immunoglobulin. *J. Immunol. Methods* 104:191-194, 1987.

5. W. Schramm, T. Yang, A.R. Midgley. Monoclonal antibodies used in solid-phase and liquid-phase assays, as exemplified by progesterone assay. *Clin. Chem.* 33:1331-1337, 1987.

6. D.G. Oliver A.H. Sanders, R.D. Hogg, J.W. Hellman. Thermal gradients in microtitration plates. Effects on enzyme-linked immunoassay. *J. Immunol. Methods* 42:195-201, 1981.

7. J.J. Langone, M.D.P. Boyle, T. Borsons. Studies on the interaction between Protein A and immunoglobulin G. II. Composition and activity of complexes formed between Protein A and IgG. *J. Immunol.* 121:333-334, 1978.

8. G.E. Scatchard. The attraction of proteins for small molecules and ions. *Ann. N.Y. Acad. Sci.* 51:660-672, 1949.

9. W.D. Zollinger, J.M. Dalrymple, M.S. Artenstein. Analysis of parameters affecting the solid phase radioimmunoassay quantification of antibody to meningococcal antigens. *J. Immunol.* 117:1788-1798, 1976.

10. W.M. Hunter. Preparation and assessment of radioactive tracers. *Br. Med. Bull.* 30:18-23, 1974.

11. R.H. Seevers, R.E. Counsell. Radioiodination techniques for small organic molecules. *Chem. Rev.* 82:575-590, 1982.

12. M.Stenberg, M.Werthen, S. Theander, H.Nygren. A diffusion limited reaction theory for a microtiter plate assay. *J. Imm. Methods* 112:23-29, 1988.

13. H.J. Trurnit. Studies on enzyme systems at a solid-liquid interface. II. The kinetics of adsorption and reaction. *Arch. Biochem.* 51:176-199, 1954.

14. J.L. Oncley, G. Scatchard, A. Brown. Physiochemical characteristics of certain proteins of normal human plasma. *J. Phys. Colloid Chem.* 51:184-198, 1947.

15. A.P.F. Turner, I. Karube, G.S. Wilson (eds.). Amperometric sensors, in *Biosensors: Fundamentals and Applications*. Oxford University Press, Oxford 1987.

11

Development of a Polypyrrole Glucose Biosensor

GUY FORTIER[1], ERIC BRASSARD and DANIEL BÉLANGER[1]. [1]Groupe de recherche en enzymologie fondamentale et appliquée, Département de Chimie, Université du Québec à Montréal, C.P. 8888, Succ. A, Montréal (Québec), Canada, H3C 3P8

1 INTRODUCTION

Currently, one of the most frequently performed analyses in biochemical laboratories is the determination of glucose in various biological fluids (1). During the last two decades, there has been a great deal of interest in the development of a device for glucose determination which will be easy to operate, portable, inexpensive, accurate and reliable. The combination of a biological catalyst along with an electrochemical transducer provides a novel and convenient approach for glucose detection (2).

The enzyme glucose oxidase reacts with glucose and, according to the following equations, generates peroxide which can be detected by an amperometric method on a platinum electrode.

$$GOD_{FAD} + \text{Glucose} \dashrightarrow GOD_{FADH2} + \text{gluconic acid} \qquad [1]$$

$$GOD_{FADH2} + O_2 \dashrightarrow GOD_{FAD} + H_2O_2 \qquad [2]$$

$$H_2O_2 \underset{+0.7V \text{ vs SCE}}{\dashrightarrow} O_2 + 2H^+ + 2e^- \qquad [3]$$

The oxidation of the peroxide (eq.3) at the surface of a platinum electrode generates a readily detected electrical current. In this study, the glucose oxidase is maintained in close contact with the platinum substrate by physical entrapment in a polymer (3,4). The immobilization process of the glucose oxidase in the polypyrrole film is achieved during the electropolymerization of pyrrole in a KCl solution (5) containing the enzyme. In this paper, data concerning the fabrication of an optimized glucose biosensor using pyrrole and glucose oxidase are given.

2 EXPERIMENTAL TECHNIQUES

2.1 Reagents

Glucose oxidase, type VII-S (E.C. #1.1.3.4), was purchased from the Sigma Chemical Co. (St-Louis, USA) and the pyrrole from Aldrich (St-Louis, USA). The pyrrole was distilled daily.

2.2 Enzyme electrode fabrication.

The platinum electrode was fabricated as previously described (6). Pt disc electrodes were cleaned according to standard procedures (7) by anodic and cathodic treatments and polished with successively finer grades of diamond polishing compounds and aqueous alumina slurry down to 0.5 µm (Buehler Ltd, USA). Electrochemical polymerization was performed in a one-compartment cell at room temperature with the platinum disc electrode (0.28 cm^2) and a platinum flag as working and auxiliary electrodes, respectively. To 2 ml of 10 mM degassed KCl solution, pH 6, was added 0.2 to 0.7 M of freshly distilled pyrrole and 2.5 to 1250 U of GOD. PP/GOD films were grown potentiostatically at +0.65 V vs SCE (saturated calomel electrode). The thickness of the films was controlled by the amount of charge passed. The electrode was washed for 3 min in PBS (phosphate buffered salts, 125 mM NaCl, 2.7 mM KCl and 10 mM phosphate buffer) solution pH 7.5, under mild stirring.

2.3 Determination of glucose.

The amperometric response to glucose was evaluated in 5 ml of 0.1 M PBS solution, pH 7, by holding the enzyme electrode at +0.7V vs SCE. The electrode was kept under gentle stirring at 200 rpm using a microprocessor-controlled stirring plate until the background current stabilized. The glucose was injected into the cell and the current-time response was recorded. The steady-state current was usually reached after 15 sec to 1 min, depending on the film thickness.

2.4 Instrumentation.

All electrochemical experiments were carried out in conventional one-compartment cells. Potentials were applied to the cell with a bipotentiostat (Pine Instruments Inc., USA) model RDE4. Current time responses were recorded on a XYY' recorder (Kipp & Zonen, USA) model BD91 equipped with a time base module.

3 RESULTS AND DISCUSSION

In order to optimize the response of the biosensor to glucose, the effect of the concentration of the pyrrole, the film thickness and the concentration of the glucose oxidase enzyme were evaluated. For all experiments, the steady state current method was used to determine the response of the enzyme electrode to a 20 mM glucose solution at pH 7.0 in a phosphate buffer. The electrode was poised at a potential of +0.7V vs SCE to oxidize the peroxide formed.

The concentration of pyrrole studied ranged from 0.1 to 0.8 M in aqueous KCl solution containing a fixed amount of the enzyme glucose oxidase (500 U/ml). The total charge deposited was kept constant at 270 mC/cm^2. The results are reported in Table 1. The optimal concentration of pyrrole was 0.3 M as indicated by the maximum current response observed. At a concentration of 0.1 M pyrrole, a non-homogeneous deposition of polypyrrole/GOD onto the platinum surface was observed. At concentrations greater than 0.7 M pyrrole, the pyrrole precipitated from the aqueous solution .

TABLE 1. Effect of pyrrole concentration in the electrodeposition solution on the response of the Pt/PP/GOD electrode to 20 mM glucose

Pyrrole (M)	Current (μA)
0.2	1.4
0.3	1.7
0.5	1.5
0.6	1.4
0.7	0.5

The effect of film thickness on the response of the glucose electrode is depicted in Figure 1. The electrodes were prepared by varying the electrodeposition time at +0.65 V (vs SCE) of a solution containing 0.3 M pyrrole, 500 U/ml glucose oxidase and 0.1M KCl, pH 6.0. The charge was evaluated from the area under the anodic current-time curve recorded during the deposition. Total charges ranging from 32 to 820 mC/cm^2 were obtained.

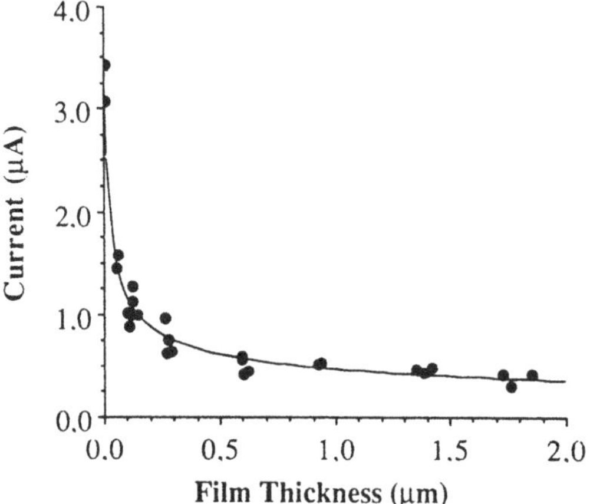

Figure 1. *The effect of film thickness on the steady-state response of the glucose electrode.* The electrodes were prepared by varying the electrodeposition time at 0.65 V of a solution containing 0.3 M pyrrole, 500 U/ml glucose oxidase and 10 mM KCl, pH 6. The electrode surface was 0.28 cm^2.

The film thickness deposited at the surface of the electrode was calculated using the relationship whereby 45 mC/cm^2 of charge is equivalent to a film thickness of 0.1 μm (8). As seen in Fig. 1, the electrode response diminished with increasing film thickness and this can be accounted for by a decreased mass transfer of the peroxide to the platinum substrate. The optimal charge was 75 mC/cm^2 , which is equivalent to a film thickness of 0.17 μm. Under these conditions, the entire surface of the electrode was homogeneously covered and the current generated by 20 mM glucose was reproducible.

The effect of glucose oxidase concentration on the response of the glucose electrode was studied in the range of 1 to 500 U/ml for charges of 50 (●) and 410 mC/cm^2 (○). The results are presented in Figure 2. Since there were large variations in the reproducibility of the response at GOD concentrations between 25 and 50 U/ml, we have arbitrarily chosen a concentration of 65 U/ml where the glucose response is still high and more reproducible.

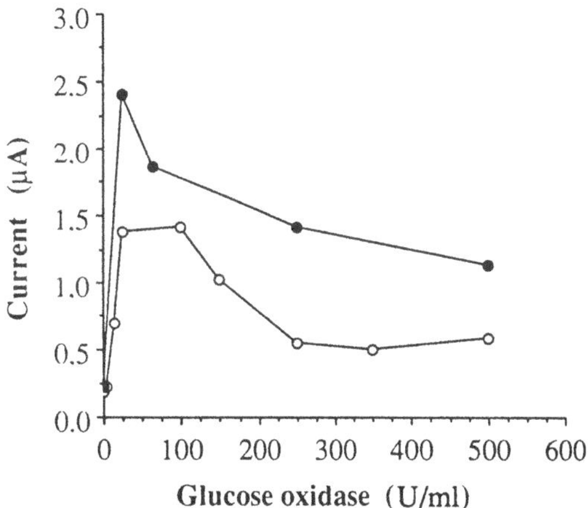

Figure 2. *The effect of glucose oxidase concentration on the steady-state response of the glucose electrode.* The electrodes were prepared by electrodeposition of 0.3 M pyrrole at 0.65 V in the presence of varying quantities of glucose oxidase (1 to 500 U/ml) in a solution of 10 mM KCl, pH 6. The charges deposited were 50 (●) and 410 mC/cm^2 (○).

In figure 3, a calibration curve for glucose obtained with the optimized Pt/polypyrrole-glucose oxidase electrode is shown. A linear response of the enzyme electrode was observed for concentrations of glucose ranging from 1 to 7.5 mM. The Km and the Imax were 33.4 mM (S.D. = 0.7) and 7.2 μA (S.D. = 0.06) respectively and were calculated by non-linear regression from the Michaelis Menten curve. The litterature value of Km for the soluble enzyme is 33 mM (9). The Lineweaver-Burk plot is given in the inset (r^2>0.999) and fitted the following equation (10):

$$1/Is = 1/Imax + 1/S \ Km/Imax \qquad [4]$$

The effect of temperature on the response of the optimized enzyme electrode to 20 mM glucose was evaluated from 4 to 50°C with (□) or without (○) stirring (200 rpm) (Fig.4). The optimal temperature for the catalytic activity of the entrapped glucose oxidase was 40°C and is similar to values obtained with other polymers (11).

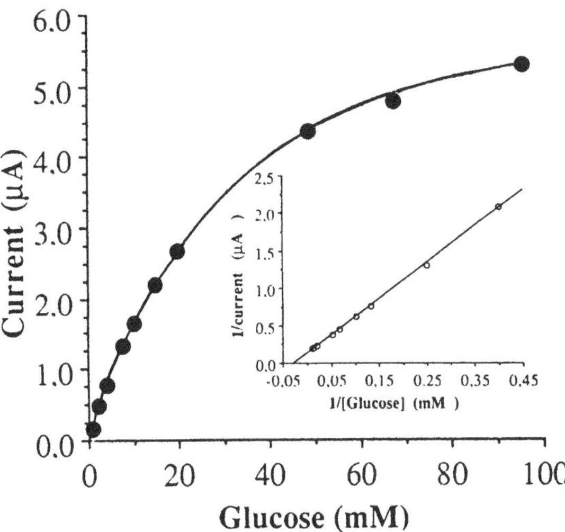

Figure 3. *Calibration curve for glucose obtained with the optimized Pt/PP/GOD electrode obtained in absence of stirring.* The electrode was prepared by electrodeposition of 0.3 M pyrrole at 0.65 V in the presence of 65 U/ml GOD in a solution of 10 mM KCl, pH 6. The charge deposited was 75 mC/cm^2. In the inset, Lineweaver-Burke-type plot is shown.

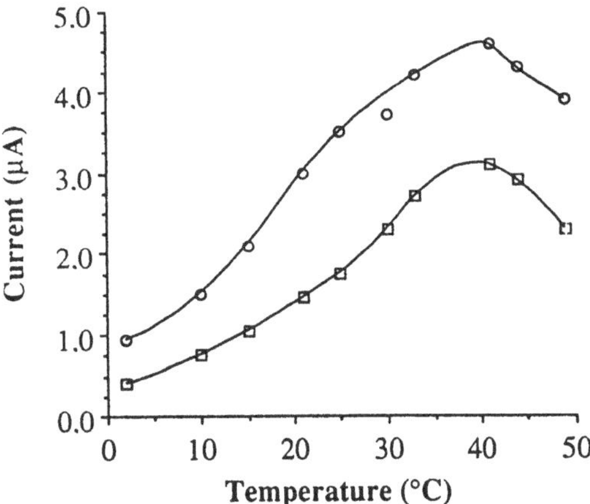

Figure 4. *The effect of temperature on the steady-state response of the glucose electrode.* The electrodes were prepared as described in Fig. 3. The effect of temperature was evaluated from 4 to 50°C with (□) or without (○) stirring (200 rpm).

ACKNOWLEDGMENTS

We would like to thank the Natural Sciences and Engineering Research Council of Canada and the "Action Structurante" program of the Québec government for financial support and also Dr D. Bates for her valuable comments and for the revision of the manuscript.

REFERENCES

1) Wingard, L.B. Jr. (1983). Immobilized enzyme electrode for glucose determination for the artificial pancreas. Fed. Proc. Fed. Am. Soc. Exp. Biol. **42**, 288-291.

2) Updike, S.J. and Hicks, G.P. (1967). The enzyme electrode. Nature, **214**, 986-988.

3) Guilbault, G.G. and Lubrano, G.L., (1973). An enzyme electrode for the amperometric determination of glucose. Anal. Chim. Acta, **64**, 439-55.

4) Fortier, G., Brassard, E. and Bélanger, D. (1988). Fast and easy preparation of an amperometric glucose biosensor. Biotechnol. Tech., **3**, 177-182.

5) Asavapiriyanont, S., Chandler, G.K., Gunawardena, G.A. and Pletcher, D. (1984). The electrodeposition of polypyrrole films from aqueous solutions. J. Electroanal. Chem., **177**, 229-244.

6) Bélanger, D., Nadreau, J. and Fortier, G. (1989). Electrochemistry of polypyrrole glucose oxidase electrode. J. Electroanal. Chem., in press.

7) Gileadi, E,., Kirowa-Eisner, E. and Penciner, J. (1975). Interfacial Electrochemistry and experimental approach, Addison-Wesley, Reading,pp. 312.

8) Holdcroft, S. and Funt, B.L. (1988). Preparation and electrocatalytic properties of conducting films of polypyrrole containing platinum microparticules. J. Electroanal. Chem., **240**, 89-103.

9) Swoboda, B.E.P. and Massey, V. (1965). Purification and properties of the glucose oxidase from Aspergillus niger. J. Biol. Chem., **240**, 2209-15.

10) Shu, F.R. and Wilson, G.S. (1976). Rotating ring-disk electrode for surface catalysis studies. Anal. Chem., **48**, 1679-1686.

11) Szajani, B., Molnar, A., and Klamar, M. (1987). Preparation, characterization and potential application of an immobilized glucose oxidase. Appl. Biochem. Biotechnol, **14**, 37-47.

12

Electrochemistry of Polypyrrole-Glucose Oxidase Electrode

DANIEL BÉLANGER, JOCELYN NADREAU and GUY FORTIER
Département de Chimie, Université du Québec à Montréal, C.P. 8888, succursale "A", Montréal, Québec, Canada, H3C 3P8.

1 INTRODUCTION

The attempt to achieve direct electron transfer between the active site of an enzyme and an electrode is an active area of research [1-6] and is of relevance to the development of an amperometric enzyme electrode. Direct electron transfer between the $FADH_2$ redox centers of glucose oxidase, GOD, and electrode has been achieved via fast redox couple [1-5]. These redox couples can be either covalently or coordinately bound to GOD [1-3], chemically bound to a flexible polymer backbone or a polycationic redox polymer [4-5]. In addition, direct electron transfer between GOD and polypyrrole, PP, has recently been claimed [6]. Electronically conductive polymers, such as PP [7-12] and poly-N-methylpyrrole [12,13] have been proposed as entrapment media for GOD.

The interest of using such conducting polymers for amperometric enzyme electrode lies in the possibility that H_2O_2 would be oxidized at the surface of the conducting polymer in addition to the underlying platinum substrate, the latter following its diffusion through the polymer layer.

In this paper we report the electrochemical behaviour of a Pt/PP-GOD electrode. Cyclic voltammetry and glucose assays with the Pt/PP-GOD electrode indicated that amperometric responses to glucose were observed only after the loss of PP electroactivity which can be induced either chemically or electrochemically. Our results allow us to conclude that PP served only as an inert immobilization matrix for GOD.

2 EXPERIMENTAL

Chemicals and sources are as previously noted [11]. The polypyrrole glucose oxidase electrodes were prepared as described previously [11]. Briefly, a Pt/PP-GOD electrode was prepared at 0.65V vs SCE using a solution containing 0.32 M pyrrole, 500 U/ml GOD and 0.1M KCl. Typically a film of 150 $mC \cdot cm^{-2}$ of charge was deposited for experiments described in this paper. Cyclic voltammograms were recorded in 0.1M KCl. The glucose assay was carried out in 0.1M PBS (phosphate buffered salts, 125 mM NaCl, 2.7 mM KCl and 10 mM phosphate buffer) solution, pH 7, under mild stirring conditions. Conventional electrochemical equipment was used [11]. All potentials were measured and are quoted against a saturated calomel electrode, SCE.

3 RESULTS AND DISCUSSION

Figure 1 shows cyclic voltammograms for the Pt/PP·GOD electrode immediately after the electrochemical deposition (——) and after glucose determinations at +0.7 V (- -) and +0.4 V (- · · -). The cyclic voltammogram for the as-deposited film was slightly different from those previously reported for the $PP \cdot Cl^-$ electrode [14] indicating that GOD incorporation had some effect on the cyclic voltammogram. Effectively a well-defined wave is now observed at -0.45 V when GOD is present. However, cyclic voltammograms recorded for PP·GOD films deposited with various amounts of GOD (100, 500 and 1000 U/mL) in the deposition solution were similar. On the other hand, an increase of the ratio of the areas under the two redox waves (-0.1V vs -0.45 V) is noticed as the thickness of the PP·GOD is increased but the area under the redox wave at -0.45 V remained constant for films of 150 and 320 mC/cm^2 of charge. Upon the application of +0.7 V to the Pt/PP·GOD electrode, the large initial background current, resulting from PP electrooxidation, decayed rapidly in the first min and then slowly reached a constant value after 1 hr. Subsequently, 20 mM glucose was added and an anodic current of 14 nA was recorded. This data point is shown in Figure 2 (—●—, at 0.7 V) where the amperometric response of the Pt/PP·GOD electrode is given as a function of potential. The data points represented as circles in Figure 2 correspond to the first glucose assay carried out at the given potential with an electrode. Following the glucose determination at 0.7 V, the electroactivity of PP was unexpectedly lost (Figure 1, - - -). The surprising result here is the fact that subsequent glucose determination gave a reproducible response despite the lack of electroactivity of PP. In addition, glucose determination was performed with the same electrode at +0.4 V. At this potential H_2O_2 oxidation is thermodynamically possible [15] and indeed the Pt/PP·GOD electrode shows a response of 12 nA (Figure 2, —■— at 0.4 V).

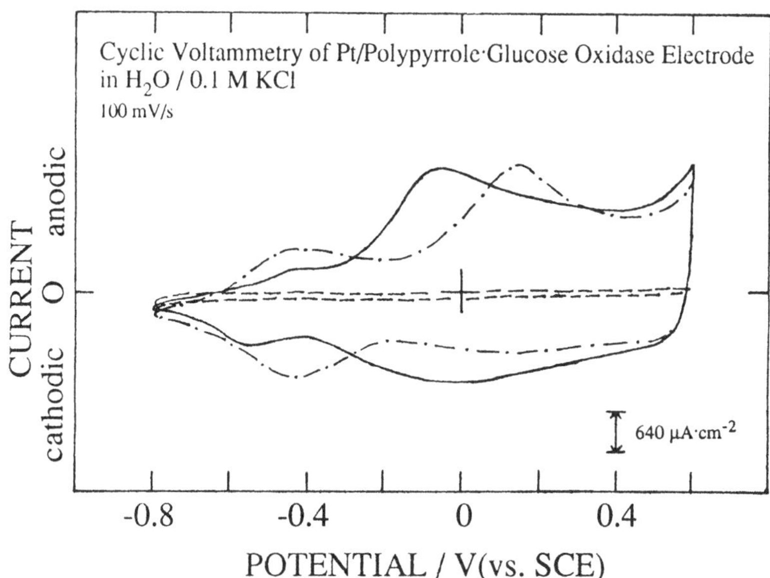

FIGURE 1 Cyclic voltammograms for a Pt/polypyrrole·glucose oxidase electrode in 0.1 M KCl; for the as-deposited film (———) after a glucose determination at +0.4 V (- · · -) and +0.7 V vs SCE (- - -) . Scan rate = 100 mV/s.

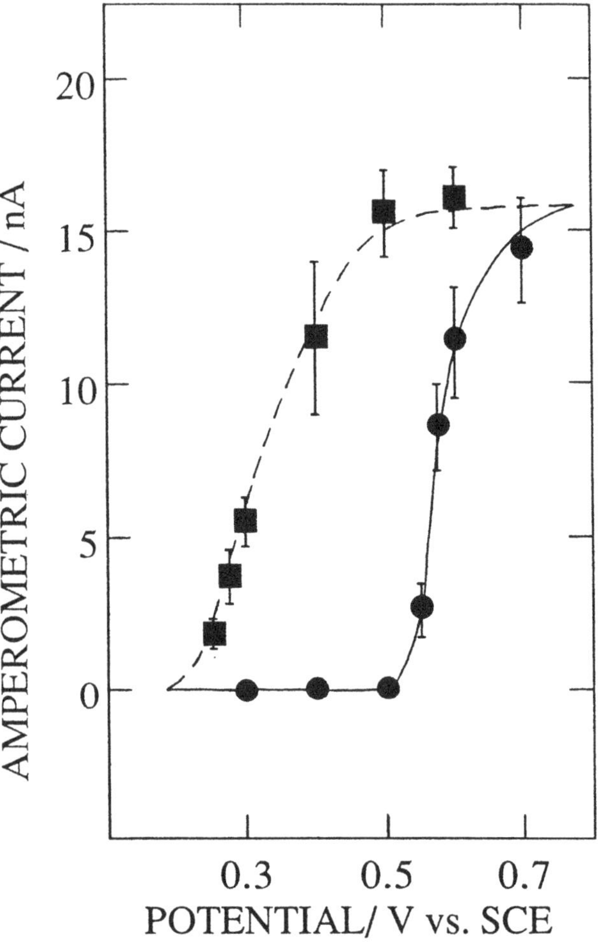

FIGURE 2 Amperometric response of a Pt/PP·GOD electrode to 20 mM glucose solution as a function of applied potential. Electrolyte: pH 7, 0.1M phosphate buffer. Initial amperometric responses (—●—) and responses after electrochemical or chemical oxidation of PP (–■–). (From Ref. 11.)

It is well known that massive oxidation of a PP film will produce an insultating film, which completely inhibits the occurence of PP redox reactions [16]. In an effort to circumvent the loss of electroactivity, the glucose determination was initially performed with a second electrode at the lower potential of + 0.4 V since at this potential overoxidation of PP is less marked. No response to a 20 mM glucose solution was noted at +0.4 V for this electrode (Figure 2, —●— at 0.4 V). Furthermore, after transferring the electrode in 0.1 M aqueous KCl, PP electroactivity was still clearly observed (Figure 1, - · · -). The cyclic voltammogram exhibited a shift of the main anodic wave from -0.1 V to +0.15 V and the growth of the redox wave at ca. -0.45 V. These modifications of the cyclic voltammogram are related to irreversible oxidation of PP and are attributed to a decrease of conjugation length [17]. Irreversible oxidation occured when the enzyme electrode was potentiostated at 0.4 V for 90 min prior to the glucose assay. Cyclic voltammogram of PP doped with immobile dopants such as sulfonate groups of Nafion shows a redox wave that is shifted to negative potential in comparaison to Cl^- doped PP [14,18]. Accordingly, the growth of the wave at -0.45 V is tentatively attributed to PP that became charge compensated with immobile irreversibly oxidized PP units. The results of the experiments described above suggest that the redox electroactivity of a Pt/PP·GOD electrode and its ability to detect glucose are closely interrelated. In order to confirm this statement, the second electrode was then used for a glucose determination at +0.7 V and an amperometric response of 14 nA was recorded for a 20 mM glucose solution. It is also important to note that a cyclic voltammogram of this electrode did not show any PP electroactivity and is similar to the one depicted in Figure 1 (dashed curve). These findings clearly demonstrate that a response to glucose was observed only when PP is not electroactive and demonstrate that PP is only an inert support for GOD. The lack of response to glucose when the analysis is initially performed at +0.4 V is related to the fact that enzymatically-produced H_2O_2 is irreversibly oxidizing the PP film rather than being detected at the platinum electrode. Chemical oxidation of PP by H_2O_2 was confirmed as PP electroactivity was lost when a Pt/PP·GOD electrode was immersed in 10 mM H_2O_2 for 5 min. When this electrode was again used for a glucose assay at 0.4 V, it effectively generated an amperometric response (Figure 2, —■— at 0.4 V).

The data of Figure 2 can be also obtained with one electrode for which glucose assays were carried out from 0.2 to 0.7 V (—●—) and subsequently back to 0.2 V

(—■—). As noticed above no amperometric response is generated at 0.4 V and for potentials lower than 0.5 V. On the other hand, when the Pt/PP·GOD electrode was completely oxidized, either chemically with H_2O_2 or electrochemically, the current-voltage curve is that expected (—■—) for the oxidation of H_2O_2 at a platinum electrode [15].

Experiments are now in progress in our laboratory to determine if other conducting polymers e.g. poly-N-methylpyrrole, behave similarly to polypyrrole in glucose oxidase-based enzyme electrode.

REFERENCES

1. Degani, Y. and Heller, A. (1987). Direct electrical communication between chemically modified enzymes and metal electrodes. 1. Electron transfer from glucose oxidase to metal electrodes via electron relays, bound covalently to the enzyme. J. Phys. Chem., **91,** 1285-89.
2. Degani, Y. and Heller, A. (1988). Direct electrical communication between chemically modified enzymes and metal electrodes. 2. Methods for bonding electron-transfer relays to glucose oxidase and D-amino-acid oxidase. J. Am. Chem. Soc., **110**, 2615-20.
3. Bartlett, P.N., Whitaker, R.G., Green, M.J. and Frew, J.J. (1987). Covalent binding of electron relays to glucose oxidase. J. Chem. Soc., Chem. Commun., 1603-4.
4. Hale, P.D., Inagaki, T., Karan, H.I., Okamoto Y. and Skotheim, T.A. (1989). A new class of amperometric biosensor incorporating a polymeric electron-transfer mediator. J. Am. Chem. Soc., **111**, 3482-84.
5. Degani, Y. and Heller, A. (1989). Electrical communication between redox centers of glucose oxidase and electrodes via electrostatically and covalently bound redox polymers. J. Am. Chem. Soc., 111, 2357-8.
6. Yabuki, S.-i., Shinohara, H. and Aizawa, M., (1989). Electro-conductive enzyme membrane. J. Chem. Soc., Chem. Commun., 945-946.
7. Foulds, N.C. and Lowe, C.R. (1986). Enzyme entrapment in electrically conducting polymers. Immobilisation of glucose oxidase in polypyrrole and its application in amperometric glucose sensors. J. Chem. Soc., Faraday Trans. 1, **82**, 1259-64.
8. Umaña, M. and Waller, J. (1986). Protein-modified electrodes. Glucose oxidase/polypyrrole system. Anal. Chem., **58**, 2979-83.

9. Fortier, G., Brassard, E. and Bélanger, D. (1988). Fast and easy preparation of an amperometric glucose biosensor. Biotechnol. Tech.,**3**, 177-182.

10. Bélanger, D., Brassard, E. and Fortier, G. (1989). Incorporation of platinum microparticles into a polypyrrole glucose oxidase electrode: Enhancement of the glucose response. Anal. Chem. Acta, in press.

11. Bélanger, D., Nadreau, J. and Fortier, G. (1989). Electrochemistry of polypyrrole glucose oxidase electrode. J. Electroanal. Chem., in press.

12. Bartlett, P.N. and Whitaker, R.G. (1987/88). Strategies for the development of amperometric enzyme electrodes. Biosensors,**3**, 359-379.

13. Bartlett, P.N. and Whitaker, R.G. (1987). Electrochemical immobilisation of enzymes. Part II. Glucose oxidase immobilised in poly-N-methylpyrrole. J. Electroanal. Chem., **224**, 37-48.

14. Hirai, T., Kuwabata, S. and Yoneyama, H. (1988). Electrochemical behaviors of polypyrrole, poly-3-methylthiophene, and polyaniline deposited on Nafion-coated electrodes. J. Electrochem. Soc., **135**, 1132-37.

15. Guilbault, G.G. and Lubrano, G.L. (1973). An enzyme electrode for the amperometric determination of glucose. Anal. Chim. Acta, **64**, 439-55.

16. Asavapiriyanont, S., Chandler, G.K., Gunawardena, G.A. and Pletcher, D. (1984). The electrodeposition of polypyrrole films from aqueous solutions. J. Electroanal. Chem., **177**, 229-244.

17. Olmedo, L., Chanteloube, I., Germain, A., Petit, M. and Geniès, E.M. (1989). Characterization of electrochemically prepared conductive polymers by in situ conductivity measurements. Synth. Met., **28**, 165-170.

18. Bidan, G., Ehui , B. and Lapkowski, M. (1988). Conductive polymers with immobilised dopants: ionomer composites and auto-doped polymers- a review and recent advances. J. Phys. D: Appl. Phys., **21**, 1043-54.

13

Amperometric Glucose Sensor Fabricated from Glucose Oxidase and a Mediator Coimmobilized on a Colloidal Gold Hydrogel Electrode

A. L. CRUMBLISS, R. W. HENKENS, S. C. PERINE, and K. R. TUBERGEN, Department of Chemistry, Duke University, Durham, NC 27706

B. S. KITCHELL and J. STONEHUERNER, Enzyme Technology Research Group, 710 W. Main Street, Durham, NC 27701

INTRODUCTION

An amperometric sensor capable of detecting glucose without the addition of exogeneous reagents has application in the hospital, laboratory, and home health care markets. There has been significant recent activity in the development of glucose oxidase (GOD) based electrodes for use in amperometric glucose sensors which can be used in various media, including whole blood. By coupling the redox activity of GOD directly to an electrode surface it is possible in principle to develop an electrode which responds to glucose concentration without interference from O_2 [1-4]. This approach requires the use of a low molecular weight mediator to act as an electron shuttle between GOD and the electrode surface. Ferrocene and its derivatives have been used as mediators for GOD [1,5,6].

Various methods have been developed to immobilize GOD and/or ferrocene at an electrode surface. Hill and coworkers have immobilized GOD through covalent attachment to an oxidized graphite surface [1]. Other groups have used entrapment in a polypyrrole film formed on an electrode surface to immobilize GOD [7,8]. Ferrocene mediators have been immobilized by two approaches. One approach involves immobilizing the ferrocene directly on the electrode surface. This has been accomplished either by entrapment of a water insoluble ferrocene in a membrane at a graphite electrode [1] or by electrodeposition of a ferrocene modified pyrrole onto a platinum electrode [8]. A second approach involves covalently binding a substituted ferrocene mediator directly to GOD [9,10].

We are currently developing an alternate approach to the preparation of an electrode based on immobilized GOD and a substituted ferrocene mediator. In designing this electrode, we have exploited the immobilization properties of colloidal gold and carrageenan hydrogel. Colloidal gold has been used extensively as a marker for electron microscopy because macromolecules adsorbed to the gold surface retain bioactivity [11-15]. Carrageenan hydrogel, an anionic polysaccharide, has been used to immobilize enzymes and microbial cells with retention of bioactivity [16].

The electrode described in this work utilizes a ferrocene mediator immobilized at the surface in a carrageenan hydrogel matrix and GOD immobilized on colloidal gold particles deposited on the electrode. This sensor electrode is a self-contained unit capable of functioning without the addition of external reagents.

EXPERIMENTAL

Fabrication of electrodes: Electrode A. A colloidal gold sol (average particle size 50 nm) [17] was added to a solution of GOD (0.17 mg/mL; Sigma Type X-S) in 0.01 M sodium citrate, pH 5.0. Bovine serum albumin (BSA) (0.10 mg/mL) was added immediately to stabilize the sol, which was then centrifuged 30 min. at 4^0C at 7 x 10^3 xg. The supernatant was removed and the pellet resuspended in 1.7 x 10^{-3} M sodium citrate, pH 6.7, and the process of centrifugation/resuspension repeated until the GOD activity of the supernatant was negligible. The

GOD/BSA/Au sol was then electrodeposited [18] onto a 52 mesh platinum gauze 1.2 x 1.9 cm. The electrode was rinsed with 2×10^{-3} M sodium phosphate and stored in this buffer at 4^{0}C.

Electrode B. A GOD/BSA/Au sol was prepared as described above and electrodeposited onto a 1.2 x 1.9 cm 52 mesh platinum gauze. This electrode was then coated with a 1.5% solution of glyoxyl (aldehyde derivatized) carrageenan (FMC Corp.) and the gel hardened 30 min in 0.1 M KNO_3. The hardened gel was reacted 89 hr. at 4^{0}C with 8×10^{-3} M ferrocenylmethylamine and 2.7×10^{-2} M $NaBH_3CN$ in 0.05 M sodium phosphate, pH 7.5, 0.1 M KNO_3 and stored as described above.

Electrode enzyme activity assay. 2,2'-Azino-bis(3-ethylbenz-thiazoline-6-sulfonic acid) diammonium salt (ABTS, Sigma) was substituted for o-dianisidine [19] as the chromophore in a GOD activity assay [20] which employs a coupled enzyme assay to measure the amount of H_2O_2 produced by the GOD catalyzed oxidation of glucose. The electrode was agitated for varying lengths of time in 2 mL 0.089 M glucose (Sigma) in 0.05 M sodium acetate, pH 5.1. At the end of the measured time interval, typically 2 to 10 min., the electrode was removed and the glucose solution mixed with an equal volume of 6.9×10^{-4} M ABTS and 2 units/mL horseradish peroxidase in the same buffer. After 5 min. at room temperature the absorbance was measured at 420 nm. One unit of GOD is defined as the amount of enzyme required to catalyze the oxidation of one μmole glucose per minute.

Electrochemical measurements. Electrochemical measurements were made with a 3-electrode (Ag/AgCl reference; A or B working; Pt wire counter) cell using normal cyclic voltammetric techniques. Sample solutions containing 0.02 M potassium phosphate (pH 7.5), 0.05 M potassium nitrate, 0.05 M sodium perchlorate and 0-50 mM glucose (and in the case of Electrode A 30 μm ferrocenylmethyl-trimethylammonium nitrate) were purged 20 min with Ar prior to measurement. All potentials are reported relative to the Ag/AgCl reference electrode.

RESULTS AND DISCUSSION

The two types of electrodes prepared in this study are designed to generate a current proportional to glucose concentration. The first (Electrode A) contains GOD adsorbed onto a colloidal gold sol which is deposited on a platinum gauze electrode. The second (Electrode B) contains similarly immobilized GOD, but in addition has a carrageenan hydrogel coating to which a substituted ferrocene mediator has been covalently attached.

Quantitative measurements of enzymatic and electrochemical activity have confirmed that colloidal gold provides a biocompatible surface suitable for immobilizing active enzymes. For example, Electrode A was found to have a total enzymatic activity of 0.069 units when freshly prepared. After use in electrochemical experiments and storage for 3 weeks at $4^{0}C$ in 2×10^{-3} M sodium phosphate (pH 7) the electrode retained over 60% of its original catalytic activity.

When Electrode A was placed in aqueous pH 7.8 buffer containing 30 μM $[Fe(Cp)(CpX)]NO_3$ ($X=-CH_2N(CH_3)_3$) a cyclic voltammogram was obtained characteristic of a reversible $Fe(Cp)(CpX)/Fe(Cp)(CpX)^+$ couple: $E_{1/2}$ = + 413 mV; ΔEpp = 55 mV (see Figure 1a). Similar observations were made for Electrode B. When placed in background electrolyte (no dissolved redox couple) the Fe(Cp)(CpX) ($X=CH_2NH_2$) covalently attached to the carrageenan hydrogel film on Electrode B exhibited a reversible redox couple: $E_{1/2}$ = +343 mV; ΔEpp = 105 mV.

When glucose was added to the solution used to obtain the cyclic voltammogram shown in Figure 1a for Electrode A, a catalytic current/voltage plot was observed (Figure 1b) which is diagnostic of a coupled electrocatalytic system [21]. Equations (1)-(3) describe the reaction sequence at the electrode surface for an electrocatalytic process capable of generating a current which is proportional to glucose concentration (GOD_O and GOD_R represent tne oxidized and reduced forms of glucose oxidase, respectively, and $FeCp_2$ represents ferrocene or one of its

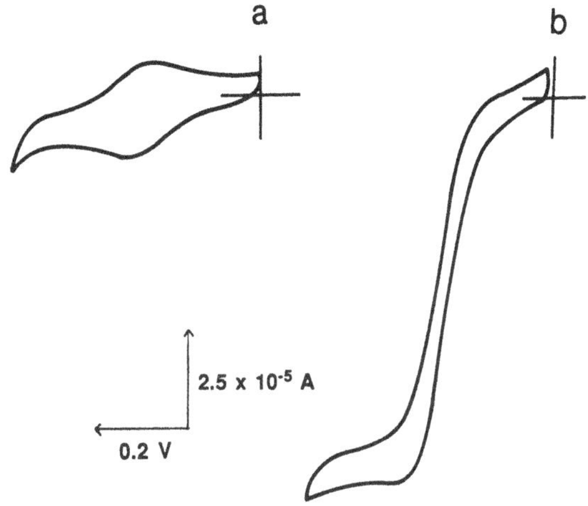

Figure 1. Cyclic voltammograms obtained with Electrode A in the absence (a) and presence (b) of glucose. Conditions: **a** $[(Fe(Cp)(Cp\text{-}CH_2N(CH_3)_3))NO_3]$ = 30 μM; background electrolyte = 0.02 M potassium phosphate buffer, 0.05 M $NaClO_4$, 0.05 M KNO_3, pH = 7.8; scan rate = 2 mV/s. **b** Same as a with [glucose] = 15 mM; scan rate = 2 mV/s.

cyclopentadienyl ring derivatives).

$$2FeCp_2 \xrightarrow[-2e^-]{\text{electrode}} 2FeCp_2^+ \quad (1)$$

$$2FeCp_2^+ + GOD_R \longrightarrow 2FeCp_2 + GOD_O \quad (2)$$

$$GOD_O + \text{glucose} \longrightarrow GOD_R + \text{gluconic acid} \quad (3)$$

Catalytic currents for Electrodes A and B were found to vary with glucose concentration and therefore demonstrate the applicability of the electrode to a glucose sensor. Figure 2 is a

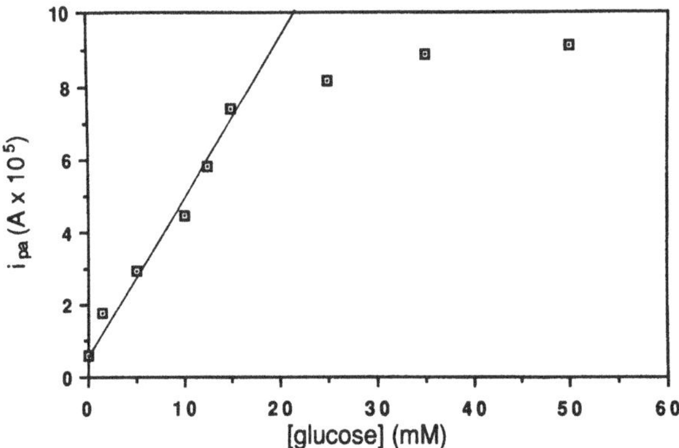

Figure 2. Catalytic peak current at 490 mV plotted as a function of glucose concentration obtained using Electrode A. Conditions: as described in Figure 1b.

graph of catalytic peak current measured at 490 mV plotted as a function of glucose concentration for Electrode A. Electrode response is rapid and linear up to a glucose concentration of approximately 20 mM. This represents an excellent electrochemical basis for an operative glucose sensor based on immobilized GOD which has a rapid response over a glucose concentration range of biological relevance.

Acknowledgements. This research was supported by DOE contract DE-AC01-86ER80351, NSF grant ISI 87-60921 and the North Carolina Biotechnology Center.

REFERENCES

1. A. E. G. Cass, G. Davis, G. D. Francis, H. A. O. Hill, W. J. Aston, I. J. Higgins, E. V. Plotkin, L. D. L. Scott, and A. P. F. Turner, Anal. Chem., **56**, 667 (1984).

2. J. E. Frew, and H. A. O. Hill, Eur. J. Biochem., **172**, 261 (1988).
3. J. E. Frew, and H. A. O. Hill, Anal. Chem., **59**, 933A (1987).
4. H. A. O. Hill, Pure Appl. Chem., **59**, 743 (1987).
5. B. W. Rockett, and G. Mar, J. Organomet. Chem., **357**, 247 (1988).
6. A. E. G. Cass, G. Davis, M. J. Green, and H. A. O. Hill, J. Electroanal. Chem., **190**, 117 (1985).
7. M. Umaña, and J. Waller, J., Anal. Chem., **58**, 2979 (1986).
8. N. C. Foulds, and C. R. Lowe, Anal. Chem., **60**, 2473 (1988).
9. Y. Degani, and A. Heller, J. Phys. Chem., **91**, 1285 (1987).
10. P. N. Bartlett, R. G. Whitaker, M. J. Green, and J. Frew, J. Chem. Soc. Chem. Commun., 1603 (1987).
11. M. Horisberger, TIBS, **8**, 395 (1983).
12. M. Horisberger, and J. Rosset, J. Histochem. Cytochem., **25**, 295 (1987).
13. W. D. Geoghegan, and G. A. Ackermen, J. Histochem. Cytochem., **25**, 1187 (1987).
14. M. Horisberger, Scanning Electron Microscopy, **2**, 9 (1981).
15. R. W. Henkens, B. S. Kitchell, J. P. O'Daly, S. C. Perine, and A. L. Crumbliss, Recl. Trav. Chim. Pays Bas, **106**, 298 (1987).
16. T. Tosa, T. Sato, T. Mori, K. Yamamoto, I. Takata, Y. Nishida, and I. Chibata, Biotech. Bioeng., **21** 1697 (1979).
17. G. Frens, Nature, **241**, 20 (1973).
18. A. R. Despic, and M. G. Pavlovic, J. Electroanal. Chem., **180**, 31 (1984).
19. W. Werner, H. G. Rey, and H. Wielinger, Z. Anal. Chem., **252**, 224 (1970).
20. Sigma Chemical Co. Data Sheet No. G-7141 (April, 1984).
21. R. S. Nicholson, and I. Shain, Anal. Chem., **36**,706 (1964).

14

Amperometric Biosensors for Glucose, Lactate, and Glycolate Based on Oxidases and Redox-Modified Siloxane Polymers

PAUL D. HALE, TORU INAGAKI, HUNG SUI LEE and TERJE A. SKOTHEIM
Department of Applied Science, Division of Materials Science, Brookhaven National Laboratory, Upton, New York

HIROKO I. KARAN Division of Natural Science and Mathematics, Medgar Evers College, City University of New York, Brooklyn, New York

YOSHI OKAMOTO Department of Chemistry, Polytechnic University, Brooklyn, New York

1 INTRODUCTION

Amperometric biosensors based on flavin-containing oxidases undergo several steps which produce a measurable current that is related to the concentration of substrate. In the initial step, the substrate converts the oxidized flavin adenine dinucleotide (FAD) or flavin mononucleotide (FMN) into the reduced form ($FADH_2$ or $FMNH_2$). Because these cofactors are located well within the enzyme molecule, direct electron transfer to the surface of a conventional electrode does not occur to a measurable degree. A common method of facilitating this electron transfer is to introduce oxygen into the system because it is the natural acceptor for the oxidases; the oxygen is reduced by the $FADH_2$ or $FMNH_2$ to hydrogen peroxide, which can then be detected electrochemically. The major drawback to this approach is the fact that oxidation of hydrogen peroxide requires a large overpotential, thus making these sensors susceptible to interference from electroactive species. In order to lower the necessary applied potential, several non-physiological redox couples have been employed to shuttle electrons between the flavin moieties and the electrode. For example, sensors based on the ferrocene/ferricinium redox couple [1,2] and on electrodes consisting of conducting salts such as TTF-TCNQ (tetrathiafulvalene-tetracyanoquinodimethane) [3,4] have previously been reported. Electron relays have also been attached directly to the enzyme molecule in order to facilitate electron transfer [5,6]. More recently, these studies have been extended to include systems where the mediating redox species are covalently attached to polymers such as poly(pyrrole) [7], poly(vinylpyridine) [8], and poly(siloxane) [9]. The present paper describes the development of amperometric biosensors based on flavin-containing enzymes and this latter family of polymeric mediators.

2 REDOX-MODIFIED SILOXANE POLYMERS

The ferrocene-modified poly(siloxane) relay systems are shown schematically in Figure 1. Although these materials are insoluble in water, their high degree of flexibility allows the ferrocene moieties to achieve close contact with the flavin centers of the enzyme, and thus serve as efficient electron transfer mediators from the reduced enzyme to the electrode. The homopolymer is comprised of approximately 35 subunits ($m=35$, $n=0$), with each containing a bound ferrocene moiety. In the copolymers, m:n ratios of approximately 1:1 and 1:2 were used, and the polymer subunits were randomly distributed (i.e. random block copolymers). Steps were taken to ensure that no low molecular weight species (which could act as freely diffusing electron transfer mediators) were present. Thin layer chromatography and high-performance liquid chromatography showed that no oligomeric materials were present in the purified materials.

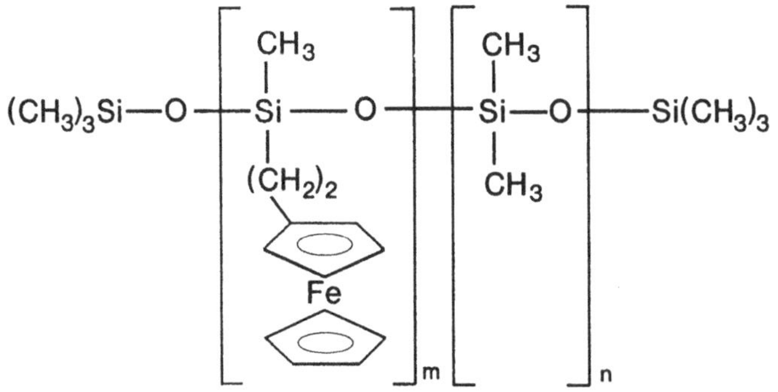

FIGURE 1 Schematic diagram of the ferrocene-modified siloxane polymers used as electron relay systems in oxidase-based amperometric sensors.

3 GLYCOLATE BIOSENSORS

Modified carbon paste for the glycolate sensors was made by thoroughly mixing 50mg of graphite powder with a measured amount of the ferrocene-containing polymer (the latter was first dissolved in chloroform), resulting in approximately 45μmole of ferrocene per gram of graphite powder. After evaporation of the solvent, 5mg of glycolate oxidase (3.8 units/mg) and 10μl of paraffin oil were added, and the resulting mixture was blended into a paste. The paste was packed into a 1.0ml plastic syringe which had previously been partially filled with unmodified carbon paste, leaving approximately a 2mm deep well at the base of the syringe. The resulting surface area of the electrode was 0.025cm^2. Electrical contact was achieved by inserting a silver wire into the top of the carbon paste. The mediating ability of the ferrocene-modified siloxane polymers can be seen in Figure 2, which shows cyclic voltammograms for the glycolate biosensors in pH 8.0 phosphate buffer solution before and after addition of glycolate.

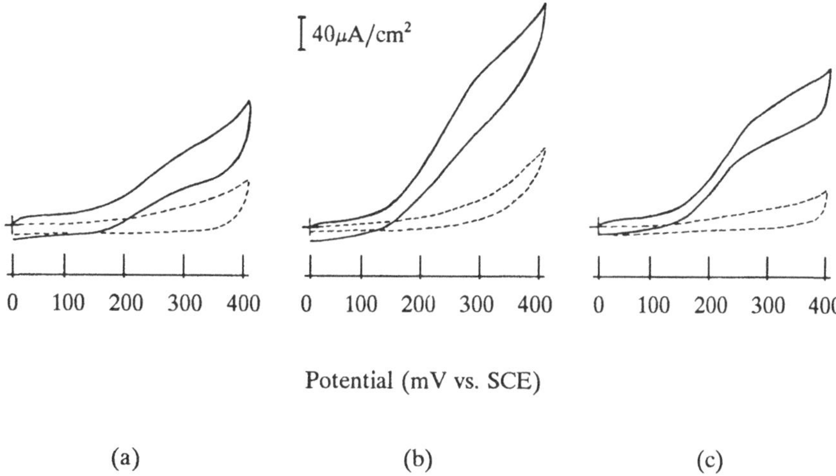

FIGURE 2 Cyclic voltammograms for the ferrocene-modified polysiloxane/glycolate oxidase/carbon paste electrodes (scan rate: 5mV/s) in pH 8.0 phosphate buffer (with 0.1M KCl) solution with no glycolate present (dashed line) and in the presence of 0.1M sodium glycolate (solid line). The electrode in (a) contained the ferrocene-modified homopolymer, while those in (b) and (c) contained the copolymers with m:n ratios of 1:1 and 1:2, respectively.

Calibration curves are shown in Figure 3 for glycolate biosensors containing the ferrocene-modified siloxane homopolymer, the 1:1 copolymer, and the 1:2 copolymer. As in the cyclic voltammetry experiments, the three polymeric relay systems display similar electron transfer mediation characteristics. The apparent Michaelis-Menten constants (K_M) for the sensors may be determined from electrochemical Eadie-Hofstee plots; K_M values range from 2 to 5mM for these sensors.

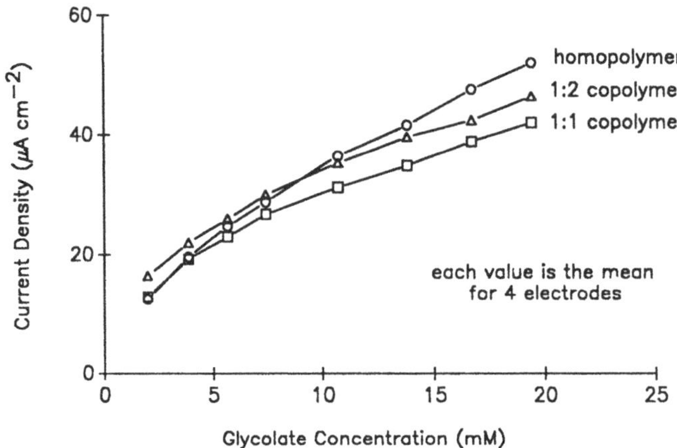

FIGURE 3 Calibration curves for the ferrocene-modified poly(siloxane)/glycolate oxidase/carbon paste electrodes at E=300mV (vs. SCE).

4 GLUCOSE BIOSENSORS: STABILITY OF THE RESPONSE

Previous studies [9] have demonstrated that these ferrocene-modified siloxane polymers work very well as electron relay systems in glucose oxidase-based biosensors. Because the relays are not free to diffuse out of the device, the sensors maintain a response to glucose over long periods of time. Figure 4 shows typical glucose calibration curves for a carbon paste electrode containing the ferrocene-modified siloxane homopolymer and glucose oxidase after storage in pH 7 phosphate buffer solution. Even after one year the sensor displays an adequate response to the addition of glucose. The decrease in response over time is most likely due to loss of enzyme into the storage solution; a simple enzyme immobilization (e.g. cross-linking) would further improve the long-term stability.

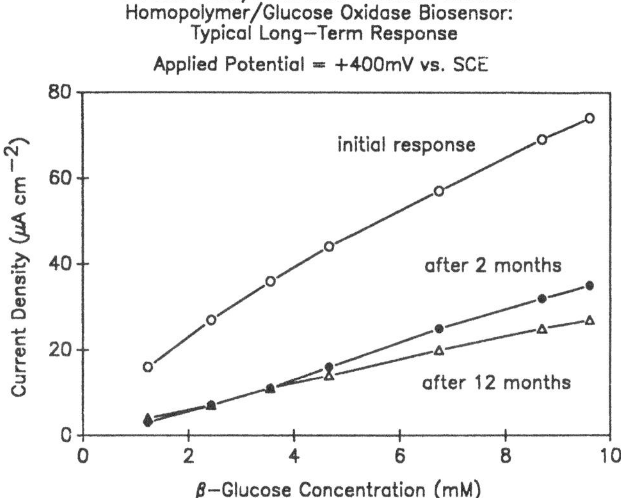

FIGURE 4 Typical glucose calibration curves for the ferrocene-modified siloxane homopolymer/glucose oxidase/carbon paste electrode after storage in pH 7 buffer.

5 LACTATE BIOSENSORS

Preliminary studies indicate that the poly(siloxane) relay systems can efficiently mediate the electron transfer from both lactate oxidase and lactate monooxygenase to a carbon paste electrode. A typical lactate calibration curve is shown in Figure 5 for a carbon paste electrode containing a dimethylferrocene-modified siloxane polymer (m:n ratio of 1:2) and lactate monooxygenase. The use of dimethylferrocene as the polymer-bound mediator allows this sensor to be operated efficiently at lower applied potential values than the sensors described above. The lactate sensors were constructed in a manner similar to the glycolate sensors described in Section 3. The constant potential experiment in Figure 5 was performed in a pH 7.0 phosphate buffer solution containing 0.1M KCl, which was deaerated by N_2 bubbling for 10min. Work is presently underway to better characterize the lactate biosensors based on the poly(siloxane) relay systems and both lactate monooxygenase and lactate oxidase.

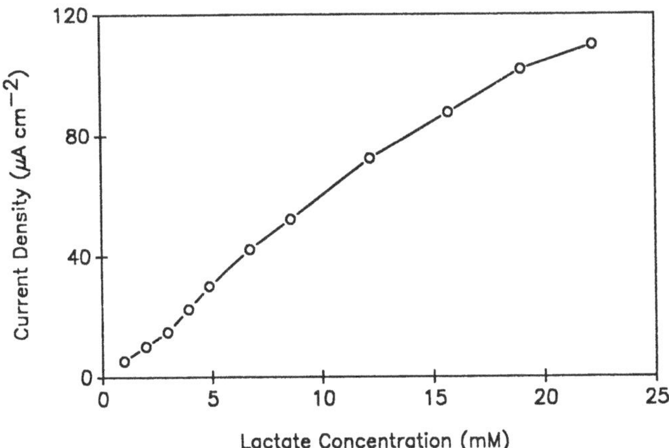

FIGURE 5 Typical lactate calibration curve for the dimethylferrocene-modified siloxane (1:2) copolymer/lactate monooxygenase/carbon paste electrode (E=200mV vs. SCE).

ACKNOWLEDGMENT

This research has been sponsored by the U.S. Department of Energy, Division of Materials Science, Office of Basic Energy Science (DE-AC02-76CH00016).

REFERENCES

1. A.E.G. Cass, G. Davis, G.D. Francis, H.A.O. Hill, W.J. Aston, I.J. Higgins, E.V. Plotkin, L.D.L. Scott and A.P.F. Turner, Anal. Chem., 56, 667 (1984).
2. J.M. Dicks, W.J. Aston, G. Davis and A.P.F. Turner, Anal. Chim. Acta, 182, 103 (1986).
3. W.J. Albery, P.N. Bartlett and D.H. Craston, J. Electroanal. Chem., 194, 223 (1985).
4. P.D. Hale and R.M. Wightman, Mol. Cryst. Liq. Cryst., 160, 269 (1988).
5. Y. Degani and A. Heller, J. Phys. Chem., 91, 1285 (1987).
6. Y. Degani and A. Heller, J. Am. Chem. Soc., 110, 2615 (1988).
7. N.C. Foulds and C.R. Lowe, Anal. Chem., 60, 2473 (1988).
8. Y. Degani and A. Heller, J. Am. Chem. Soc., 111, 2357 (1989).
9. P.D. Hale, T. Inagaki, H.I. Karan, Y. Okamoto and T.A. Skotheim, J. Am. Chem. Soc., 111, 3482 (1989).

15

Transition Metal Encapsulation by "Metallocrown" Ethers

MYOUNG SOO LAH and VINCENT L. PECORARO Department of Chemistry, University of Michigan Ann Arbor, MI 48109-1055

MARTIN L. KIRK and WILLIAM E. HATFIELD Department of Chemistry, University of North Carolina Chapel Hill, NC 27599-2390

Organic molecules designed to bind cations selectively have been important components of metal ion detection systems. The crown ethers and derivatives (1-3), the paradigm of this molecular class, include ether oxygens as metal donor atoms and confer enhanced specificity by tailoring the cavity of the ligand to the optimal size and coordination number of the cation to be sequestered. The primary targets of crown ethers are mono and divalent alkali and alkaline earth cations and trivalent lanthanide ions. Crown ether complexes of transition metal ions are very rare, presumably because the donor capacity of a neutral oxygen atom to a transition metal atom is poor. Furthermore, while crown ethers are selective cation coordination compounds, they are not well suited for anion binding. In this contribution we provide an entry into a possible new class of sequestration agents called metallocrown ethers. These novel clusters are conceptually related to 9-crown-3 and 12-crown-4. A ring structure of ethereal like oxygen atoms are linked by two atom bridges of nitrogen and transition metal ions. This distinction leads to altered metal binding character and may provide an entry into selective anion detection agents.

The concept of metallocrowns arises from a marriage of synthetic inorganic chemistry and microbial metal ion sequestration agents. The siderophores are a group of low molecular weight metal ion chelating agents that employ hydroxamate or catecholate moieties to sequester and transport ferric ion into bacterial cells (4). This suggests a biomimetic approach to trivalent transition metal binding using phenolate, catecholate and hydroxamate ligands (5). Indeed, such specificity has been exploited in iron decorporation therapy in the treatment of β-thallesemia (6). One might expect metal selectivity using a ligand, such as salicylhydroxamic acid shown below, that contains two of these functional groups. Furthermore, salicylhydroxamic acid is particularly interesting as three protonation states are available (7): the singly deprotonated hydroxamate (B), the doubly deprotonated hydroximate (C) and the triply deprotonated hydroximatophenolate (D). It is this last form which can be converted into a crown ether analogue.

A B C D

A demetalated metallocrown (8) is illustrated in the structure of $[V(V)=O(SHI)(CH_3OH)]_3$ {**1**, 9-$C_{(VO)N}$-3}. This vanadium cluster mimics the conformation of 9-C-3 by forming a 9 membered ring with an endo configuration of three ethereal oxygen atoms. While these oxygen atoms are joined by ethylene groups in the crowns, metallocrowns are constructed through M^{3+}-N linkages. In this case, the metal position is occupied by the complex ion, VO^{3+}. Naively, one might expect that the difference between metal heteroatom bonds (V-N= 2.02 Å; V-O= 1.86 Å) and typical carbon bonds (C-O= 1.35 Å; C-C= 1.45 Å) would lead to a significant alteration of the metal binding cavity. Yet, the cavity radii of 9-C-3 and 9-$C_{(VO)N}$-3 are 0.25 Å and 0.35 Å, respectively. This similarity is a result of the large changes in bond angles in the linking atom of the 9-C-3 and 9-$C_{(VO)N}$-3 molecules. Standard C-C-O and C-O-C angles are approximately tetrahedral (109.5°), while V-N-O, N-O-V and O-V-N angles are 120°, 118° and 86°, respectively.

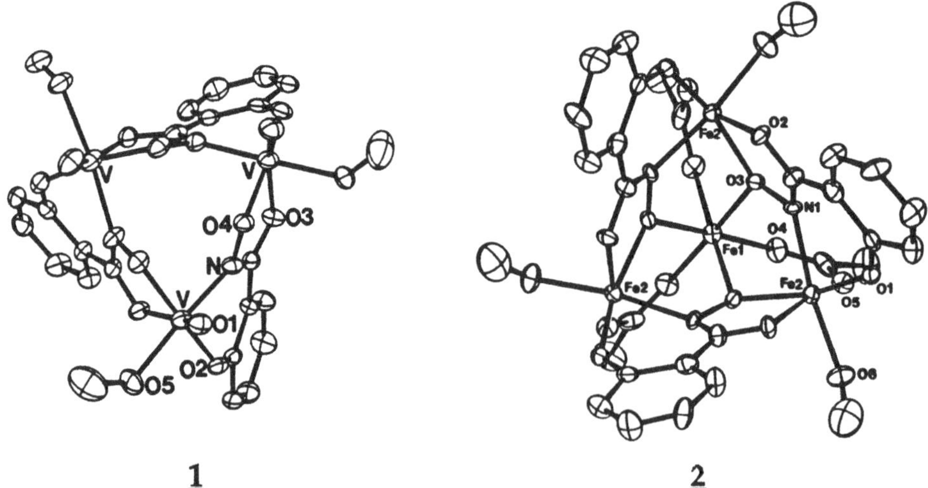

1 **2**

Although neither 9-C-3 nor 9-C_{VN}-3 have been shown to bind transition metal ions, a slight modification of the 9-$C_{M^{3+}N}$-3 assembly successfully leads to this result. The Fe(III)[Fe(III)(SHI)(OAc)(CH_3OH)]$_3$ {2, Fe(9-C_{FeN}-3)} differs from the 9-C_{VN}-3 in three significant ways (9). First, the three ethereal oxygen atoms form a facial chelate for a capping, octahedral, high spin Fe(III). Second, the remaining three coordination sites of this iron are filled by carboxylate oxygen atoms from bridges between the capping ion and the ring metal ions. The third difference is that the ring iron does not contain a terminal oxo group, leaving this coordination site available for the oxygen atom in the bridging acetate which stabilizes the capping iron(III). Note, however, that the cavity radius of 0.25 Å is identical to 9-C-3. In 2, we see the two advantages of the metallocrowns over their organic relatives. First, *the basicity difference between an ether oxygen and the coordinated oxime makes the latter a better ligand for hard transition metal anions.* Second, *the incorporation of ring metal ions leads to stabilization of transition ion coordination through bidentate bridging moieties.* Metal complexation by the 9-C-3 or 9-$C_{M^{3+}N}$-3 is too weak to be observed without such stabilization.

The metallocrowns are not limited to a 9-C-3 structure as demonstrated by [Fe(III)[Fe(III)(SHI)(μ_2-SO_4)$_{0.5}$(CH_3OH)$_{1.5}$]$_4$]$^-$ {3, Fe(12-C_{FeN}-4)} (10) which would be expected to be isostructural with M^{3+}(12-C-3) if such transition metal crowns could be prepared. The cavity radii of 3 and 12-C-4 are 0.6 Å. Once again, the difference in oxygen basicity between the metallocrowns and crowns and the ability to stabilize transition metal ions through bridging moieties leads to metal sequestration unprecedented in simple crown ether complexes. Furthermore, we now see *the potential for anion selectivity* as sulfate forms

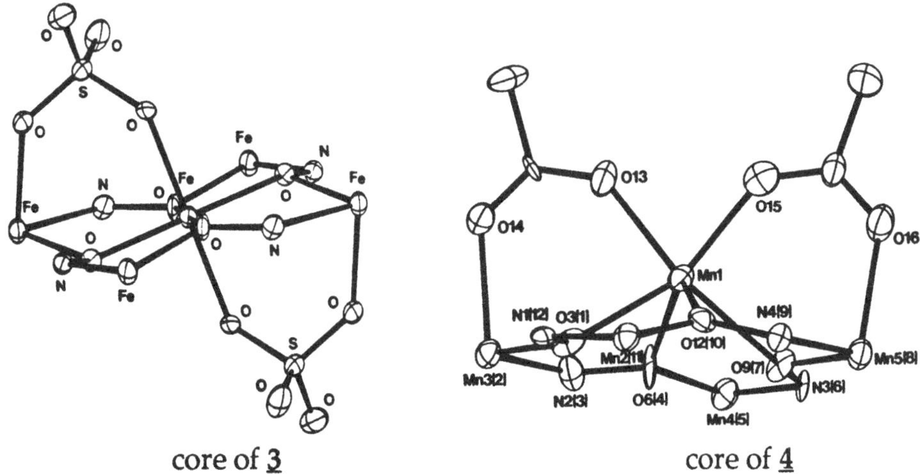

core of 3 core of 4

the bridge between ring and captured iron(III) atoms. We will discuss strategies to enhance this selectivity below.

As illustrated by $Mn(II)[Mn(III)(SHI)(OAc)_{0.5}(DMF)_{1.5}]_4$ {**4**, Mn(12-C_{MnN}-4)}, which contains Mn(II) in the capping position (11), transition metal encapsulation by metallocrowns can be extended to ions other than iron(III) . This mixed valent manganese pentamer adopts a 12-C-4 structure which is very similar to **3**. The ring structure is stabilized by four Mn(III) ions. The separation of metals in the rings are 4.85 Å (**3**) and 4.64 Å (**4**) and the cavity radii are 0.6 Å (**3**) and 0.5 Å (**4**). However, the Mn(II) coordination environment in **4** is distinct from the Fe(III) in **3**. Besides the obvious charge difference, the Mn(II) lies 1.2 Å above the best least squares plane of the four ring oxygen atoms while **3** is a centrosymmetric structure with the Fe(III) rigorously in this 4-atom plane. Two acetate anions form bridges from the Mn(II) to ring Mn(III), while sulfate dianions satisfy this requirement in the iron complex. Thus, **4** is neutral while **3** is an anion. In addition, the acetates of **4** are in a *syn* configuration (same face of crown ring) while the sulfates of **3** are in an *anti* orientation (opposite faces of crown).

The behavior of **3** and **4** is reminiscent of metalloporphyrin compounds where, depending on the size and spin state of the metal, one can see significant displacements of the bound ion from the porphyrin ring. The size restriction imparted by the metallocrown ring structure may lead to selective metal sequestration. For example, we would expect that Mn(II) could be displaced from the core of **4** by Fe(III) in the presence of sulfate leading to a mixed metal metallocrown of structure $Fe(III)[Mn(III)(SHI)(\mu_2\text{-}SO_4)_{0.5}(DMF)_{1.5}]_4$. With the ability to prepare mixed metal metallocrowns, the possibility of selective anion sensors becomes more attainable. Specificity for salicylate has been reported with Sn(IV) porphyrins (12). The metallocrowns have the potential for similar anion binding interactions. Additionally, anion selectivity may be achieved by a combination of parameters that include ring and capping metal type, anion charge and denticity, and metallocrown ring size. We have observed that acetate and sulfate have much greater affinities for the metallocrowns than trifluoro- or trichloroacetates. We are presently examining the association of other anions such as phosphate.

Because of the large number of transition metal ions in these compounds, the metallocrowns have a number of physical properties that distinguish them from organic crowns. Complex **1** is a deep blue, **2** and **3** are reddish and **4** is green-brown. Many are electroactive, For example, a quasi-reversible one electron reduction of the capping Fe(III) in **2** is observed in DMF at -330 mV vs SCE. Thus, direct electrochemical or spectrophotometric detection of coordinated ions are possible. The magnetic properties of these materials are also extraordinary. Magnetization measurements on solid samples of **2** were made at 4.2 K in fields up to 15 kOe. These data strongly suggest the presence of an S=5 ground state. Variable temperature magnetic susceptibility data were collected at 1 kOe in a region where the magnetization varied linearly with the applied field. The data indicate both intra- and inter cluster antiferromagnetism. Analysis using Heisenberg exchange theory gave best fit values g=2 (fixed), J_1= -4.92 cm^{-1} (capping Fe-ring Fe), J_2= -0.47 cm^{-1} (ring Fe-ring Fe) and J'= -0.16 cm^{-1} intercluster interaction. The magnetic behaviors of **3** and **4** are being examined. Compound **1** is diamagnetic which may make it a useful probe in NMR experiments.

To be useful analytical reagents, the metallocrowns must retain their integrity in the solvents or ion permeable membranes containing the desired analyte. We have shown that compounds **1**-**4** are soluble in THF, acetonitrile and DMF. The X-band epr spectrum of **4** in DMF at 110 K shows a six-line signal, the hallmark of uncomplexed Mn(II); however, a standard curve indicates that this signal arises from 20 ± 10% of the Mn(II) in the sample. Acetonitrile solutions of **1** contain an additional broad derivative shaped resonance centered at g=2 that underlies a very weak six line signal. The intensity of this broad feature is slightly greater at 4 K than at 110 K suggesting that it arises from the electronic ground state. Thus, we believe that this poorly resolved signal is associated with the intact cluster while the small amount of six line signal corresponds to less than 5% of the overall spin. These conclusions are supported by the ^{1}H NMR of **4** in different solvents. In d^6-DMF, coordinated acetate resonances are observed at +56.1 ppm and resonances from the phenolate ring protons are at -14.1, -15.5, -22.4 and -23.0 ppm. The same peaks are observed at -16.4, -17.6, -21.4 and -22.0 ppm (phenolate) and +60.6 ppm (acetate) in d^3-acetonitrile. The acetate resonances were confirmed by obtaining spectra of **4** prepared using d^3-acetate. Similar solution chemistry is observed for complexes **1**- **3** in these solvents. In methanol, however, complexes **1**, **2** and **4** dissociate completely. The behavior of **3** is unique in this regard as ^{1}H NMR spectra confirm that the pentameric structure is retained even in methanol, suggesting that additional stability is imparted to the cluster by its negative charge. The most promising observation is that **3** can be trapped in a poly(vinylchloride) membrane using THF as the solvent for the polymerization (13). The resulting membrane can be placed in water for days without any discoloration, indicating that the metallocrowns are stable in ion permeable membranes that are in direct contact with water for long periods. This suggests the possibility that these metal clusters may form the basis for stable potentiometric anion sensors.

In this article, we have described a new class of metal chelating agents that have strong affinity for high valent transition metal cations. Specificity of transition metal ion sequesteration can be achieved at two levels by the metallocrown ethers. The first is selectivity for trivalent metals or complex ions in the ring system. The second is for di- or trivalent metals in the capping positions. Furthermore, because of the ability to form bridges between capping and ring metals, the potential for anion detectors which might distinguish bidentate chelating groups such as sulfate, phosphate, acetate or salicylate is envisioned. These new materials have unique spectral, electrochemical and magnetic properties that may be used in detection systems. Finally, the compounds are stable in a variety of organic solvents and in ion permeable membranes, an important prerequisite for any future commercial application.

ACKNOWLEDGEMENTS

This work was supported by the National Institutes of Health (GM-39406) and the Alfred P. Sloan Foundation (VLP) and by the National Science Foundation (CHE8807498) (WH).

REFERENCES

1. C. J. Pedersen J. Amer. Chem. Soc., 89, 2495 (1967).
2. R. M. Izatt, J. S. Bradshaw, S. A. Nielson, J. D. Lamb, J. J. Christensen and D. Sen Chem. Reviews,, 85, 271 (1985).
3. G. A. Melson, ed. Coordination Chemistry of Macrocyclic Complexes, (1979), Plenum Press, New York.
4. J. B. Nielands, ed. Microbial Iron Transport: A Comprehensive Treatise, Academic Press, New York, (1974).
5. K. N. Raymond, V. L. Pecoraro, and F. L. Weitl Development of Iron Chelators for Clinical Use, A. E. Martell, W. F. Anderson and D . G. Badman, eds., Elsevier/North Holland, New York, 165 (1981).
6. A. Jacobs, Br. J. Haematol., 43, 1 (1979).
7. Actually, there are many different tautomeric structures for B and C since the acidities of phenolate and hydroxamate groups are similar. This scheme shows two of these tautomers, one as the monoanion and one as the dianion, for illustration.
8. V.L. Pecoraro Inorg. Chim. Acta., 155, 171 (1989).
9. M. S. Lah, M.L. Kirk, W. Hatfield and V.L. Pecoraro J. Chem. Soc., Chem. Comm., 111, 7258 (1989).
10. M. S. Lah and V.L. Pecoraro Comments Inorg. Chem., submitted.
11. M. S. Lah and V.L. Pecoraro J. Amer. Chem. Soc., 111, 7258 (1989).
12. N. A. Chanotakis, S. B. Park and M. E. Meyerhoff Anal. Chem. 1989.
13. S. B. Park and M. E. Meyerhoff, personal communication.

IV

Optical and Acoustic Wave-Based Sensors

16

Optical Fiber Electrodes for Electrochemical Luminescence-Based Homogeneous Immunoassay

Masuo Aizawa Department of Bioengineering, Tokyo Institute of Technology, Ookayama, Meguro-ku, Tokyo 152, Japan

1 INTRODUCTION

Striking demands of immunoassay have urged many investigators to develop immunosensors provided with such requisites as (1) high selectivity, (2) high sensitivity, (3) simplicity, and (4) reproducibility. Since the concept of immunosensors was proposed in the early 1970's[1,2], a considerable numbers of papers on immunosensors have been published[3-5]. These immunosensors are categorized into (1)immunosensors without labels and (2) immunosensors with labels. The principles of these immunosensors are schematically illustrated in Figs. 1 and 2. All of these immunosensors depend on molecular recognition of antibody for their high selectivity. Non-label immunosensors are characterized by simple operation, but may not attain sufficiently high sensitivity. In contrast, label immunosensors may provide high sensitivity, although they suffer from lack of simplicity in operation.

Immunoassay with label immunosensors is performed in a heterogeneous manner which requires B/F separation process. Few label immunosensors, however, provide homogeneous immunoassays which are free from B/F (bound and free forms) separation.

A novel homogeneous immunoassay has been developed on the basis of the findings that electrochemical luminescence(ECL) of pyrene-labeled antigen is extremely inhibited by immunochemical complexation with the corresponding antibody[6]. An optical fiber electrode fabricated with an optically transparent electrode on the edge surface of an optical fiber has proved sensitive enough to detect ECL of labels for homogeneous immunoassay[7-10]. Although ECL of labels can be electrochemically generated by applying both negative and positive potentials to an electrode, luminol was found

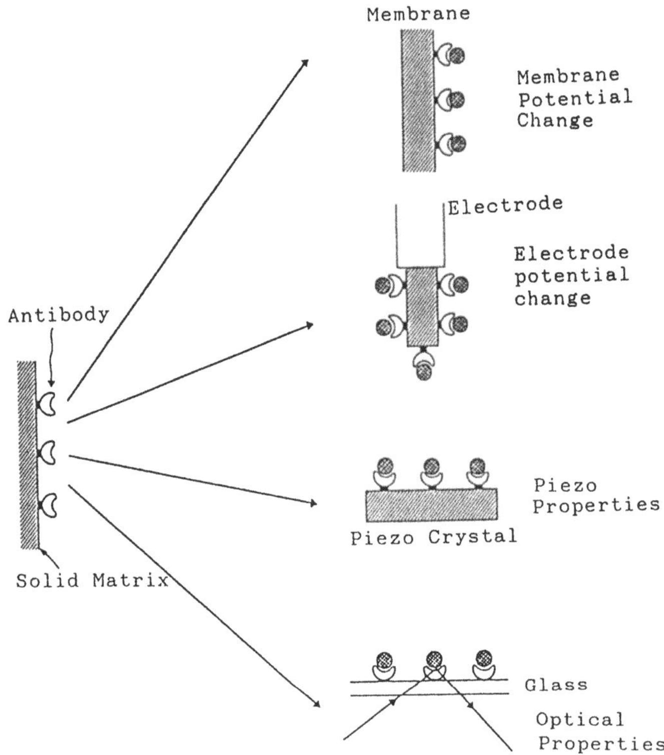

Fig.1 Principle of non-labeled immunosensors

to luminesce only if the electrode potential was shifted positive enough to generate a cation radical in the presence of hydrogen peroxide. A highly sensitive and simple homogeneous immunoassay has thus been performed using an optical fiber electrode as a signal transducer and luminol as a label.

2 HOMOGENEOUS IMMUNOASSAY

Since homogeneous immunoassay requires no B/F separation process, intensive research has been made to search for suitable labels which sensitively change their characteristics in association with immunochemical reactions. Schematic illustration of a homogeneous immunoassay procedure is presented in Fig.3. Labeled

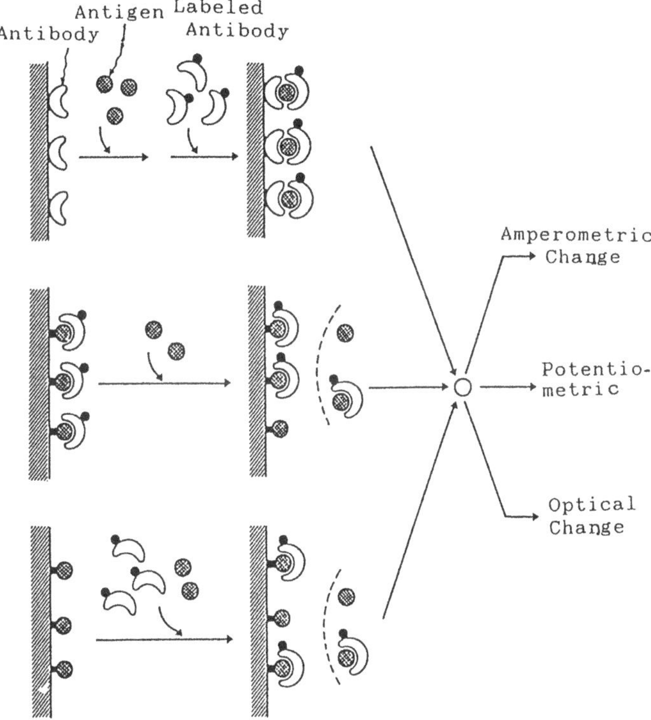

Fig.2 Principle of labeled immunosensors

antigen is complexed with the corresponding antibody in the presence of analyte (non-labeled antigen). Immunochemical complexation results in the coexistence of labeled antigen/antibody complex, non-labeled antigen/antibody complex, free labeled antigen, free non-labeled antigen, and free antibody. The labeled antigen/antibody complex may be discriminated from free labeled antigen in the measurement, if the immunochemical complexation causes a change in a measurable characteristic of the label.

Glucose-6-phosphate dehydrogenase (G-6-PDH) is one enzyme label that can be used for homogeneous immunoassay. Enzyme activity of G-6-PDH is considerably inhibited by immunochemical complexation. The problem is, however, that a sophisticated reagent system for colorimetric determination of the enzyme activity is required. It is therefore difficult to construct an immunosensor for homogeneous immunoassay using G-6-PDH as label.

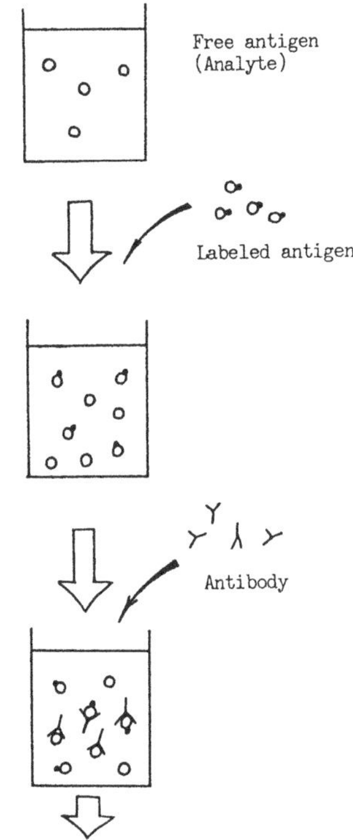

Fig.3 ECL-based homogeneous immunoassay

Electrochemically luminescent substances were found promising as labels for homogeneous immunoassay. Labeled antigen generates luminescence by electrochemical reaction at the electrode surface. The ECL-generated photons can be quantitated with a photon counter. The immunochemical complex of the labeled antigen with the corresponding antibody generates no appreciable luminescence. The analyte (non-labeled antigen) is thus quantitatively determined by detecting photons derived from electrochemical luminescence after immunochemical complexation.

3 PRINCIPLE OF ECL-BASED HOMOGENEOUS IMMUNOASSAY

The principle of electrochemical luminescence-based homogeneous immunoassay is schematically depicted in Fig.3. Known amounts of labeled antigen and the corresponding antibody are added to a test solution containing non-labeled antigen to be determined. The solution remains incubated at a constant temperature to achieve immunochemical complexation.

The solution is then assayed for its electrochemical luminescence. The number of emitted photons correlates with the concentration of free labeled antigen in solution. The concentration of analyte may be determined referring to a standard curve which is obtained for standard solutions of analyte.

4 ELECTROCHEMICAL LUMINESCENCE OF PYRENE-LABELED ALBUMIN

The feasibility of pyrene-labeling for ECL homogeneous immunoassay has been studied using human serum albumin as a model analyte. Aminopyrene dissolved in dimethylsulfoxide was incubated in a phosphate buffer containing glutaraldehyde. Human serum albumin (HSA) was added to react with the pyrene. The coupling reaction was terminated by the addition of sodium borohydride. The reaction mixture was then dialyzed and chromatographed on Sepharose CL-6B. The fraction of the main product (pyrene-labeled HSA) was collected for further use.

Electrochemical measurements were performed in a three-electrode cell installed with an optical fiber. The working and counter electrodes were platinum plate (0.5 x 1 cm^2) ; the surfaces of these electrodes were aligned perpendicular to the cell bottom. A silver/silver chloride (Ag/AgCl) reference electrode was used. The ECL was measured through an optical fiber, which was positioned the vicinity of the working platinum electrode, in conjunction with a photon counter.

The main fraction of the pyrene-labeled HSA was spectrophotometrically assayed for its pyrene moiety. The molar ratio of pyrene to albumin was nearly 8 for the main fraction.

ECL of the pyrene-labeled HSA was studied in phosphate buffer (PB). The electrode potential was cyclically scanned in the range from +1.4 V to -2.25 V vs. Ag/AgCl. Figure 4 illustrates a typical cyclic voltammogram and light intensity vs. potential profile. The reduction (or oxidation) currents of the pyrene moiety and water were overlapped. ECL intensity increased with an increase in the concentration of the labeled HSA.

ECL in this system decreased after immunoreaction between the labeled HSA and antibody, whereas in the presence of goat serum control, little change in luminescence was observed. A relation of the amount of antiserum to the luminescence intensity was

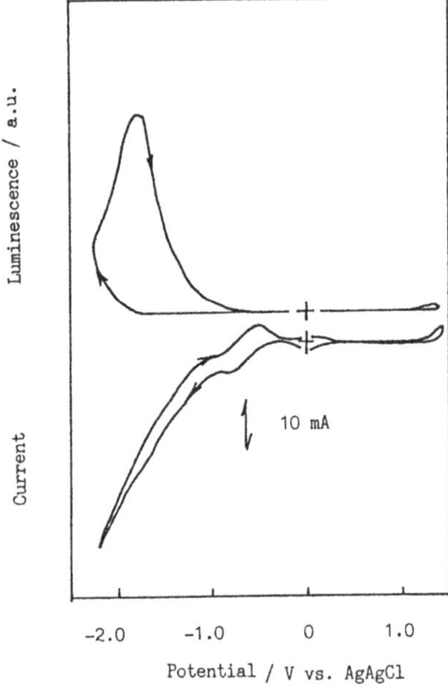

Fig.4 Cyclic voltammetry with ECL of pyrene

studied under a constant concentration of pyrene-labeled HSA. The luminescence intensity decreased with an increase in the antibody concentration, reaching a minimum. This result correlates to a typical immunoprecipitation curve between multivalent antigen and divalent antibody (immunoglobulin G).

Homogeneous immunoassay was performed by competitive binding of HSA and the labeled-HSA (constant) with anti-HSA serum (constant) in 2 mL PB. These components underwent competitive binding at 37 °C for 1 h, followed by ECL measurement in the cell. The potential of the working electrode was swept from +1.4 V to -2.25 V vs. Ag/AgCl. A standard curve for determination of HSA was obtained in the concentration range 3-25 x 10^{-6} M. The minimum detectable concentration was approximately 10^{-6} M.

Although the immunochemically induced inhibition mechanism of ECL has not been clarified, it is noted that fluorescence of the pyrene-labeled HSA is enhanced by the immunochemical complexation. blueshift in peak wavelength and an increase in fluorescence intensity were markedly induced by the immunochemical reaction of the labeled HSA with the corresponding antibody.

have insufficient sensitivity in the homogeneous immunoassay. The authors seached for other labels that would result in attain highly sensitive homogeneous immunoassays. Of these labels, luminol was found to be promising.

The ECL of luminol was measured using an optical fiber electrode in an aqueous solution. An optically transparent platinum thin layer electrode was formed on the top of an optical fiber, and a counter electrode was fabricated around the optical fiber (Fig.5). The potential of the transparent electrode was controlled against a Ag/AgCl reference electrode with a potentiostat/function generator. The optical fiber electrode was routed to a photon counter which was connected to a digital storage oscilloscope, computer, and printer. Luminol was initially dissolved in a small amount of dimethyl sulfoxide (DMSO) and then diluted with 0.1 M phosphate buffer solution (pH 7.0). The final concentration of DMSO was adjusted to 0.1%. Dissolved oxygen was purged by nitrogen gas bubbling before the measurement. ECL was simultaneously measured in conjunction1 with cyclic voltammetry using a potential scanning rate of 100 $mV \cdot s^{-1}$. For 1mM luminol at the optical fiber electrode, the onset potential of ECL was

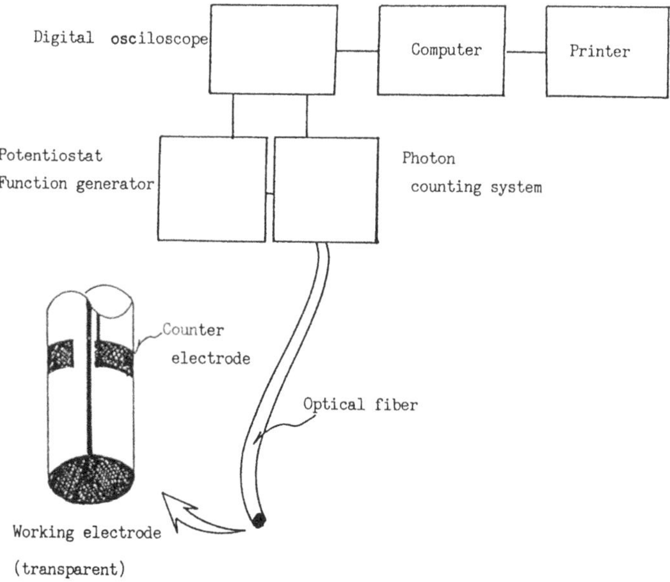

Fig.5 Optical fiber electrode

around 0.5 V vs. Ag/AgCl. Although no distinctive peak of oxidative current of luminol appeared around 0.5 V vs. Ag/AgCl in cyclic voltammetry, differential pulse voltammetry showed a very sharp anodic peak at 0.495V vs. Ag/AgCl as presented in Fig.6. The electrochemical luminescence of luminol should be derived from the electrochemical oxidation of luminol at this potential.

Cyclic voltammetry of luminol suggested that both anodic and cathodic electrochemical processes were required for ECL of luminol. Two electrochemical processes were initiated by a double potential step application. For the anodic process 0.65V vs. Ag/AgCl was determined to be optimum, and for the cathodic process -1.5V vs. Ag/AgCl was optimum. These two potentials were sequentially applied to the optical fiber electrode to generate ECL of luminol. As shown in Fig.7 it should be optimum that the potential is initially controlled at -1.5V vs. AgAgCl for 5 sec and then at 0.65V vs. AgAgCl for 15 sec.

ECL was determined under the optimum conditions at various concentrations of luminol. Luminol was determined in the concentration range of 10^{-8} -10^{-3}M. The minimum limit of detection was 10^{-8}M, which resulted primarily from improvement due to the optical fiber electrode.

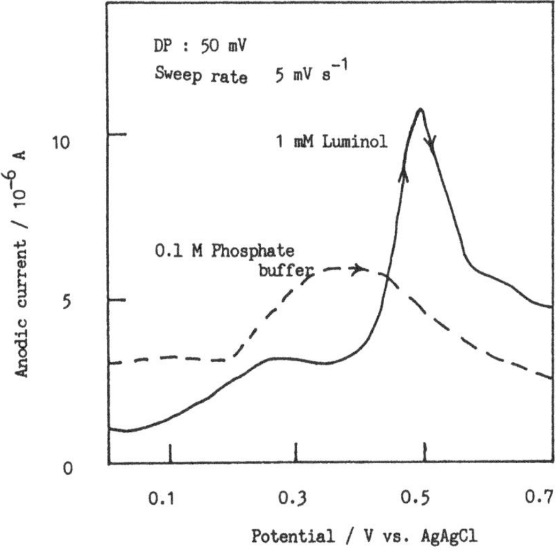

Fig.6 Differential pulse voltammetry of luminol

6 ENHANCED ECL OF LUMINOL BY HYDROGEN PEROXIDE

During the investitigation of the reaction mechanism of luminol ECL, an enhanced effect of hydrogen peroxide on luminol ECL was found. The hydrogen peroxide was generated by electrochemical reduction of dissolved oxygen. These findings led us to generate ECL of luminol by single potential step in the presence of hydrogen peroxide.

In the presence of hydrogen peroxide luminol generated ECL resulted from a single potential step to +0.65V vs. Ag/AgCl. No cathodic potential application was required. The sensitivity of ECL determination of luminol has been improved enormously by the enhancement effect of hydrogen peroxide. The minimum limit of luminol detection was improved to 10^{-11}M.

7 ECL HOMOGENEOUS IMMUNOASSAY WITH LUMINOL LABEL

ECL homogeneous immunoassay has also been demonstrated using luminol as label. ECL of luminol labeled antigen was inhibited by the immunochemical complexation. The concentration of antigen (analyte) was determined by measuring ECL of the luminol label after immunochemical reaction. In the case of immunoglobulin G as analyte, the limit of detection was 10^{-13} g·mL^{-1}.

8 CONCLUSION

Immunochemically induced inhibition of ECL has made a sensitive homogeneous immunoassay possible. Luminol is a promising label for ECL homogeneous immunoassay. An optical fiber electrode has tremendously enhanced the sensitivity of ECL measurement.

9 REFERENCES

1) M.Aizawa, A.Morioka, H.Matsuoka, S.Suzuki, Y.Nagamura, H. Shinohara, I.Ishiguro, J.Solid-Phase Biochem. 1.319-326
2) J.Janata, J.Am.Chem.Soc. 97, 2915-2916 (1976)
3) M.Aizawa, Phil.Trans.Roy.Soc.London B316 121-134 (1987).
4) M.Aizawa, Tanpakushitsu Kakusan Koso (No.31) 272-279 (1987).
5) T.T.Ngo, ed., "Electrochemical Sensors in Immunological Analysis" Plenum, New York (1987)

6) Y.Ikariyama, H.Kunoh, M.Aizawa, Biochem.Biophys.Res.Commun. 128, 987-992 (1985).
7) M.Aizawa, Y.Ikariyama, K.Emoto, Proc. 2nd Intl Meeting Chemical Sensors, Bordeaux, 622-625 (1986)
8) M.Aizawa, Y.Ikariyama, M.Tanaka, H.Shinohara, Proc. ECS Symp. Chemical Sensors 362-369 (1987)
9) M.Aizawa, Y.Ikariyama, M.Tanaka, H.Shinohara, Tech.Digest 8th Sensor Symp. 7-12 (1989)
10) M.Aizawa, M.Tanaka, Y.Ikariyama, R.W.Murray, "Chemical Sensors and Microinstrumentation" (R.E.Murray, R.E.Dessy, W.R.Heineman, J.Janata, W.R.Seitz, eds.), Am.Chem.Soc., Washington,DC, 129-138 (1989)

17

Immunosensors: Remaining Problems in the Development of Remote, Continuous, Multi-Channel Devices

J.D. Andrade, J.-N. Lin, V. Hlady, J. Herron, D. Christensen, and J. Kopecek, Department of Bioengineering, University of Utah, Salt Lake City , Utah, 84112

1 GOALS AND OBJECTIVES

The goals and objectives of the Immunosensors Program at the University of Utah are to develop the science and engineering basis for optically based immunosensors. This includes the development of sensors for proteins and other antigens, the development of multi-channel sensors (including built-in calibration and reference channels), the development of sensors which are capable of remote on-line and continuous or semi-continuous function and the development of sensors which are biocompatible and stable. This chapter will serve as a 1989 progress report on these various goals and objectives.(1)

Figure 1 summarizes these goals. An animal or patient is shown, which could also represent a bioreactor or biochemical reactor. An extracorporeal loop is shown, for example, the extracorporeal blood pathway in hemodialysis or cardiopulmonary bypass during open-heart surgery. A connector is shown in that loop which contains a multi-channel immunosensor. Outputs of the various channels are appropriately referenced, ratioed, and otherwise processed to permit the quantitative analysis of the analytes of interest. The output is shown on a continuous or semi-continuous plot of analyte concentration as a function of time.

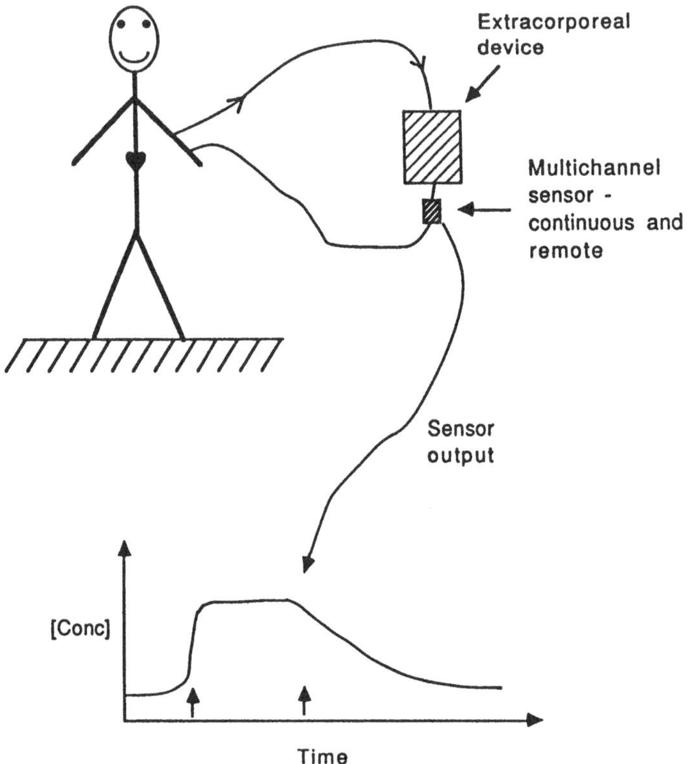

FIGURE 1
On line, continuous, remote sensing is the long-range goal of the Utah program. An array of such sensors can be applied in extracorporeal blood circuits for the monitoring and control of cardiovascular devices, in process control in the biotechnology and biochemical engineering industries, and for water monitoring in environmental engineering. Our focus is on immunoassay technologies for proteins, hormones, and drugs.

Application areas include:

1. Biochemical engineering and biotechnology, primarily for process control;
2. Medical diagnostics;
3. Extracorporeal device monitoring and control (Figure 1);
4. Implanted device monitoring and control;
5. Biomedical research, such as the monitoring of analyte concentrations in experimental animals and in cell cultures;

6. Water and waste-water monitoring of environmental pollutants and contaminants.

Our approach is based largely on immunoassay; thus, we are interested in applying these sensors to the assay of the following general classes of antigens/haptens:

1. Coagulation proteins
2. Complement proteins
3. Antibody levels
4. Lipoproteins
5. Enzymes
6. Enzyme inhibitors
7. Hormones
8. Growth factors and regulators
9. Drugs
10. Viruses and bacteria

Coagulation proteins are our current applications focus.

2 INTRODUCTION AND BACKGROUND

Most of our work is based on the use of antibody or antigen immobilized on a quartz or amorphous silica surface.(2) Silica is used because of its optical properties, specifically its high optical transmission, low fluorescence, and relatively high refractive index. The latter permits one to use total internal reflection optics and the interfacially bound evanescent wave as a means to excite fluorescence on the solution side of the solid liquid interface without exciting bulk fluorescence in the solution phase.(3)

This approach has been studied by a large number of groups for its possible immunosensor application.(4-8) In our case, we have used principally a flat quartz plate excited by a single total internal reflection geometry. This so called total internal reflection fluorescence (TIRF) method has been widely used by us and others for the fundamental study of protein adsorption and immobilization at solid liquid interfaces as well as for fluorescence immunosensor development.(1,3) We have also used silica optical fibers and developed a sensing region in the fiber by the appropriate removal of cladding and coating (4), as have others.(4,5)

In Figure 2 a conventional silica core fiber is shown, but with the end stripped to remove the cladding and protective coating. The distal end of the fiber has been coated with a black rubber or epoxy to prevent light from propagating from the end of the fiber into the bulk solution. The stripped fiber surface is shown to contain immobilized Immunoglobulin and, after exposure to specifically bound antigen, the fluorescence intensity plot demon-

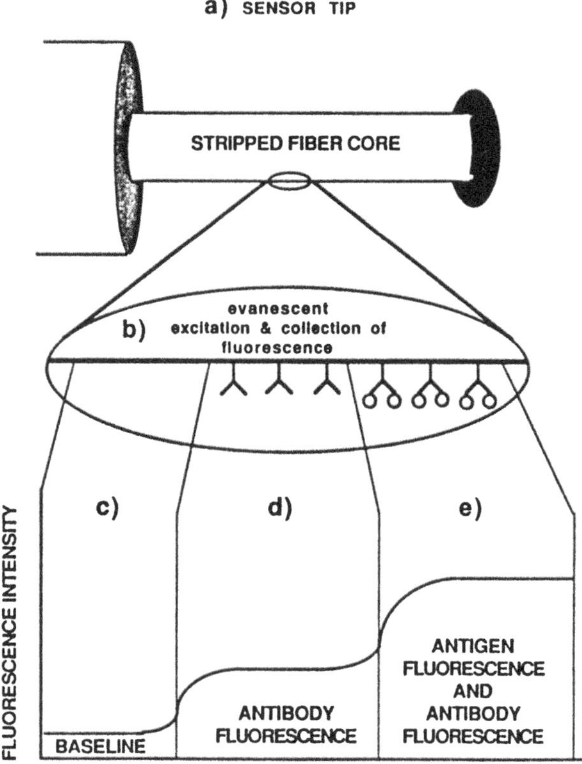

FIGURE 2
A typical optical fiber evanescent immunosensor design. From Reichert et al. (Ref. 16)

strates that the same fiber can be used to excite interfacial fluorescence as well as to collect a portion of the fluorescence generated. If the excitation wavelength is in the range of 280-290 nanometers, the intrinsic UV fluorescence of proteins is detected.(3) Thus, the immobilization of an unlabeled antibody can be directly probed and monitored.(6) In addition, if the antigen is fluorescent or if a fluorescently labeled antigen is added as a reagent to compete with unlabeled antigen for the antibody binding sites, then a conventional competitive fluoroimmunoassay is produced, and the visible fluorescence of the labeled antigen can be readily detected and measured.

More recently we have been working with multi-channel detection primarily through the use of a two-dimensional CCD (charge coupled device) camera.(7) We have demonstrated that various channels, ie., different spatially distinct regions of immobilized antibody, can be readily detected. Figure 3 demonstrates the optical geometry for such an experiment.

3 ANTIGEN-ANTIBODY BINDING

The sensitivity and specificity of an immunosensor is based on the sensitivity and specificity of the interaction of specific antibodies with a particular antigen.

Figure 4 presents the basic antibody antigen equilibrium equation and the plot based on the assumed reversibility of these interactions. The plot shows antigen binding as a function of antigen concentration. The dynamic range of an immunoassay or immunosensor is usually considered to be roughly from 10 to 90% saturation of the antibody used, or about two orders of magnitude in antigen concentration.(8) If one wishes to sense a much wider range of concentrations, then two or more antibody channels are required each with a different antibody with the appropriate binding constant.

In the case of a multi-epitope antigen it may be desirable to use an array of channels, each containing a different monoclonal antibody. In this way, the dynamic range could be enhanced

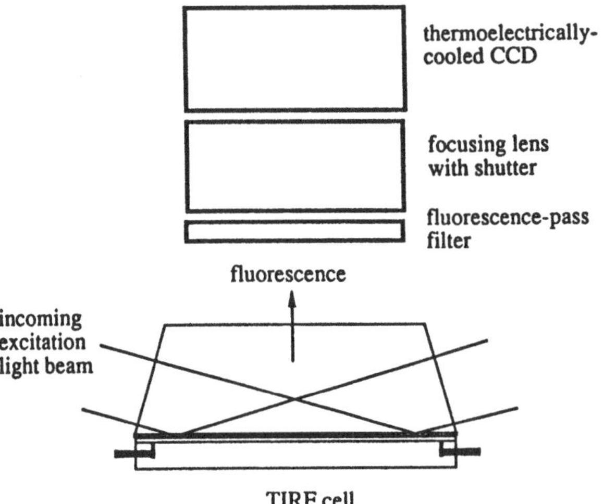

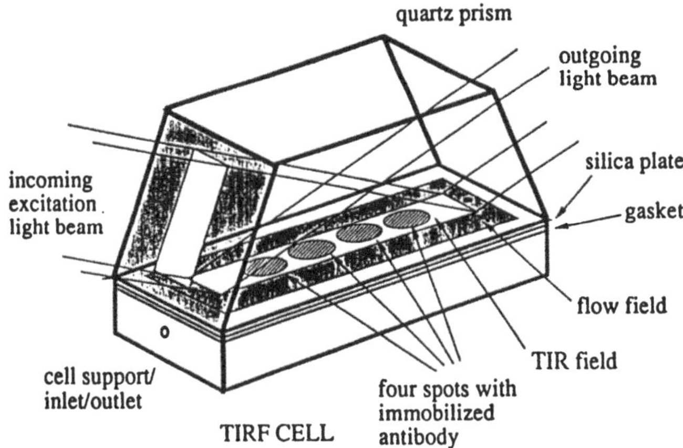

FIGURE 3
Use of the single reflection TIRF geometry for the development of multi-channel immuno sensors. A cooled CCD is used as a position and wavelength sensitive detector. Four different immobilized Ab regions are detected. (From Ref. 7)

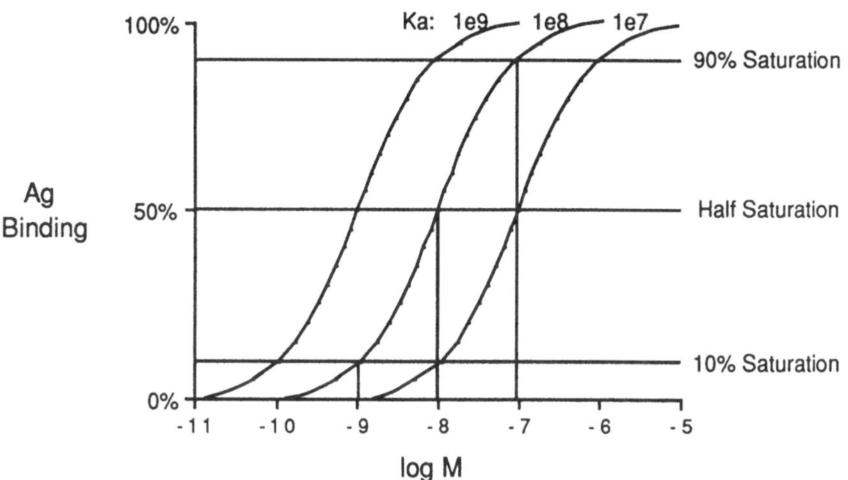

FIGURE 4
Bound Ag - Bulk Ag equilibrium curves, based on a reversible Ag-Ab interaction:

$$\text{Ab} + \text{Ag} \underset{K_2 \text{ off}}{\overset{\text{on } K_1}{\rightleftarrows}} \text{Ab-Ag}; \qquad K_a = K_1/K_2 = \frac{[\text{Ab-Ag}]}{[\text{Ab}][\text{Ag}]}$$

when $K_a \sim 1/[\text{Ag}]$, Ab sites are ~ 50% saturated.

Range of immunoassay is usually defined as:

$$\frac{0.1}{K_a} < [\text{Ag}] < \frac{10}{K_a},$$

i.e. 10 to 90% saturation results in two orders of magnitude range for [Ag].

and discrimination against nonspecific binding could be improved as well.

For much of our work, we have chosen to work with a model system of anti-fluoroscein monoclonal antibodies developed by Voss and coworkers at the University of Illinois.(9) The binding thermodynamics of this system have been studied and presented by Herron et al.(10) The overall association constant as a function of temperature for three different anti-fluoroscein monoclonals is given in Figure 5. This is bulk solution data and demonstrates that the overall association constant can vary by up to two orders of magnitude over a temperature range of some 40 to 50 degrees centigrade. It was this behavior that led to the concept of the thermal regulation of antigen antibody binding which our group is now studying.(8)

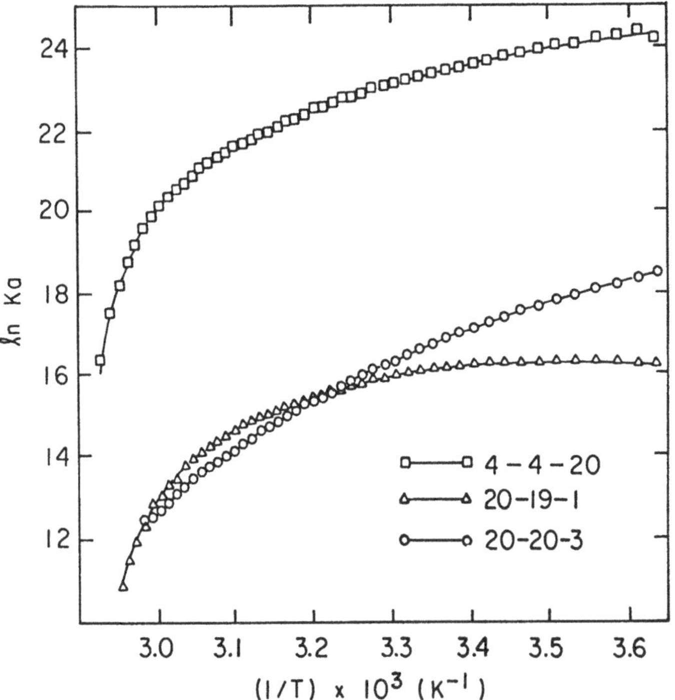

FIGURE 5
Association constants, Ka, as a function of reciprocal temperature for 3 antifluorescyl monoclonal antibodies. (from Ref. 10)

Table 1 presents the binding kinetics for five of the anti-fluoroscein monoclonals, ranging in overall association constant from 5 X 10^7 to 3 X 10^{10} moles $^{-1}$. The table shows that the association rate constant is relatively constant (of the order of 5 X 10^6) while the dissociation constant or its reciprocal, the dissociation lifetime, changes by a factor of 500. It is clear, therefore, that the overall association constant of an antigen-antibody complex can be governed almost entirely by the dissociation rate constant. The dissociation lifetime is the response time of an immunosensor as it attempts to respond to changes in circulating analyte concentration. Therefore, for the development of a truly reversible, continuous immunosensor, the dissociation lifetime issue has to be addressed and considered.

TABLE 1
Ag-Ab binding data for 5 antifluorescyl monoclonal antibodies. The "sensitivity" of a sensor is best indicated by Ka, the overall affinity or association constant. The sensitivity of 50% Ab saturation is shown at the far right. The response time is given by the dissociation lifetime, which is the reciprocal of the off-rate constant (from Ref. 10).

Clone	Association Rate	X	Dissociation Lifetime	=	Affinity Ka	[Ag] at 50% Saturation
	M^{-1} s^{-1}		s		M^{-1}	[M]
4-4-20	6.28 x 10^6		5376		3.38 x 10^{10}	3.10^{-11}
20-19-2	1.28 x 10^6		454		5.81 x 10^8	2.10^{-9}
20-20-3	1.08 x 10^7		38		4.10 x 10^8	2.10^{-9}
6-10-6	5.33 x 10^6		14		7.46 x 10^7	1.10^{-8}
20-4-4	4.67 x 10^6		11		5.14 x 10^7	2.10^{-8}

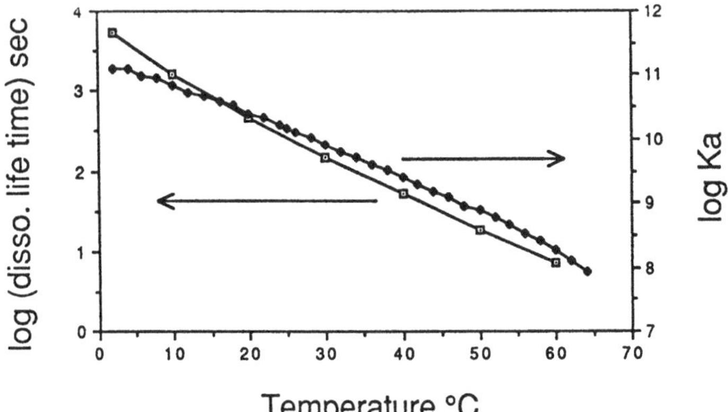

FIGURE 6
The dissociation lifetime (on the left) for the 4-4-20 antifluorescyl monoclonal antibody as a function of temperatures. Log Ka data is given on the right axis. Note that Ka decreases an order of magnitude with a 20° increase in temperature. (from Ref. 10)

Figure 6 presents the dissociation lifetime data for one of the antibodies, the 4-4-20 clone, as a function of temperature. Here one can readily see that the response time of a sensor can be improved by an order of magnitude with a 20 degree change in local temperature.

This discussion of antigen/antibody binding, however, has used data taken in bulk solution. Under those conditions, antigen/antibody interactions are reversible. However, the situation may change significantly when one of the components in the binding reaction is immobilized at a solid liquid interface. We will next discuss the question of antibody immobilization followed by the issue of the reversibility of antibody/antigen interactions at interfaces.

4 ANTIBODY IMMOBILIZATION

A wide range of immobilization methods have been developed and applied. We have experimented with: (11)

- surface modification by the use of silane chemistries;

- the use of cross-linking and coupling agents, including glutaraldehyde;
- the use of a precursor film of protein (such as bovine serum albumin);
- the use of proteins which may help to at least partially orient the immobilized antibodies, such as protein A.

In our case the reactions are constrained by the fact that we need to immobilize at an interface which is optically compatible with the total internal reflection/evanescent wave optical separation method previously described. In addition to the detailed immobilization chemistry, it is important to consider the collision and adsorption of the antibody to the interface, a precursor step to the covalent chemistry employed in the immobilization process.(12) Thus, it is important to understand the collision, orientation and adsorption of antibody at the solid/liquid interface.

An up-to-date, although qualitative, picture of protein adsorption is presented in Figure 7. The protein must first approach and collide with the surface, given by an overall adsorption rate constant. It may also desorb from the surface, given by the desorption rate constant. When these two processes are equal, then we say we have an equilibrium amount of protein adsorbed on the surface. However, Langmuir adsorption does not generally apply to the adsorption of macromolecules because a variety of other processes and interactions are present. One of the most interesting is the fact that the protein may conformationally change and the degree of that change may be a function of residence time at the surface. This is indicated by the time dependent conformational change depicted in Figure 7.

Another problem is that antibodies, in addition to being large macromolecules, have different, distinct domains. The domains may have their own particular interface activity characteristics. This is indicated at the bottom right of Figure 7 which shows a two-domain protein interacting with a surface by one of its domains.

If there is more than one type of protein present in the solution, then there are multi-component, competitive adsorption and immobilization processes which also occur. This is illustrated at the bottom left of Figure 7.

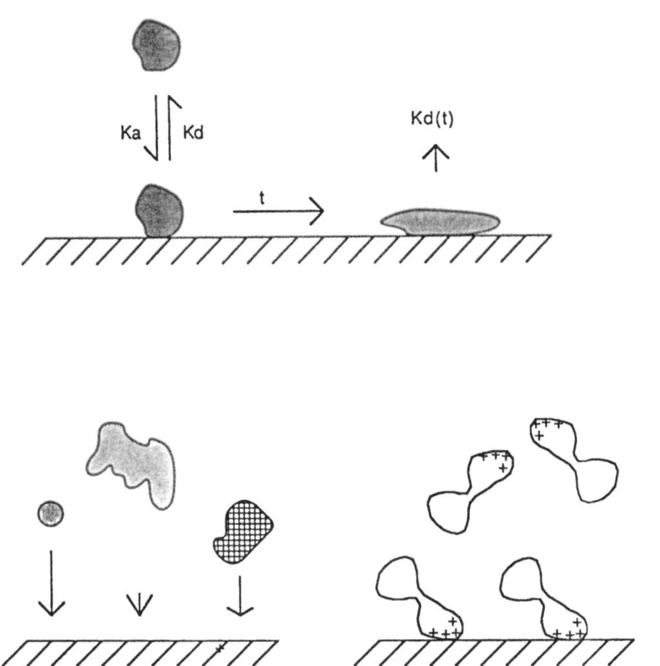

FIGURE 7
Top: Adsorption from a single protein solution can be described in terms of adsorption (Ka) and desorption (Kd) rate constants at initial contact (t=0). With increasing residence time, t, at the surface the adsorbed protein may conformationally change or denature, generally resulting in a greatly decreased desorption rate, represented by Kd(t).

Bottom Left: Adsorption from a multi-component protein solution can be treated in terms of the concentrations and diffusion coefficients of each component--ie. in terms of the collision rate of each component--and a measure of the affinity of each component for the interface and the denaturability of each component. (17,18)

Bottom Right: The adsorption of complex, multi-domain proteins may be dominated or controlled by the interface activity of one key domain, such as the positively charged binding domains in the heparin-binding plasma proteins. (19,20)

Immunoglobulins are highly complex proteins with a variety of distinct functional and structural domains. There are hinge regions and switch regions, the function of which might depend on the local micro-environment and mode or mechanism of adsorption and immobilization. These regions, in turn, may affect the binding constant of the active site in ways which are not fully understood at present. Intentionally denaturing IgG prior to its adsorption at a solid/liquid interface (12) can result in a significant increase in the surface antigen binding capacity. Lin, et al. demonstrated that it is possible to engineer the immobilization of antibodies to optimize their properties at the interface by control of their structure in solution.(12) This work is continuing with a detailed investigation of the solution, denaturation and structural characteristics of model antibodies in the hopes of optimizing means to adsorb and then immobilize these molecules with enhanced antigen binding characteristics.

5. ANTIGEN/ANTIBODY REVERSIBILITY

A true immunosensor requires that the sensor respond to changes in the circulating analyte concentration. Most immuno "sensors" developed to date are not true sensors but rather are detectors. They are designed to measure the analyte concentration and then either are discarded or regenerated by some process.

Our goal is to develop immunosensors which are inherently reversible and can continuously sense circulating analyte concentration. The problem is illustrated briefly in Figure 8. The bottom half basically demonstrates immobilized antibody interacting with its antigen and shows that although the on-rates in the bulk solution and interface case may be similar, the off-rate constant is much smaller in the case of immobilized antibody, meaning that the dissociation lifetime is much longer, which means then that the response of the sensor is very slow. The question is why?

This issue has been addressed briefly by several authors (15) and more completely by Lin et al. in a recent paper which presents six general hypothesis for the observation of partial irreversibility in immobilized antibody systems.(2)

1. Diffusion and *mass transport* effects. In many systems, particularly highly porous particulate systems, these effects can be very pronounced and indeed dominate the system, so that the irreversibility is only apparent. When proper account is taken of concentration, diffusion, and mass transport effects, the system may be behaving reversibly or similarly to its behavior in bulk solution.

Solution:

$$\mathrm{Ab} + \mathrm{Ag} \underset{K_2}{\overset{K_1}{\rightleftharpoons}} \mathrm{Ab\text{-}Ag}$$

$$Ka = \frac{K_1}{K_2} \sim 10^6 - 10^{12} \quad M^{-1}$$

Surface:

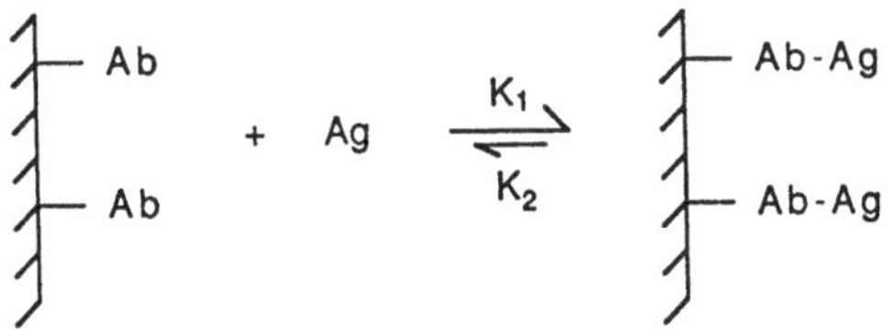

$$\begin{matrix} \mathrm{Ab} \\ \mathrm{Ab} \end{matrix} + \mathrm{Ag} \underset{K_2}{\overset{K_1}{\rightleftharpoons}} \begin{matrix} \mathrm{Ab\text{-}Ag} \\ \mathrm{Ab\text{-}Ag} \end{matrix}$$

$$(Ka)_{surface} \gg (Ka)_{solution}$$

$$(K_2)_{surface} \ll (K_2)_{solution}$$

FIGURE 8
Bulk solution Ab-Ag equilibria (left) are not generally observed when Ab or Ag is immobilized at an interface (right)--see Ref. 3.

2. The <u>immobilized antibody</u> is in a different <u>conformation</u> than the antibody in solution, thus influencing the nature of the antibody/antigen interaction. This is very difficult to directly measure, other than through on and off rate constants, because the conformational change of the antibody need not necessarily be a gross or very major change. Protein conformational changes are normally detected by changes in the circular dichroic spectra, infrared or Raman spectra, or by tryptophan fluorescence emission. All of these are relatively global measures of protein structural conformation. There could be a significant alteration in the Fab antigen binding site without a global conformational change. Such a local conformational change would not be detected by common techniques.
3. Antibody/<u>antibody lateral interactions</u>. The concentration of antibody at an interface is generally significantly higher than the concentrations used in bulk solution studies. Antibodies are known to readily aggregate, particularly under elevated concentration conditions. It may well be that two dimensional aggregation, perhaps due to lateral interactions at an interface, may significantly affect the antigen binding characteristics, which could result in a slow off-rate.
4. Change in <u>solution micro-environment</u>. It is well known that a change in local solution environment can change the nature of antigen/antibody interactions. For example, in affinity-chromatography columns immobilized antigen is normally released through the use of eluents which change the local solution environment and therefore the nature of the antigen/antibody binding. Although this is not fully understood, it is well known that low pH, eluents containing chaotropic salts, and eluents containing substances which minimize hydrophobic interactions are particularly effective in the removal of bound antigen from immobilized antibody columns.

5. Non-specific adsorption. The antigen may bind to the antibody through its particular epitope interacting with the Fab region of the antibody, but it may also bind by non-specific mechanisms to perhaps other parts of the immobilized molecule and to regions of the surface which are not covered with antibody. Such non-specific binding is a particular problem in the case of protein antigens, which are large macromolecules and can undergo non-specific interactions by a variety of mechanisms. This was illustrated nicely by Lin et al. (2) and also by Schram et al.(15)
6. Multi-valent binding. This is particularly important for larger antigens. If the antigen can be bound by more than one binding site, then it is a cooperative binding process. If there are two or more distinct and perhaps even independent binding events or binding sites holding down the antigen, then even if the antibody-antigen bond is released, the non-specific bond to the surface at that instant in time is maintained. This increases the probability that the antigen antibody bond will reform or reassociate. That makes it almost impossible to ever completely desorb or remove a bound antigen. This is exactly the mechanism believed to be responsible for the irreversibility of physical adsorption processes of proteins and other macromolecules. The multiplicity of binding sites means that the probability that all of the binding sites would be released at the same time is zero; thus, desorption does not occur. This would be expected to be observed in the case of large antigens, but not necessarily in the case of a very small antigens or haptens.

It is clear that all six of the above hypotheses and mechanisms are operable, some more so than others, in a particular experimental situation. It will be very difficult to isolate and sort out the individual components responsible for the irreversibilty of antigen/antibody interactions at interfaces. Lin et al. have summarized the variables affecting the behavior of immobilized antibody/antigen interactions.(2)

6. OTHER ISSUES

A truly remote fluoro-immunosensor will require some means to deliver fluorescently labelled antigen, as the basic principle of such a sensor is that a fluorescently labeled antigen competes with unlabeled circulating antigen for the finite number of antibody binding sites. We have previously described a number of approaches to solve this problem. Those studies are ongoing. Dr. J. Kopecek and co-workers are continuing the development of controlled delivery methods for fluorescent antigens.(21)

Earlier it was noted that it might be possible to regulate the antigen/antibody binding constant by changes in temperature or even by other means. We have performed a number of studies along these lines. However, it is necessary to immobilize antibody by means that permit the reversibility of the antibody/antigen interaction, before one can expect to regulate the nature of the binding constant. Our studies on binding constant regulation are continuing, based on the assumption that we will indeed develop methods to solve the "irreversibility" problem described above.

Non-specific binding is, of course, a problem which must be minimized. Although certain aspects of the problem can be overcome by the use of appropriate reference channels, it is clearly desirable to minimize the problem as much as possible. In our case, this is done through the use of polyethylene oxide as a "protein-repulsive" coating to minimize protein adsorption. This has been discussed extensively elsewhere.(22) We are also developing methods to immobilize antibody through the use of polyethylene oxide tethers or spacers in the hopes of minimizing non-specific adsorption to the spacer or to the chemical linkage itself.

Finally, there may be another problem with the development of truly remote sensors based on immobilized antibodies, particularly in blood and related environments. Blood is known to contain a variety of protease pro-enzymes, which can become activated under appropriate conditions to produce proteolytic activity. If protease activity is indeed generated locally at the surface of an immunosensor, perhaps due to non-specific binding of coagulation or complement proteins, and if such proteases attack the immobilized antibody, then the sensor surface will degenerate with time and will eventually cease to function. That is one of the reasons why it is so important to build multi-channel devices with the appropriate calibration and reference channels to account for decrease or change in immobilized antibody concentration or activity. It is also why the non-specific adsorption problem is so important to eliminate and not simply to reference or calibrate out, as noted earlier. If we minimize the non-specific adsorption of all proteins then we also minimize the possibility of interfacially induced protease activation. Again, our approach to this problem is through the polyethylene oxide surface approach. Studies on the stability of immobilized antibodies are only now being initiated in our laboratory.

7. CONCLUSIONS

The development of truly remote, continuous, high sensitivity and specific immunosensors, capable of functioning remotely in blood or in other biological environments, is still in its early stages. There are a number of important technologies which must be developed. As the work progresses, one can envision the development and eventual production of multichannel biosensors based on microintegrated devices incorporating biochemical, optical and even electronic functions.

This paper has briefly reviewed the general concept and at least one approach to each of the major problems.

ACKNOWLEDGEMENTS

We acknowledge discussions and assistance from many colleagues and coworkers, including; A.Edmundson, M.Block, D.Gregonis, J.Ives,

M.Reichert I.Skurnik, P.Suci, D.Tirrell, R.VanWagenen and E.Voss. The early phases of the work were funded by the Office of Naval Research, Biomolecular Engineering Program. Application to coagulation proteins was funded via NHLBI grant HL37046. Biocompatibility and reagent delivery aspects are supported in part by the Center for Biopolymers at Interfaces and by the National Science Foundation (Grant ECE86-02107). Studies dealing with Ag-Ab binding constant regulation are funded by the U.S. Army Research Office. The authors thank Ms. Carol Felis for skillful and personable preparation of the manuscript.

REFERENCES

1. Andrade, J.A., Herron, J., Lin, J-N., Yen, H., Kopecek, J., Kopeckova, P. (1988). On-Line Sensors for Coagulation Proteins: Concept and Progress Report, Biomaterials, 9: 76.
2. Lin, J-N., Herron, J., Hlady, V., and Andrade, J.D. (1989). Dissociation of Ab-Ag Complexes on Solid Surfaces: An Overview, Biosensors: in press.
3. Hlady, V., Reinecke, D.R., and Andrade, J.D. (1986). Fluorescence of Adsorbed Protein Layers. I., J. Coll. Interface Sci. 111, 555.
4. Block M.J., and Hirschfeld, T.B. (1987) US Patents 4 558 014 (1984), 4 447 546 (1984), 4 582 809 (1986), 4 654 532 (1987).
5. Place, J.F., Sutherland, R.M., and Dahne, C. (1985). Biosensors 1: 321.
6. Andrade, J.D., and Van Wagenen, R.A. (1983). Process for Conducting fluorescence Immunoassays Without Added Labels and Employing Attenuated Internal Reflection, US Patent 4 368 047.
7. Hlady, V., Lin, J-N., and Andrade, J.D. (1989). Spatially Resolved Detection of Ab-Ag Reactions at S/L Interfaces Using Total Internal Reflection Excited Ag Fluorescence and CCD Detection, Biosensors, in press.

8. Andrade, J.D., Lin, J-N., Herron, J., Reichert, M., and Kopecek J. (1986). Fiber Optic Immunodetectors: Sensors or Dosimeters, Proceedings of SPIE 718: 280.

9. Kranz, D.M., Herron, J.N., Voss, E.W. (1982). Mechanisms of Ligand Binding by Monoclonal Anti-fluorescyl Antibodies, J. Biol. Chem. 257: 6987

10. Herron, J.N., Kranz, D.M., Jameson, D.M., Voss, E.M. (1986). Thermodynamic Properties of Ligand Binding by Monoclonal Anti-fluorescyl Antibodies, Biochem. 25: 4602.

11. Lin, J-N., Herron, J., Andrade, J.D., and Brizgys, M. (1988). Solid Phase Immobilization of Antibodies for Optical Biosensor Application, IEEE Trans. Bio-Med Eng. 35: 466.

12. Lin, J-N., Chang, I-N, Herron, J., Andrade, J.D. (1989). Influence of Adsorption of Native and Modified Ab on Their Activity, J. Immunologic. Methods, in press.

13. Andrade, J.D. and Hlady, V. (1986). Protein Adsorption and Materials Biocompatibility, Adv. Poly. Sci., 79: 1.

14. Norde, W. (1986) Proteins at Solid Interfaces, Adv. Colloid Interface Sci. 25:, 267.

15. Schramm, W., Yang, T., and Midgley, A.R. (1987). Surface Modification with Protein A for Uniform Binding of Monoclonal Antibodies, Clin. Chem., 33: 1338.

16. Reichert, W.M., Bruckner, C.J., Joseph, J. (1987). L-B Films and Black Lipid Membranes in Biospecific Surface-Selective Sensors, Thin Solid Films, 152: 345.

17. Andrade, J.D. and Hlady, V. (1987). Plasma Protein Adsorption - The Big Twelve, Ann New York Academy Science 516: 151.

18. Andrade, J.D. and Hlady, V. (1987). Protein Adsorption -- The Denaturation Correlation, Croatica Chemica Acta 60: 495.

19. Andrade, J.D., Hlady, V., and Wei, A-P. (1990). A Structural and Functional Domain Approach to Protein Adsorption, Croatica Chemica Acta, submitted.

20. Ho, C-H. (1990). Adsorption of Plasma Proteins Detected by 2-D Gel Electrophoresis, MSc Thesis, in preparation, University of Utah.

21. Yen, H-R., Kopecek, J., Andrade, J.D. (1989). Optically Controlled Ligand Delivery, 1, Makromol. Chem. 190: 69.

22. Lee, J-H., Kopecek, J., Kopeckova, P., and Andrade, J.D. (1989). Surface Properties of PEO-Containing Polymeric Surfactants: Protein-Resistant Surfaces, J. Biomedical Materials Res. 23: 351.

18

Direct Observation of Immunoglobulin Adsorption Dynamics Using the Atomic Force Microscope

J.-N. Lin, B. Drake[†], A.S. Lea, P.K. Hansma[†], and J.D. Andrade
Dept. of Bioengineering and the Center for Biopolymers at Interfaces, University of Utah, Salt Lake City, Utah 84112
[†]Dept. of Physics, University of California, Santa Barbara, California 93106

Abstract

Atomic force microscopic images of a murine antifluorescyl monoclonal antibody (IgG 4-4-20) depositing from solution onto freshly cleaved mica were observed in real time. These images clearly indicate a cooperative adsorption process, not a random one. Only IgG aggregates formed stable deposits, whereas isolated molecules desorbed readily from the surface. Subsequent adsorption occurred adjacent to the aggregates, forming ridges and eventually a near monolayer was produced. Additional layers deposit only after the initial monolayer adsorption was nearly complete. Desorption of the IgG molecules in a distilled water medium was not observed.

Introduction

Some of the more common methods[1] to study proteins at interfaces are radiolabelling, ellipsometry, total internal reflectance fluorescence (TIRF), infrared (IR), Raman, and X-ray photoelectron (XPS) spectroscopies, and scanning electron microscopy (SEM). While each of these techniques is capable of providing critical information regarding the adsorbed species, this information is actually a measure of the average properties of all the adsorbed proteins in a micron sized (or greater) area.

No technique is available with which to characterize individual adsorbed proteins. In addition, SEM and XPS are normally used in a vacuum environment which is radically different from an aqueous one in which protein adsorption is occurring. So, the information may not be representative of the actual events. The atomic force microscope (AFM), however, can be operated in an aqueous environment and is capable of providing real time images of protein adsorption with a resolution sufficient to see individual molecules.

The AFM[2] can be used to obtain atomic scale images of surfaces[3-7]. The surface to be imaged is mounted onto a (xyz) piezoelectric crystal and is rastered beneath a sharp tip attached to a cantilever. The tip rides across the surface and the forces between the surface and the tip cause deflection of the cantilever. This deflection can be monitored using a scanning tunneling tip[2,3] or more easily, it can be monitored by movement of a laser beam that is reflected off the back of the cantilever [8,9]. Since the cantilever is sensitive to the intermolecular forces between the tip and the surface, the sample need not be a conductor to be imaged. Images have not only been obtained from graphite[3-5] and metals[6], but also from semiconductors[4,7] and insulating polymers[10-12]. Magnetic fields[13] and charged regions in materials[14] have been imaged as well. More detailed reviews of the AFM theory are presented by Marti et al. and Hansma et al.[15,16].

The AFM has already been used to image surfaces in an aqueous environment[17]. Underwater images of crystalline mica and polyalanine on mica have been obtained. One advantage of using water as a scanning medium is the minimization of general adhesion forces that result between the tip and the surface[18]. Such forces dominate the interaction between the tip and the sample and prohibits the possibility of obtaining high-resolution images. In addition, scanning surfaces in aqueous environments enables one to realistically image biological systems. The AFM can obtain new images within a few seconds and can therefore monitor biological processes in real time. Recently, Hansma et al.[17] were able to follow the formation of a polymerized fibrin network on a mica surface by adding thrombin to a solution of fibrinogen. These images showed fibrin oligomers aggregating to form a single polymer strand. Formation of additional strands occurred adjacent to first.

This paper discusses the images obtained from the adsorption of a murine anti-fluorescyl monoclonal immunoglobulin G (4-4-20 IgG_2 (κ))[19] from solution onto clean mica surfaces. This protein was chosen because it is easily crystallized and has self-aggregating properties. We hoped that some unique ordering upon adsorption to the mica surface might occur and, if so, this ordering could be imaged with the AFM. We felt that desorption could be observed as well.

Methods

The AFM experimental apparatus has already been described and can be found elsewhere[16]. Movement of the microfabricated cantilever[20] is detected by the positioning of a laser light beam that has reflected off the back of the cantilever and is detected by a pair of photodiodes. The AFM images are continuously recorded on video tape for later review. A flow cell has been set-up across the surface of the mica that allows rapid exchange of the fluid.

Mica (Asheville-Schoonmaker) was affixed to the piezoelectric crystal stage and cleaved *in situ.* The flow cell was constructed around the stage and distilled water was injected onto the mica surface. The microcantilever was advanced until the force between the tip and the surface approximated 10^{-9} N. The mica was then imaged continuously in the feedback mode with a scan area of 1800 Å by 1800 Å and a constant scan speed of 16 msec/line.

The AFM tip was retracted from the mica surface and a solution of 18 µg/mL IgG 4-4-20 (a gift from J. N. Herron) in phosphate buffered saline (pH 7.4) was injected into the flow cell. The tip was advanced to the mica surface which was then imaged continuously in the feedback mode over a scan area of 1800 Å by 1800 Å. After 4 minutes, the scan area was increased to 4500 Å by 4500 Å (full scale). After another 1 1/2 minutes, the AFM was switched to variable force mode for the remainder of the imaging[21]. The adsorption process was imaged continuously for 40 minutes. During this time, the scan area was decreased to 1800 Å by 1800 Å, to 900 Å by 900 Å, and then returned to full scale.

Immediately after the 40 minute IgG adsorption, the tip was retracted and the flow cell was flushed with distilled water. The surface was scanned for 10 minutes at full scale, at 1800 Å by 1800 Å, and then at 900 Å by 900 Å.

Results

The image obtained of the mica surface underwater is flat and featureless indicating a pristine surface.

Within the first two minutes after injection of the IgG into the flow cell, a continuously growing aggregate was observed in the lower right-hand corner of the screen. This image was obtained in feedback mode and had dimensions of 1800 Å by 1800 Å. This aggregate appeared on top of the featureless mica background. After five minutes, the scan area was increased to 4500 Å by 4500 Å and 'ridges' appeared (A). The AFM was then switched to variable force mode (B) and and the same image appeared (different contrast) indicating that either mode could be used. As time progressed, it was clear how the adsorption was taking place. Molecules that landed adjacent to these ridges would adhere resulting in two-dimensional growth in the plane of the surface (C). Yet most molecules that landed by themselves would desorb readily as evidenced by the disappearance of these isolated molecules. The size of these molecules roughly matched the known size of an IgG molecule. The deposited IgG appeared as mounds and subsequent frames showed smearing of these images.

The ridges continued to spread (D,E) along the surface until a monolayer covered the surface of the mica. Although it is difficult to obtain accurate height dimension in variable force mode, the monolayer thickness was approximated at 50 Å, which is consistent with the dimensions of an IgG molecule. Near the end of the monolayer formation, a second layer started to appear. This second layer arose from many different sites on the first layer since protein interactions could occur from anywhere on the surface (F). Upon growth of the second layer, most IgG

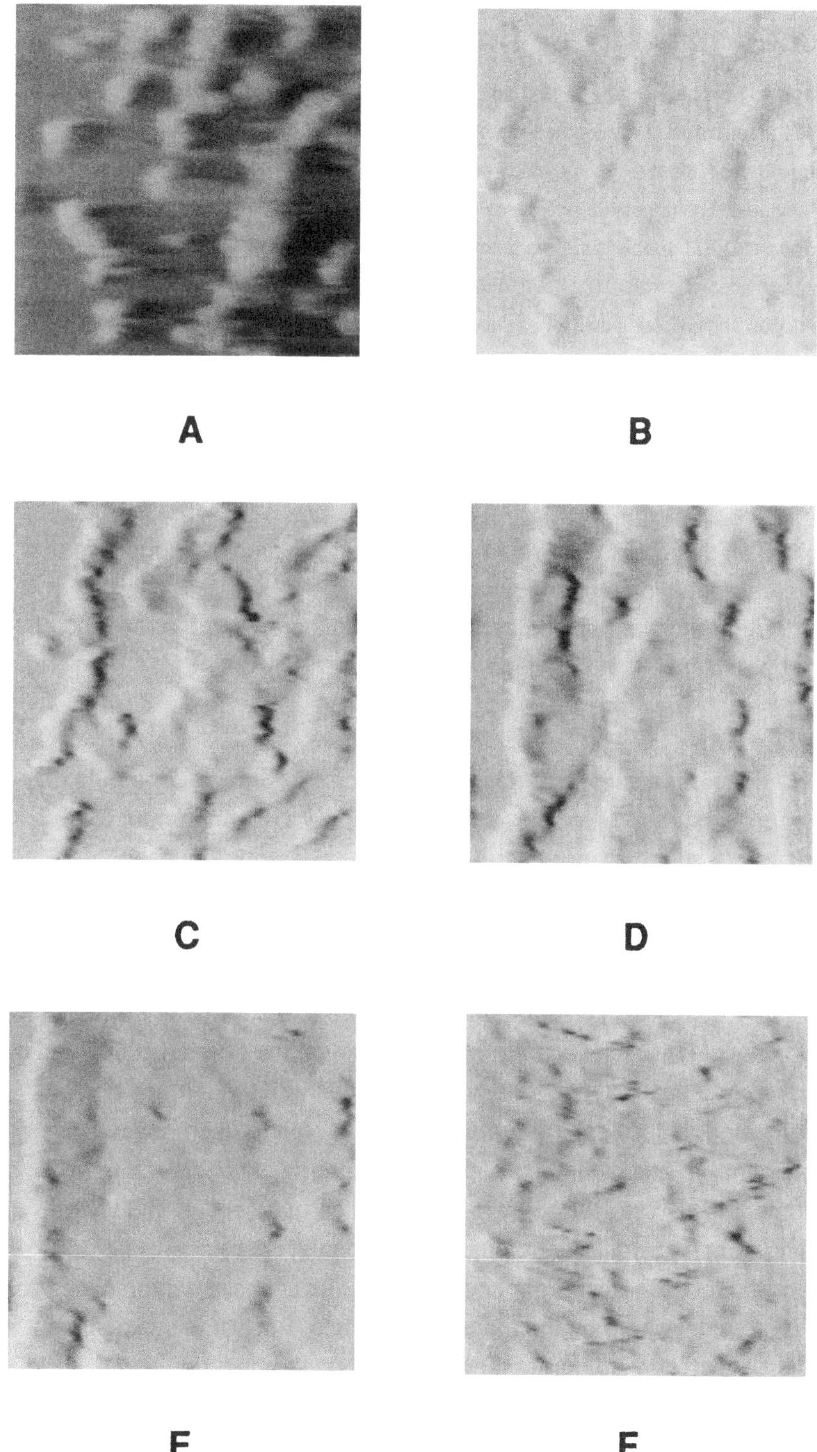
A
B
C
D
E
F

Image A. Feedback image of 18 μg/mL IgG 4-4-20 in PBS on clean mica after 5 minutes. Note the formation of aggregate 'ridges'. The scan area is 4500 Å by 4500 Å.
Image B. Variable force mode image of 18 μg/mL IgG 4-4-20 in PBS on clean mica after 5 1/2 minutes. The ridges are now resolved better. The scan area is 4500 Å by 4500 Å.
Images C,D,E. Variable force mode images of 18 μg/mL IgG 4-4-20 in PBS on clean mica. Times of adsorption are 15, 17 1/2, and 20 minutes. Growth of the monolayer centers about the ridges and proceeds until a near monolayer is formed. The scan areas are 4500 Å by 4500 Å.
Image F. Variable force mode image of 18 μg/mL IgG 4-4-20 in PBS on clean mica. Adsorption time is 37 minutes. After a near complete monolayer is formed, a second layer begins to deposit. The scan area is 4500 Å by 4500 Å.

molecules that deposited would adhere, but then smear, suggestive of a rapid conformational change.

After the water flush, the surface exhibited altered features, but there was no evidence that IgG desorption was taking place.

Discussion

The observations of deposited IgG on the surface appearing only as aggregates and of individual mounds rapidly desorbing from the surface are suggestive of lateral interactions occurring between the adjacent IgG molecules, which appear to be important for formation of a stable protein layer. These lateral interactions are not unexpected, since this protein has some self-aggregating properties. What is interesting is the necessity of lateral interactions for adherence to the surface. Perhaps, an IgG molecule by itself can only get a toe-hold on the surface at first and can be desorbed easily. Once it has multiple holds with the surface and neighboring molecules, the probability of desorption decreases significantly[1]. This would explain the phenomena we observed here. This argument is also supported by the observation of a second IgG layer arising from many different areas on the monolayer surface. Here, the deposited IgG can arise from any number of places, since interactions can occur from anywhere on the monolayer surface. Prior to this experiment , a protein adsorption isotherm on mica was obtained using ^{125}I-labelled IgG.

The isotherm showed Langmuir-like behavior and at a concentration of 18 µg/mL, the mica surface was only 40% covered (less than a monolayer).

After the water flush, IgG desorption was not observed. Perhaps, desorption was slower than the observation time (minutes) due to the strength of interaction between the adjacent IgG molecules. Previous data has shown[22] that IgG does desorb from a silica surface, but that study was performed using polyclonal IgG and may behave differently from the present system.

Certainly, these observations were not solely a consequence of simple adsorption phenomena. A number of times, protein mounds would be displaced parallel to the rapid scanning direction only to be returned to its original position upon subsequent images. It is clear that the tip of the probe is 'massaging' or pushing the molecules on the surface. The extent to which this occurs, however, is not known and any conclusions can only be made keeping this in mind. For example, maybe the formation of aggregates results from the probe pushing the molecules over to a small cluster of molecules. The probe may not be able to displace this cluster laterally because of the strength of interaction it has with the surface and can only 'hop' over it. In this manner, the probe may behave as a gathering device which sweeps the molecules into piles. This phenomena may explain the discrepancy between the AFM images and the isotherm data. In addition, the desorption of individual molecules from the surface may be a result of tip interaction. Thus, the probe may sweep these molecules off the surface as well.

The authors would like to emphasize that this experiment is a preliminary one done at one protein concentration. The effect of concentration on the adsorption pattern is yet unknown, but is the subject of ongoing studies. Furthermore, the issue of protein adsorption on the probe itself was not addressed here. This issue is important and merits further detailed study and consideration.

Conclusion

Using an atomic force microscope, real time imaging of IgG deposition on flat mica was accomplished. While IgG adsorption may occur anywhere on the surface, only those molecules with sufficient lateral interactions had the capability to remain on the surface. Isolated molecules desorb readily. A second layer could be observed after 35 minutes of adsorption. It was hoped that unique ordering of the IgG on the surface could be visible, but this was not evident. Although, restructuring of the surface had occurred in the desorption experiment, desorption was not conclusive.

While it is exciting that individual molecules could occasionally be seen, it is not clear how much the probe affects molecular conformation. When more sensitive cantilevers and more sophisticated detection systems are developed, it may be possible to operate the AFM using forces of 10^{-10} to 10^{-11} N and image biomolecules unperturbed by the probe.

Acknowledgements:

We thank J. N. Herron for supplying the IgG, Y. S. Lin for surface preparation, and C. Prater and A. Weisenhorn for assistance in conducting this experiment. We also thank A. Pungor, C-Z Hu, and S. Mohanty for assistance and helpful discussions. This work was supported by the Center for Biopolymers at Interfaces, NIH Grant HL 37046 and the Office of Naval Research.

References

1. Andrade, J. D. In *Surface and Interfacial Aspects of Biomedical Polymers*; Andrade J. D. Ed.; Plenum Press: New York, 1985; Vol. 2, pp. 1-80.
2. Binnig, G.; Quate, C. F.; Gerber, Ch. *Phys. Rev. Lett.* **1986**,*56,* 930-3.
3. Binnig, G.; Gerber, Ch.; Stoll, E.; Albrecht, T. R.; Quate, C. F. *Europhys. Lett.* **1987**, *3,* 1281-7.
4. Albrecht, T. R.; Quate, C. F. *J. Appl. Phys.,***1987**, *62*, 2599-602.
5. Marti, O.; Drake, B.; Hansma, P.K. *Appl. Phys. Lett.* **1987**, *51*, 484-6.
6. Alexander, S.; Hellemans, L.; Marti, O.; Schneir, J.; Elings, V.; Hansma, P. K.; Longmire, M.; Gurley, J. *J. Appl. Phys.* **1989**, *65*, 164-7.
7. Kirk, M. D.; Albrecht, T. R.; Quate, C. F. *Rev. Sci. Instrum.* **1988**, *59*, 833-5.

8. Amer, N. M.; Meyer, G. *Bull. Am. Phys. Soc.* **1988**, *33*, 319.
9. Meyer, G.; Amer, N. M. *Appl. Phys. Lett.* **1988**, *53*, 1045-7.
10. Albrecht, T. R.; Dovek, M. M.; Lang, C. A.; Grütter, P.; Quate, C. F.; Kuan, S. W. J.; Frank, C. W.; Pease, R. F. W. *J. Appl. Phys.* **1988**, *64*, 1178-84.
11. Marti, O.; Ribi, H. O.; Drake, B.; Albrecht, T. R.; Quate, C. F.; Hansma, P. K*Science* **1988**, *239*, 50-2.
12. Gould, S.; Marti, O.; Drake, B.; Hellemans, L.; Bracker, C. E.; Hansma, P. K.; Keder, N. L.; Eddy, M. M.; Stucky, G. D. *Nature* **1988**, *332*, 332-4.
13. Martin, Y.; Wickramasinghe, H. K. *Appl. Phys. Lett.* **1987**, *50*, 1455-7.
14. Stern, J. E.; Terris, B. D.; Mamin, H. J.; Rugar, D. *Appl. Phys. Lett.* **1988**, *53*, 2717-9.
15. Marti, O.; Gould, S.; Hansma, P. K. *Rev. Sci. Instrum.* **1988**, *56*, 836-9.
16. Hansma, P. K.; Elings, V. B.; Marti, O.; Bracker, C. E. *Science* **1988**, *242*, 209-16.
17. Drake, B.; Prater, C. B.; Weisenhorn, A. L.; Gould, S. A. C.; Albrecht, T. R.; Quate, C. F.; Cannell, D. S.; Hansma, H. G.; Hansma, P. K. *Science* **1989**, *243*, 1586-9.
18. Weisenhorn, A. L.; Hansma, P. K.; Albrecht, T. R.; Quate, C. F. *Appl. Phys. Lett.* **1989**, *54*, 2651-3.
19. Gibson, A. L.; Herron, J. N.; He, X.-M.; Patrick, V. A.; Mason, M. L.; Lin, J.-N.; Kranz, D. M.; Voss, Jr., E. W.; Edmundson, A. B. *Proteins* **1988**, *3*, 155-60.
20. Albrecht, T. R.; Quate, C. F. *J. Vac. Sci. Technol.* **1988**, *A 6*, 271-4.
21. Variable force mode for an AFM is analogous to constant height mode for an STM. Hansma, P. K.; Tersoff, J. *J. Appl. Phys.* **1989**, *61*, R1-R23.
22. Hlady, V.; Van Wagenen, R. A.; Andrade, J. D. In *Surface and Interfacial Aspects of Biomedical Polymers*; Andrade J. D. Ed.; Plenum Press: New York, 1985; Vol. 2, pp. 81-119.

19

A Comparison of Three Thermal Sensors Based on Fiber Optics and Polymer Films for Biosensor Applications

Raymond Dessy, Larry Arney,
Lloyd Burgess, and Eric Richmond

Virginia Polytechnic Institute and State University
Chemistry Department, Blacksburg, Virginia 24061

Three novel thermal sensors for biosensor applications are described. Two of these employ fiber optic interferometers, the other uses piezo/pyroelectric polyvinylidene fluoride films. The strengths and weaknesses of each system are explored and applications to urease, catalase, and metal catalyzed reaction systems are described.

INTRODUCTION

Biosensors based on the heat produced by enzyme/substrate reactions have traditionally used microcalorimeters (1), thermistors (2), and Peltier or other macro devices (3,4). The area has been reviewed by Guilbault (5). The size, response time, and thermal mass of these detectors suggest that thermally responsive microsensors based on modern technologies need to be explored.

This article examines three types of new temperature sensitive transducer systems suitable for biosensors. In each case the approach employs a substrate that can respond to the temperature generated by a catalyzed reaction occurring on the surface of the sensing device. A number of important criteria must be met in a useful thermal biosensor; (A) the device must be extremely sensitive to temperature, (B) it must be pressure insensitive, (C) the final system must respond to small samples, and involve low dead-volume in a flow cell, (D) the sensing device must be chemically inert with respect to biological samples, (E) it must not degrade under normal chemical operating conditions, and (F) it must be rugged and inexpensive.

Following are reports on (A) a pyroelectric sensor based on poly(vinylidene fluoride) films, (B) a two-arm Mach-Zehnder interferometer based on monomode fiber optics, and (C) a single arm fiber optic interferometer based on a birefringent optical fiber.

A. POLYMER FILM BASED ENTHALPIMETER

Modern flow systems place unusual constraints on sensor configuration. Rugged, inexpensive sensors that can easily adapt to the geometries and inherent pressure pulses imposed by FIA systems are essential. It is of interest to explore the possibility of fabricating a useful enthalpimetric sensor from films of piezo and pyroelectric (6) organic polymers. These materials are thin enough that simple cutting and molding allow the sensor material to conform to the required geometry of the sample cell, rather than designing the cell geometry around a fixed sensor. The films are inexpensive, and available from several sources.

Piezo and pyroelectric materials are derived from substances with non-centrosymmetric crystal lattices. The seven groups of crystal lattices occurring in nature are comprised of some 32 classes possessing characteristic symmetry elements. Chemists would be familiar with these in terms of the point groups to which molecules are assigned based on the planes and axes of symmetry that they contain. Of these 32 classes of crystal structures, all show electrostriction; changes in dimension upon application of an electrical field. However, these changes are insensitive to field polarity.

Some 20 classes may exhibit piezoelectric characteristics, and of these a subset of ten may show pyroelectric behaviour. The requirement for either effect is that one of the crystal axes must have "polarity". This term defines the property of being able to develop a charge distribution with a predetermined orientation upon application of a stress that is either pressure (piezoelectricity) or temperature (pyroelectricity).

If only one of the major crystal axes is polar the material may be pyroelectric; if more than one is polar the material may be piezoelectric. Thus all potential pyroelectric materials are also potentially piezoelectric. Whether a material shows either of these effects to a useful degree depends on the magnitude of the induced charge distributions that result from pressure or heat.

Pyroelectricity is often complicated by contributions that may be elicited by (A) primary pyroelectricity described above, (B) an electrostrictive effect that causes a piezoelectric lattice distortion giving rise to what is often called secondary pyroelectric effects, and (C) the application of non-uniform temperature gradients along a crystal axis which gives rise to tertiary pyroelectric effects. In practice all three may be significant contributors to the overall pyroelectric effect observed.

Polyvinylidene fluoride (PVDF) films, ranging in thickness from a few microns to a millimeter, can be made piezo- and pyroelectric by special treatment after manufacture (7). The materials are simultaneously subjected to an increased temperature, elongation stress along one or two axes, and a high DC field potential. As the material is allowed to cool, with the stress and electrical field applied, orientation effects occur that result in a residual polarization of the film, rendering it piezo/pyroelectric.

Chemically, charge injection probably occurs during this process. Physically, alignment of the electronegative fluorine atoms associated with the CF bonds toward the positive pole occurs, leading to a large amount of beta phase PVDF which forms crystallites. There is some controversy about the actual phenomena involved in the observed piezo/pyroelectricity, and several effects may be concurrently responsible (8-11). Such materials show electrostriction. The Poisson ratio of the films is high (differential axial thermal coefficients of expansion). Finally, the crystallite concentration is temperature dependent. Regardless of the source, the films find application in sonar transducers, audio speakers, and microphones because of their piezoelectric behaviour. Their pyroelectric properties have led to imaging device applications.

In principle a biosensor could be fabricated from the material by immobilizing an enzyme on one surface, and flowing a substrate solution past the film sensor. A simple charge amplifier might be used to measure the difference between the two surfaces of the sensor. In turn, this could be related to concentration. In practice a somewhat different approach needs to be taken.

INSTRUMENT DESIGN

Films of PVDF 40 microns thick from Solvay were used throughout most of the study. These films have a thin metal coating that is vapor deposited on each surface to facilitate the electric field orientation process. This coating may also be used to make electrical contact for sensor applications. For the present studies these films were configured as a bimorph, or double laminate, by placing like surfaces of two pieces of film face-to-face. The bimorph was pressure mounted in an FIA flow cell made of Plexiglas (Figure 1). The intent of the bimorph architecture is to partially eliminate piezoelectric effects that occur from the mounting process and pressure surges that

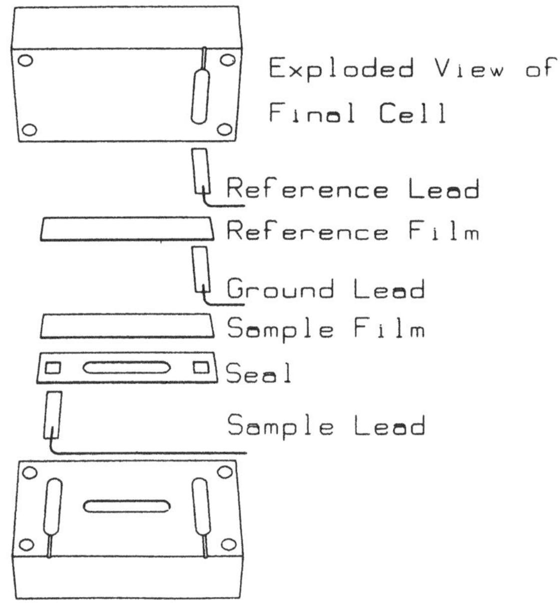

1. Exploded view of polyvinylidene fluoride film based enthalpimeter.

occur during sample flow, to reduce electromagnetic interference, and to help compensate for ambient temperature changes.

The bimorph has three electrical points of contact; the mating interior surfaces of the bimorph, and the two exterior surfaces. The interior surfaces shared a common ground. The other surfaces provided a contact for a reference and sample side. The sample side formed the floor of a flow channel that was machined into the Plexiglas mount. The channel was 25mm x 5mm x 0.5mm. The enzyme was immobilized onto the roof of the channel using stand-

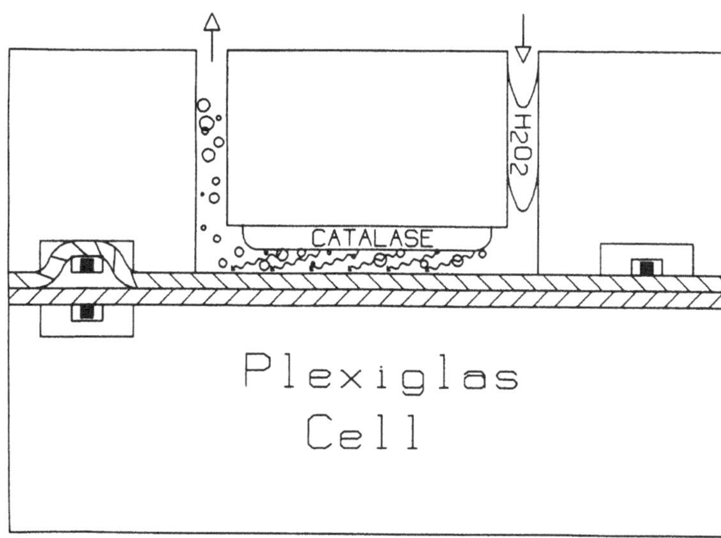

2. Cross-section of polyvinylidene fluoride film based enthalpimeter.

ard gluturaldehyde copolymerization procedures (Figure 2). Attempts at placing the enzyme directly onto the sample film surface led to poorer response, both in signal level and noise level. This is presumably due to the poor thermal transport characteristics of the hydrated biopolymer.

The signals from the sample and reference surfaces were first buffered via the non-inverting inputs of two electrometers, AD515s, which had very high input impedance and low input bias currents. The output of the two electrometers were used as inputs to an instrument amplifier, AD625. Output from the instrument amplifier was digitized with a 25 usec successive approximation ADC, and noise reduced by use of a 21-point Savitzky-Golay weighted digital filter (12). Several approaches to quantization were made. The best results were obtained by simple peak height measurements. All control and manipulation software was written in PolyForth. The computer was a DEC LSI-11 attached to the laboratory network.

RESULTS AND DISCUSSION

The peroxide/catalase system was selected for study. The FIA carrier contained Triton-X as a surface active agent to reduce bubble formation. Typical FIA flow characteristics were 4 ml/min, and a sample loop of 80 uL. Typical sensor output is shown in Figure 3. The calibration curve developed for the peroxide/catalase system is linear from

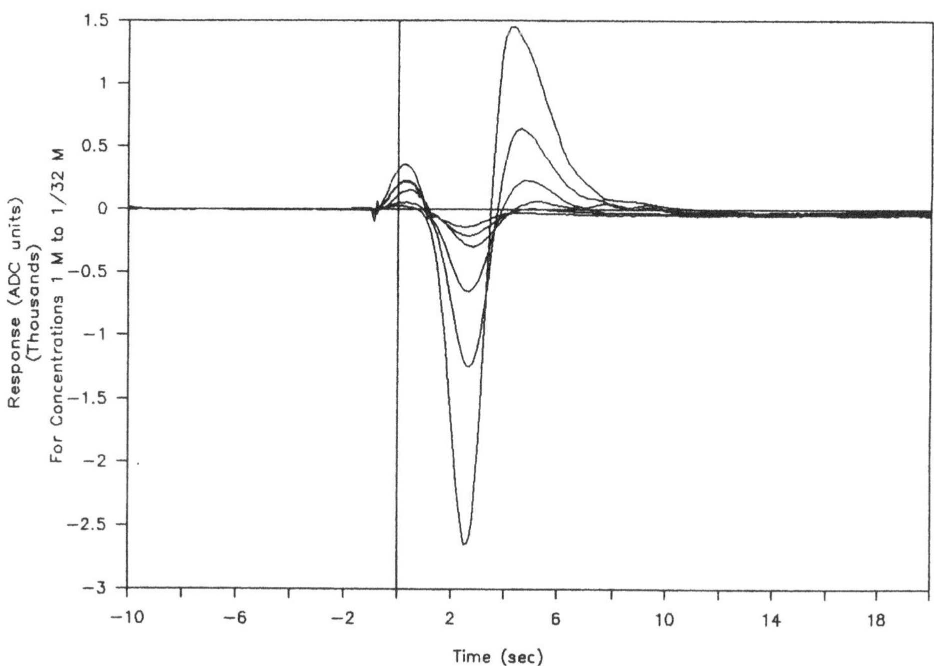

3. Polymer film enthalpimeter output for various concentrations of hydrogen peroxide passing over a catalase bed immobilized on the roof of the flow channel.

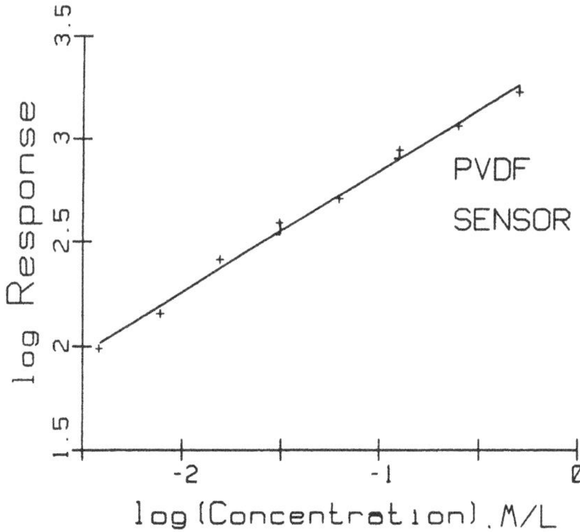

4. Typical calibration curves for a polymer film enthalpimeter using the peroxide/catalase system.

0.005M to 1.0M (Figure 4). The error bars shown in the calibration curve were calculated by multiplying the standard deviation by the 95% confidence limit for a set of data with four degrees of freedom. The correlation coefficient of the line is 0.995.

The thermal flux from the enzyme/substrate reaction crosses the aqueous layer and rapidly diffuses through the 200 Angstrom thick aluminum coating on the top layer of the bimorph. Modelling of the heat transport within the film, to be published elsewhere, shows that the thermal transport process may be treated as a semi-infinite solid; i.e., an infinitely thick solid with one surface. This is reasonable since the PVDF and Plexiglas have quite similar heat transfer properties, with the thermal diffusivity of Plexiglas being somewhat higher. The model produces thermal time gradients in agreement with those experimentally observed, and satisfactorily predict the timing and amplitude of the phase change observed as the thermal boundary passes from one layer of the bimorph to the other.

The shape of each response curve is easily explained. There is an initial small "upward going" excursion that is caused by piezoelectric effects within the film resulting from the pressure surge in the stream injected by the FIA valve switching process. As this pressure surge passes the sensor the amplifier output returns to baseline. This peak, which is artificially broadened by the Savitzky-

Golay filter, can serve the same function as the air peak in a GC trace. Subsequently, as the thermal front generated by the chemical reaction moves into the first layer of the bimorph that layer becomes hotter than the reference side, and a "downward going" excursion is observed. As the thermal diffusion process continues a point is reached where both films of the bimorph are the same temperature, and a "zero-crossing" occurs. Then the reference film becomes warmer than the sample film, as the latter is cooled by the flowing FIA stream, causing an "upward going" excursion. Finally, both film layers return to ambient temperature, and the output of the amplifier returns toward zero baseline. The pyroelectric signal can be enhanced by placing a thermal insulator between the bimorph layers. However, this results in a concomitant increase in the piezoelectric noise contribution and the observed S/N ratio does not improve.

The poly(vinylidene fluoride) pyroelectric sensor has interesting potential. It is easy to build, and involves inexpensive support electronics. On the other hand, to achieve modest sensitivity one must use a detector with a rather large surface area. The piezoelectric response of the device contributes a large amount of noise to the temperature signal. This can be partially compensated by bimorph construction, or could be achieved by running side-by-side sample and reference detector systems.

Unpublished studies have explored this route (13). However, the large piezoelectric component to the signal in flowing streams will always be a problem. Finally, the metal coatings on the commercial films used in this study degrade under exposure to biological buffer conditions.

B. A TWO-ARM FIBER OPTIC-BASED ENTHALPIMETER

Although there is currently great interest in the application of fiber optics as chemical sensors most of these applications have involved the extrinsic properties of the waveguide materials. In these applications the fibers are used as light pipes for the conduction of guided optical waves employed in absorbance and fluorescence measurements. However, changes in the intrinsic properties of such fibers offers a new realm for the development of microsensors. Such phenomena have been investigated by physicists in their development of acoustic, magnetic, thermal, and pressure sensors (13-16). Following is a report on the successful application of this approach to a biosensor based on a two arm fiber optic thermal sensor.

The instrument, Figure 5b, involves a two-arm Mach-Zehnder interferometer constructed from mono-mode fiber optic waveguides. One arm of the interferometer is coated with an immobilized enzyme, while the other is used as a reference. Both arms of the interferometer are firmly

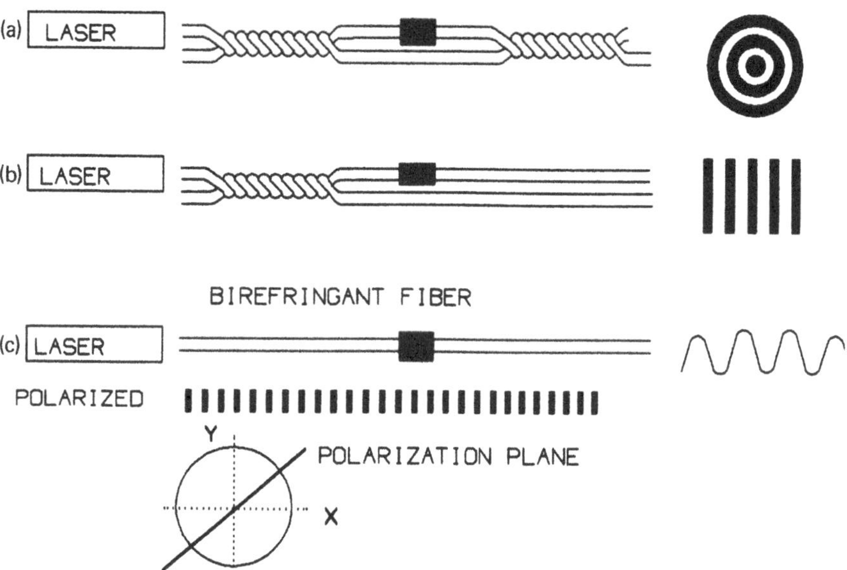

5. Three types of interferometers constructed from optical fibers: (a) Mach-Zehnder, (b) an interferometer based on Young's dual slit principle similar to the one reported on in this article, and (c) a single arm interferometer based on a birefringent fiber, also discussed in this article.

held in the middle of a conduit that is incorporated into a flow injection analysis (FIA) system, serving as a substitute for the normal absorbance, fluorescence, pH, or electrochemical detectors.

An inexpensive He/Ne laser source of phase coherent light is used to launch a beam down both arms of the interferometer. The exit beams from both fibers are superimposed in the far field on a linear photodiode array optical detector. This superposition produces the classical two-slit pattern of light and dark bars due to interference. As sample boluses containing substrates specific to the enzyme pass the sensing area, heat is produced around one fiber. This heat, partitioned between the flowing stream and the fiber, produces a thermal and stress/strain effect on the coated fiber which changes its light propagation characteristics. Although shifts in the resulting bar pattern can be detected by a single optical detector, a linear array has many advantages. If an integral number of periods of the bar pattern, n, illuminate the active area of the array a Fourier transform of the data from the scanned array will produce a new real and imaginary data set. The ratio of the real and imaginary values at the spacial frequency n yields the phase angle difference between the two beams and simultaneously eliminates noise contamination since this is commonly found at other spacial frequencies. The phase angle difference can be related to sample concentration.

INSTRUMENT DESIGN

An inexpensive Spectra-Physics Model 120 HeNe laser was used as a source of coherent radiation. This radiation was equally divided between the two arms of the interferometer by use of a 3 dB coupler (18). This was constructed from two lengths of ITT T-1601 single mode optical communication fiber. This fiber exhibits a numerical aperture of 0.10 and will operate at single-mode propagation down to 580 nm. These fibers have an outer sheath of DuPont Hytrel 7246, and an inner sheath of General Electric RTV 615 (Figure 6). These may be stripped off by mechanical and chemical means in the coupler area. The residual glass fiber consists of a 4 micron core surrounded by an 80 micron glass cladding. If the two fibers are twisted together under tension the outer cladding can be largely stripped away in an HF bath. This stripping is continued until about 50% of the light launched down one fiber evanescently couples into its companion waveguide. Standard fiber positioners and microscope objectives may be used to deploy these fiber optic components.

Downstream, the unstripped sections of fiber were held in a Plexiglas channel 20mm x 1mm x 1mm in dimension.

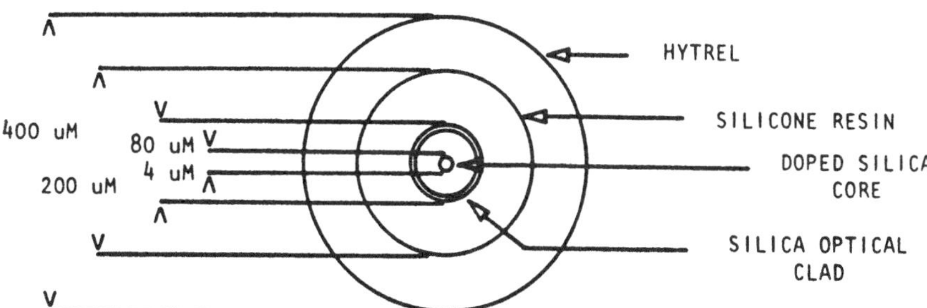

6. Cross-section of ITT T-1601 optical fiber

One arm of the interferometer was coated over a 10mm length with the desired enzyme immobilized in a gluteraldehyde copolymer (5, 19). The channel was covered with a Plexiglas plate and the fiber entrances sealed with RTV silicone. The channel was incorporated in a FIA system.

The exit beams of the two arms were optically combined onto the surface of a Reticon S-series 512 element linear array. A Reticon RC-1024SA interface board provided signal control, clocks, and integrate/sample-hold circuitry for the processing of the pulse packets emerging from the common video line of the detector chip. A 25 usec successive approximation analog-to-digital converter (ADC) was used to digitize this data stream. Each data set was subjected to Fourier transform using software extracted from Digital Equipment Corporation's Laboratory Applications package. All other control and data manipulation was written in PolyForth (Forth, Inc.). The computer was a DEC LSI-11 connected to a laboratory network hosted by PDP-11/23's.

Purified enzymes were obtained from Sigma Chemicals; catalase (E.C.1.11.1.6) and urease (E.C.3.5.1.5). They were immobilized on the fiber using gluteraldehyde (Fisher). Phosphate buffers (0.1 M) were used for fiber storage and as carriers in the FIA system. Thymol (50 mg/L) was used to inhibit bacterial and fungal growth in the buffer.

RESULTS AND DISCUSSIONS

Changes in the light propagation characteristics of a fiber due to temperature arise from (A) thermally induced length changes, (B) the temperature dependence of the core refractive index, and (C) elasto-optic changes in the core due to thermally induced stress/strain changes.

Plots of phase angle difference in the interferometer arms vs. time are related to heat-production vs. time, and this in turn is related to the concentration of the species responsible for heat production. Typical instrument output for the urea/urease system is shown in Figure 7.

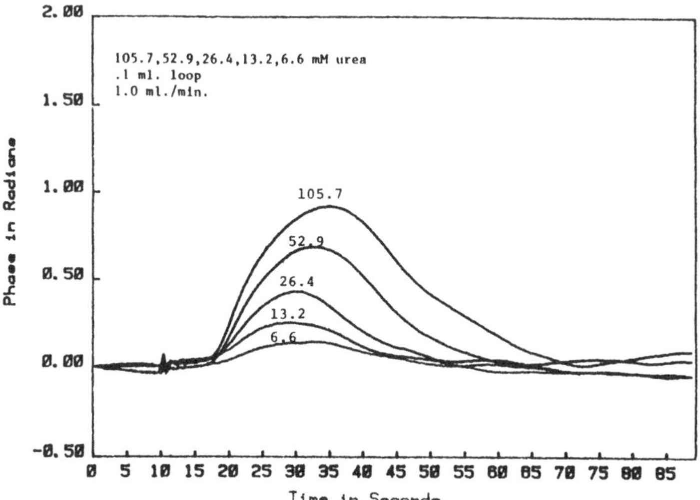

7. Interferometer output for various urea concentrations passing over a urease bed immobilized on one arm.

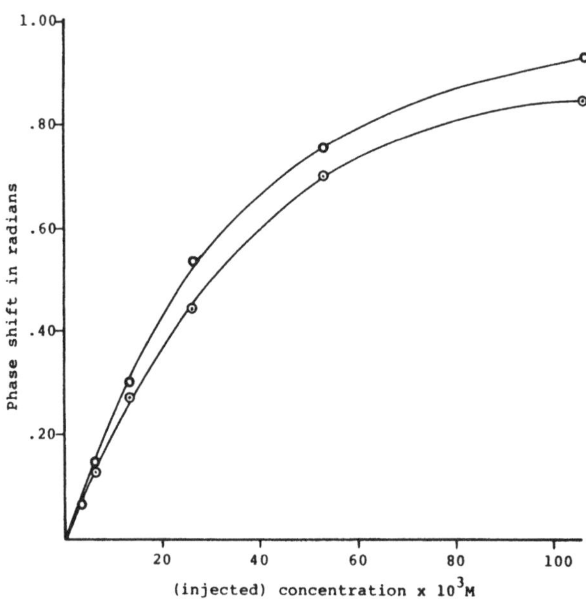

8. Calibration curve for urea/urease system at 0.8 and 1.0 ml/min.

Calibration curves can be constructed as shown in Figure 8. The system is reasonably sensitive. Minimum detectable levels of urea are 5 mM. Over extended time periods (7 days) the relative standard deviation at 5 mM concentrations is better than 5%. The optimum FIA conditions were around 1.0 ml/min flow rate, with a sample loop of 0.1-0.25 ml.

Detailed modelling studies on heat transport in such systems, to be published elsewhere, are easy to develop since the thermal conductivity, thermal diffusivity, and the heat capacities of the various fiber components are known. The stress/strain effects are almost completely asserted in a thin surface layer of the Hytrel, because of the poor conductivity of this sheath, and the underlying viscoelastic insulating RTV layer. However, Hytrel has an extremely high thermal expansion modulus, which helps compensate for this deficiency (15). The jacketing does protect the detector system from effects due to interaction of the evanescent field, associated with the guided wave, with the environment due to absorbance or refractive index changes in the solution. The response time of the system is limited by the insulating characteristics of the jacket materials. Obvious extensions of the concept would involve different jacket configurations to enhance the stress/strain action, and/or coating with aluminum to enhance heat transport to the fiber surface. Simple calculations show that about half of the generated heat is lost to the surrounding water medium in the present configuration.

Studies on the peroxide/catalase system yielded response curves with poorly defined maxima, and badly drifting base lines. The source is presumably the bubbles of gaseous oxygen produced by the reaction. These develop in the later stages of the reaction. Clinging to the fiber, these bubbles apparently result in mechanical and/or thermal effects that distort the expected profile.

Although the addition of surface active agents (ethoxylated lauryl alcohol) moderates the distortion and improves base line performance, the ill-defined peaks did not respond to peak-height or area measurements. The peaks were broad, did not return to any reliable base line position, and were typified by low signal/noise ratios. It proved impossible to derive consistent area or height information from repeat runs using either visual methods, or standard peak-picking algorithms. Reliable quantitative calibration curves could only be derived from evaluation of the slope of the phase angle difference curve as a function of time at a fixed arbitrary point near the beginning of the heat evolution.

These fiber optic sensor systems are extremely sensitive to environmental noise. Pneumatically supported optical tables were required. Pressure fronts developed from droplets falling from the exit of the FIA tubing are easily sensed by the interferometer. Care is required in mounting the fibers in the FIA channel. Diminished response, or even inversion of the signal response, is easily induced by improper tensioning. The radial and axial stresses resulting from the fixing of the two ends of the sensor area within the flow-cell compete with the heat induced stresses. Heat may subsequently increase or decrease the total signal observed. The manufacture of reproducible fiber detector heads is a difficult task.

C. A ONE ARM FIBER OPTIC BASED INTERFEROMETER

The two arm Mach-Zehnder type interferometer described above is extremely sensitive to both pressure and temperature. Unfortunately, in many chemical applications the two are hard to decouple and separate. Flow injection analysis is a good example. Even with the best of care pump oriented systems have pressure pulses in the stream that easily mask temperature effects. Even pumpless systems are prone to pressure pulses created as drops of liquid fall from the end of the waste tubing. These are large enough to elicit a response from a two arm interferometer.

It is possible to build a fiber optic interferometer that only employs a single arm (Figure 5c), and experiments have been undertaken to explore this avenue, with the goal being the development of a temperature sensitive, but pressure insensitive detector. The basic concept involves two guided waves in the same fiber which permit compensation for isotropic pressure changes around the fiber. In addition it is possible to configure these sensors in such a way that source intensity flucuations are not important.

Conventional fiber optic waveguides have a refractive index profile across their face that is centrosymmetric. It is possible, using very clever chemistry, to construct a fiber in which the refractive index profile is different along the two Cartesian axes meeting at the fiber's center point. Such fibers demonstrate the phenomenon of birefringence, and allow what loosley might be called a "sample" and "reference" beam to share the same fiber.

These "bow-tie" fibers (Figure 9) are manufactured by beginning with a conventional fluorophosphate doped glass tube blank. The inner surface of this tube is successively layered with different materials that eventually create the bow-tie refractive index profile shown in Figure 9. First, a layer of heavily boron oxide doped glass is laid down. This will eventually become the bow-

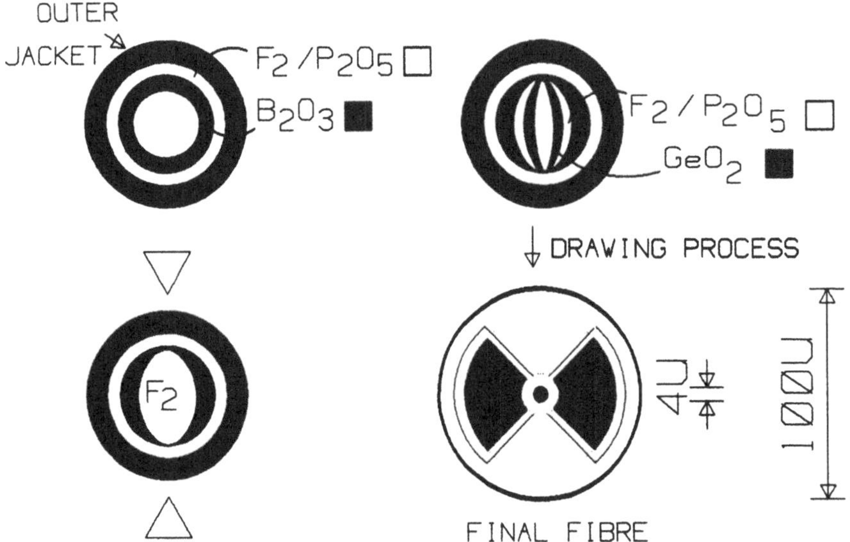

9. Construction of a "bow-tie" fiber.

tie, a characteristically shaped section of higher refractive index glass. At this point the inner cylinder of boron oxide doped glass is chemically machined so that its exposed surface is ellipsoidal in shape. This is done by passing fluorine into the tube, and heating the tube from the outside at opposite points on the surface. The thermally induced etching process leaves the desired ovoidal shape. Then a layer of fluorophosphate glass, and finally a germanium oxide doped glass layer are laid down. The latter eventually becomes the very high refractive index core. The tube is then collapsed under high temperature and pulled in a drawing tower to produce a monomode birefringent fiber optic. The core is 4 micron in diameter, and the total diameter of the unjacketed fiber is 125 micron.

INSTRUMENT DESIGN

If a beam of plane-polarized coherent light is launched through a quarter wave plate down such a bow-tie fiber at a 45 degree angle to the main refractive index axes, the fiber will guide two beams of circularly polarized light (Figure 10). With a quarter wave plate in front of the waveguide these beams will originally be 90 degrees out of phase with respect to one another. As these two beams pass through the fiber they will be differentially retarded by the birefringent nature of the fiber, and will be

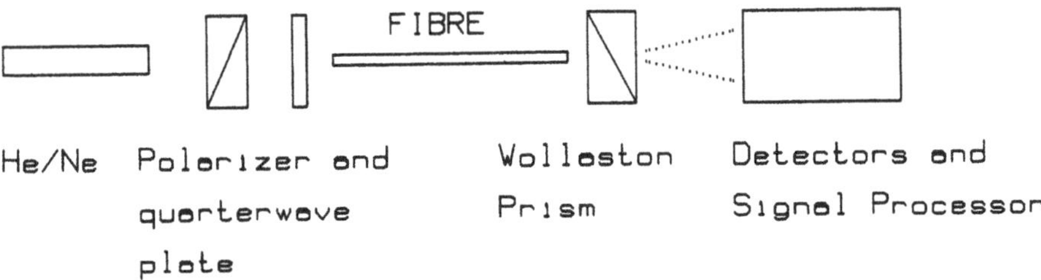

10. Typical single arm interferometer instrument.

subjected to further differences in retardation due to the different temperature coefficients of the elastooptic properties of the non isotropic fiber. There will be interaction between these modes, and they will beat against one another, creating an interference pattern along the longitudinal axis of the fiber. From the side this will appear as beads of brilliance, much like pearls threaded on a string (cf. Figure 5). The distance between the pearls is called the beat distance, and is used as a figure of merit for such birefringent fibers. Good fibers have beat distances of a few mm.

Theoretical studies have indicated that although the temperature sensitivity of the devices is less than the standard Mach-Zehnder, the single arm bow-tie fiber interferometer rejects pressure effects over 170 time better than the isotropic fiber based double arm interferometer (20). This is the driving force behind investigating the application of such fibers to chemical studies involving the measurement of temperature change in flowing stream systems.

If one looks into the exit of such a bow-tie fiber, as the temperature changes a sinusoidal periodicity in light intensity will be observed (cf. Figure 5). Unfortunately, such a simple detector would be subject to effects created by source instability. A more useful detection system for such a single arm interferometer splits the light exiting from the fiber into its components using a Wollaston prism. This involves two calcite crystals cemented together, with their optical axes orthogonal to one another. The two beams strike identical photodiodes, creating signals called Ix and Iy. These two signals are complex functions of the source intensity and phase angle shifts related to the temperature coefficients of the two birefringent axes. One of these functions involves a sin(2) function, the other a cos(2) function that are initially 90 degrees out of phase with respect to each other. Ix and Iy can then be treated electronically, with analog components, to produce the function (Ix-Iy)/(Ix+Iy). Simple geometric considerations will show this to be equal to the cosine of theta, that indicates the change in the state of polarization between the two modes (Figure 11). This function is independent of any fluctuations in the source intensity. In this configuration the system is

Wolloston SiPD Signal-Processing

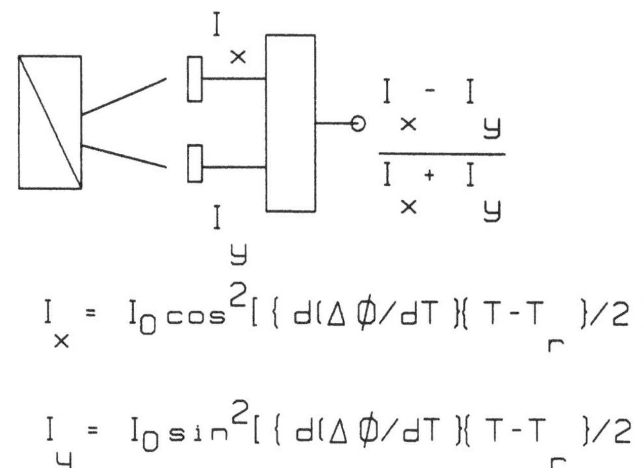

(a)

$$\left.\begin{aligned}\phi_x &= k\,n_x L\\ \phi_y &= k\,n_y L\end{aligned}\right\} \quad \phi_x - \phi_y = k L\,(n_x - n_y)$$

$$\Delta\phi = k L \Delta n$$

o

o

o

(b) $$\frac{1}{L}\frac{d(\Delta\phi)}{dT} = -\left(\frac{k\,\Delta n}{T_s - T_a}\right)$$

11. Single arm interferometer detector output mathematical relationships.

(a). Basic signal equations; Phi is the phase angle, T is the temperature, and Tr is a reference temperature.

(b). Transduction Equations: Phi is the phase angle, L is length, n is refractive index, k= 2 Pi/lambda, Ts is the softening point of the core and Ta is ambient temperature.

said to operate in quadrature, making the measured response nearly linear for small temperature changes.

RESULTS AND DISCUSSION

This single arm interferometer has been used to examine the temperature changes that accompany the reactions of hydrogen that occur on a thin catalyst film deposited on the surface of the fiber. This film was composed of an undercoat of palladium 60 Angstrom thick, covered with an overcoat of platinum 300 Angstrom thick. The fiber was laid down in a channel 1mm x 1mm in cross section and several centimeters long. The fiber was held in place at either end of the flow channel by high temperature viscoelastic gels to prevent induced strain from affecting the sensor response. This mounting procedure made it possible to build scores of sensors that were very reproducible in characteristics. The hydrogen was introduced in a flowing air stream that had velocities around 1 liter per minute. This chemical system was chosen in order to allow experiments that could demonstrate temperature sensitivity and pressure insensitivity. It was also chosen to demonstrate the differences between this thin film sensor and a very thick film sensor study (a 10 micron thick palladium film) using a two arm Mach-Zehnder configuration reported by Butler (21).

This thin film system is easily capable of reliably detecting hydrogen concentrations between 1 and 100 mM

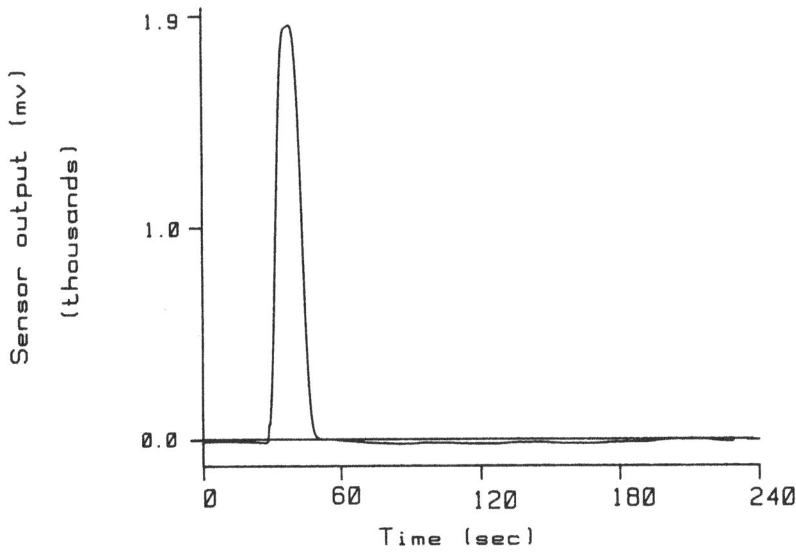

12. Typical signal from single arm interferometer.

(Figure 12). These samples were introduced as boluses 0.5 to 10 seconds wide into a flowing air carrier stream with a flow velocity approximately 1000 ml/min. The resident time of a sample cross-section in the sensor area is typically a few milliseconds. Acceptable detector response statistics were obtained (Figure 13). At the upper limit of hydrogen concentration sensor degradation occurs over long time periods. A lower limit is imposed by the difficulties of making, maintaining, and detecting low hydrogen concentrations.

The system shows a sensitivity of 0.3 radian/K-m, very close to the theoretical limit of the 0.9 radian/K-m

% IN AIR	X	SD	RSD
6.7	1.97	0.16	7.9%
2.8	0.86	0.05	6.2%
1.4	0.62	0.02	4.0%

13. Response characteristics of single arm interferometric hydrogen sensor,

reported by Eickhoff (20). Theoretical studies have also shown that the sign of the temperature sensitivity in such birefringent fibers should be opposite from any pressure effects that might be observed. Standard temperature measuring semiconductor devices imbedded in the block surrounding the fiber indicate that the response being measured is temperature. Thick film studies (21) are reported to respond by effects due to pressure stresses as the palladium lattice is affected. This suggests that thin biomaterial films should be employed. The enzyme structures required may be immobilized on the cylindrical surface of the fiber, replacing the metal catalysts sytem reported in this study.

Flow studies where the gas stream passing the fiber is jumped instantaneously from 1.0 to 1.2 L/second demonstrate no change in the output signal, supporting the expected lack of pressure sensitivity. Subjecting the sensor system to deliberate increases in internal pressure of 2 psig led to decreases in signal response of 1%, while temperature elevation increased the observed signal. Such pressure changes are far in excess of those to be encountered in normal flow systems. The fact that these pressure effects are experimentally opposite in direction to those induced by temperature confirm again that the basic effects reported here are due to temperature, and not isotropic pressure effects.

The optical components involve a small 1 mw He/Ne laser, and common silicon photodiodes. The only moderately expensive component is the Wollaston prism. The electronics associated with the optical portions of the sensor are quite inexpensive and simple. They involve standard operational amplifiers and a AD538 analog math processing element. With the advent of inexpensive solid state lasers and hybrid optical components it would be possible to make small, rugged versions of this instrument employing planar waveguide assemblies with almost all the signal processing units on the same carrier.

CONCLUSIONS

Rough comparisons of the three systems are shown in Figure 14. Although each is functional and useful, these results suggest that for thermal biosensor applications the single arm interferometric design involves the simplest, most

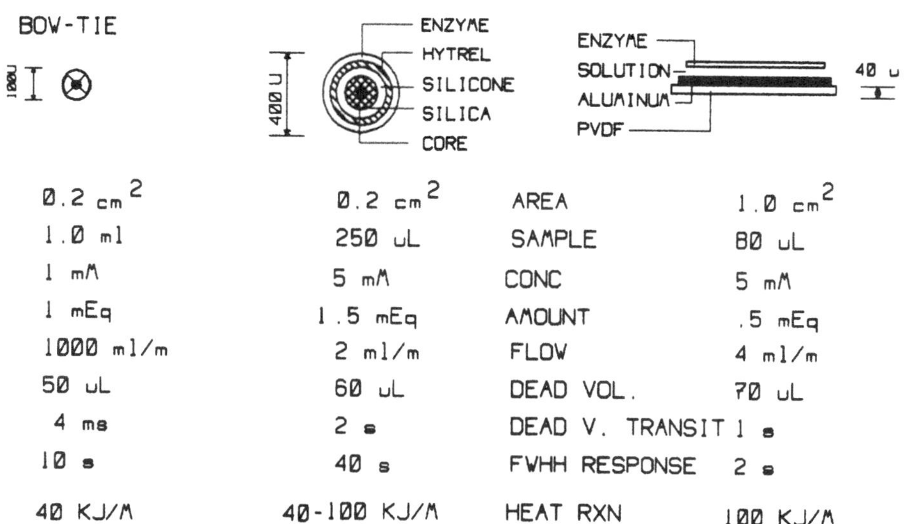

BOW-TIE	Fiber optic		PVDF
0.2 cm^2	0.2 cm^2	AREA	1.0 cm^2
1.0 ml	250 uL	SAMPLE	80 uL
1 mM	5 mM	CONC	5 mM
1 mEq	1.5 mEq	AMOUNT	.5 mEq
1000 ml/m	2 ml/m	FLOW	4 ml/m
50 uL	60 uL	DEAD VOL.	70 uL
4 ms	2 s	DEAD V. TRANSIT	1 s
10 s	40 s	FWHH RESPONSE	2 s
40 KJ/M	40-100 KJ/M	HEAT RXN	100 KJ/M

14. A comparison of the fiber optic and PVDF film enthalpimeters.

chemically inert, sensitive detector system that provides the degree of immunity from pressure noise required in flowing systems.

ACKNOWLEDGEMENTS: The figures in this article are used with the permission of Virginia Polytechnic Institute and State University and the authors, the copyright owners.

REFERENCES:

1. Johansson, A., Lundberg, J., Mathiason, B. Mosbach, K., Biochim. Biophys. Acta, 304, 214 (1973).

2. Pennington, S., NSF/RA 760032 Enzyme Technology Grantees-Users Conference; PE 256 584 (1975).

3. Cooney, C., Weaver, J., Tannenbaum, S., Faller, D., Shields, A., Jahnke, M., "Enzyme Engineering", Vol. 2, Plenum Press, New York (1974).

4. Rich, S., Ianello, R.,Anal. Chem., 51(2), 204 (1979).

5. Guilbault, G., Danielsson, B., Mandenlus, C., Mosbach, K., Anal. Chem., 55(9), 1582 (1983).

6. Cady, W. G., "Piezoelectricity", McGraw Hill Book Co., New York(1946).

7. Kawai, H., Japanese Journal of Applied Physics, 8, 975 (1969).

8. Anderson, R., Kepler, R., Ferroelectrics, 33, 91 (1984).

9. Bergman, J., McFee, J., Crane, G., Applied Physics Letters, 18, 203 (1971).

10. Kepler, R., Anderson, R., Journal of Applied Physics, 49, 4918 (1978).

11. Kepler, R., Anderson, R., Lagasse, R., Ferroelectrics, 57, 151 (1984).

12. Savitzky, A., Golay, J., Anal. Chem., 36, 1627 (1964).

13. Mark Malmros, Ohmicron Corporation, Personal Communication, May, 1989.

14. Hocker, G., Applied Optics, 18(9), 1445 (1979).

15. Lagakos, N., Bucaro, J., Jarzynski, J., Applied Optics, 20(13), 2305 (1981).

16. Aaurer, G., Cole, J., Optics Letters, 7(11), 561 (1982).

17. Schuetz, L., Cole, J., Jarzynski, J., Lagakos, N., Bucaro, J., Applied Optics, 22(3), 478 (1983).

18. Sheem, S., Giallorenzi, T., Optics Letters, 4(1), 29 (1979).

19. Attiyat, A., Christian, G., Biotechnology Laboratory, 2(2), 8 (1984).

20. Eickhoff, W., Optics Letters, 6(4), 284 (1981).

21. Butler, M., Ginley, D., J. Appl. Phys. 64(7), (1988)

20

Fiber Optic-Based Biosensors Utilizing Immobilized Enzyme Systems

Abdel-Latif, M.S. and Guilbault, G.G. University of New Orleans, Department of Chemistry, New Orleans, Louisiana 70148

ABSTRACT

Biosensors are attracting the attention of many investigators in the field of biotechnology related research. A biosensor is a device that combines the specificity of a biomaterial (enzymes, antibodies, receptors or even whole cells) with the sensitive and well established bioassays. Biosensors are of potential use in many fields including clinical and biotechnology monitoring. An important class of enzymes results in H_2O_2 production, after the reaction with a suitable substrate, and O_2 is consumed. Either H_2O_2 generation or O_2 depletion can be monitored to follow the enzymatic reaction and thus determine the substrate level. Other enzyme systems, like urease and penicillinase, result in a pH change which can be followed using a pH sensitive device. For the many advantages of fiber optic sensing, extensive research efforts have been devoted for the production of reliable, self-contained and sensitive fiber optic biosensors which are capable of in situ monitoring. An overview of the possibilities and challenges associated with the construction of such sensors are discussed.

INTRODUCTION

Enzymes have been known to catalyze specific reactions with suitable substrates. The enzymatic reaction is usually very specific for the substrate or a group of substrates with a common functional group. It also requires a very small amount of the substrate. According to specificity, enzymes are classified into two major categories:

a. Enzymes that have molecular specificity, like urease.
b. Enzymes with group specificity like L-amino acid oxidase.

The enzymatic reaction is also efficient in product formation, yielding products which are, in most cases, easy to detect by electrochemical or spectroscopic techniques. Alternatively, the uptake of a certain reactant can be used to follow the reaction.

Because of the great sensitivity and excellent selectivity provided by biological systems, biosensor research has been very active recently in the development of an analytical device that can sensitively detect and quantify a substrate. This device has a biological component, like an enzyme, antibody, receptor or even a whole cell, held in an immobilized state so that the sensor is reusable and provides very high specificity. The second part of the biosensor is the transducer, which measures the progress of the biological reaction. These sensors can be electrochemical (electrode), optical (optrode) or piezoelectric.

There are many reasons for using immobilized enzymes in a biosensor. These include economics, stability and convenience, especially in combination with flow injection systems.

1. Methods of Enzyme Immobilization

Many methods for immobilizing enzymes have been reported in the literature (1). These methods use either physical or chemical means. The physical means involve:

a. Adsorption

There are many types of supports that have the ability to adsorb other materials. For example, ion exchange resins, polystyrene, silica gel, alumina and activated carbon are known to adsorb a variety of substances, like enzymes. The adsorption may occur through ionic, hydrogen bonding or hydrophobic interactions. In all cases, the enzyme adsorbed is subject to desorption which makes the enzymatic preparation difficult to use.

b. Entrapment

Some polymers such as polyacrylamide are known to entrap biological compounds. The entire enzyme, or a whole cell, can be entrapped in the pores of the polymer. Other polymers which have been used in the entrapment of enzymes include collagen, agar, and alginate.

c. Encapsulation

Enzymes can also be encapsulated in nylon or other materials by placing the enzymatic solution in a medium that, upon reaction, results in the formation of capsules. For example, nylon capsules are formed according to the following equation:

$$NH_2(CH_2)_6NH_2 + Cl\text{-}\overset{\overset{\displaystyle O}{\|}}{C}\text{-}(CH_2)_8\text{-}\overset{\overset{\displaystyle O}{\|}}{C}\text{-}Cl \longrightarrow \text{nylon}$$

Chemical methods produce more stable immobilized product than physical methods, since the enzyme is tightly held to the solid support or, in some cases, is a part of it. Chemical immobilization can be achieved by the following methods:

a. Covalent attachment

Direct covalent immobilization can take place if the solid support contains aldehyde groups and the enzyme contributes an amino group that reacts with the aldehyde group to form a strong imine bond. Chemical techniques are usually used to create the aldehyde group on the surface of the solid support. For example, the immobilization of enzymes to collagen membranes is shown below

Collagen

$$\vdash COOH \xrightarrow{CH_3OH\ /\ 0.2\ N\ HCl} \vdash COCH_3$$

$$\vdash COCH_3 \xrightarrow{1\%\ NH_2NH_2} \vdash CONHNH_2$$

$$\vdash CONHNH_2 \xrightarrow{0.5\ M\ NaNO_2\ /\ 0.3\ N\ HCl} \vdash CON_3$$

$$\vdash CON_3 \xrightarrow{H_2N\text{-}ENZYME} \vdash CONH\text{-}ENZYME$$

b. Crosslinking

Crosslinking reagents can also be used to link the enzyme to a high molecular weight protein like bovine serum albumin (BSA). Glutaraldehyde has been extensively used as the crosslinking agent (see equation below). The two aldehyde groups present in the glutaraldehyde molecule react with the amino groups of the enzyme and the BSA forming a viscous thick gel which solidifies when the solvent evaporates.

$$
\begin{array}{c} CHO \\ | \\ (CH_2)_3 \\ | \\ CHO \end{array}
\;+\;
\begin{array}{c} H_2N\text{- ENZYME} \\ \\ \\ \\ H_2N\text{- ALBUMIN} \end{array}
\longrightarrow
\begin{array}{c} HC{=}N\text{-ENZYME} \\ | \\ (CH_2)_3 \\ | \\ HC{=}N\text{-ALBUMIN} \end{array}
$$

2. Enzyme Electrodes

These sensors combine the high specificity of one or more enzymes, for a certain substrate, or a group of substrates with a amperometric or potentiometric base sensor used as the transducer (1). The enzyme, which is fixed on the membrane of an electrode, reacts with the substrate. Either the product of the enzymatic reaction, or a reactant (e.g., O_2) can be measured by the base sensor. For example, urea can be determined by immobilizing urease on an ammonium selective electrode. The generated ammonium ions will change the potential difference between the reference electrode (usually an Ag/AgCl electrode) and a working electrode. The amount of the change in potential is related to the concentration of urea where

$$E = E^o - 0.059 \log [NH_4^+]$$

A major problem of these enzyme electrodes is the selectivity of the membrane for other ions. For example, the ammonium ion selective electrode is also responsive to K^+ and Na^+. Also, in amperometric sensors, electroactive compounds that can be oxidized or reduced at the potential applied will cause an error. An excellent advantage of electrode based systems is the ability to do turbid and colored samples, which are difficult to do using spectroscopic techniques.

3. Fiber Optic Biosensors

Transparent fiber strands can transmit light with very low losses. The theory of light transmission through the fiber is dependent on the internal total reflection concept within the core of the fiber, which is covered by a cladding of different refractive index (2). Light has to enter the fiber core through an angle called the acceptance or core angle, a,

$$\text{Sin } a = \frac{1}{n_o} \sqrt{n_1^2 - n_2^2}$$

where n_o is the refractive index of the medium at the light entrance into the fiber, n_1 and n_2 are the refractive indices of the core and the cladding respectively.

The acceptance angle is dependent on the critical angle (the angle at which light is totally reflected when exceeded), d, given by the ratio of the cladding and core refractive indices

$$\sin d = \frac{n_2}{n_1}$$

Another descriptive feature of an optical fiber is a term known as the numerical aperture (NA) where

$$NA = n_o \sin a$$

NA indicates the range of angles that can be accepted by the fiber.

a. **Fiber Bundles (cables)**

Light input, and hence output, is dependent on the diameter of the fiber. Since a very small diameter is required for flexible fibers, this size is a limiting factor in the fabrication of fibers . For this reason, fibers are made from bundles which have the advantage of efficient light collection and flexibility. Also, the arrangement of fibers into bundles is of significant importance since bifurcated and multi cable construction becomes feasible. Fiber bundles of 8, 16, or more fiber strands are known. The process of reflection within a fiber optic bundle can be explained if the bundle (Fig. 1) is viewed as a single fiber (which is true since only the outer surface of the bundle is cladded). As light exits from the cable, it hits the reagent phase at the core-reagent interface, therefore, it is totally reflected if the angle of reflection is greater than the critical angle defined by the refractive indices of both the core and the reagent phase. In the case of a bifurcated fiber optic cable, 50% of the reflected light is lost since there is a 50% probability that light will follow the correct direction towards either terminal of the bifurcated cable.

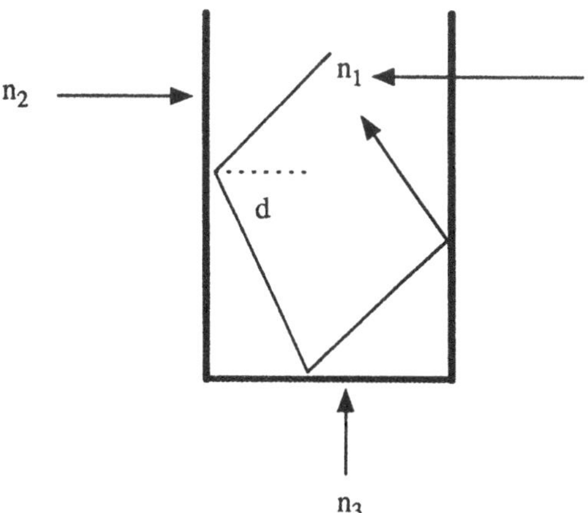

Figure 1. Schematic of the fiber optic. n_1 n_2 n_3 are the refractive indices of the core, cladding and the reagent phase, respectively.

The material from which fibers are manuafactured depends on the application, since glass fibers can be used to transmit light in the wavelength range from 400 nm to about 1000 nm. Fused silica based fiber optics can be used in the range from 250 nm to about 1000 nm. However, below 400 nm and 250 nm glass and fused silica, respectively, will have much less radiation transmission. A great change in light transmission is observed as the wavelength is changed.

b. Biosensor Development

Fiber optic biosensors for various biological compounds use available bioassay methodology. Enzymes can be immobilized on the end of a bifurcated fiber optic bundle. These react with the appropriate analyte producing a species that alters the absorption or fluoresence of a dye or fluor present in the vicinity of the fiber end. The generated species may, upon reaction with some other substances, result in light production and CL is observed. In all cases, the extent of spectral change is related to the analyte concentration. In this respect, fiber optic biosensors are very similar to enzyme electrodes. In fact they are called optrodes or optical electrodes. The ultimate goal of the development of optrodes is to obtain an all immobilized dip sensor, that can sense one or more analytes and give precise analytical information.

c. Features of Optical Biosensors

There are many important advantages for optical biosensors including:

a. Optical biosensors are highly specific since an enzyme, antibody or a receptor is an integral part of the sensor.

b. Since fibers can have a very small cross section, miniaturization of the sensor is possible.

c. Problems associated with reference cells and liquid junction potentials in potentiometric measurement are eliminated.

d. In situ measurements using optical fibers are possible. Thus analysis can be performed in real time.

e. Inaccesible or dangerous samples can be analyzed, since remote sensing is possible due to the ability of fibers to transmit light for more than 1000 meters with little loss of signal.

f. An important direction in biosensor research is the development of biosensors for in vivo measurements. Since the signal is optical, such biosensors offer an advantage of safety. Also, the optical nature of the signal eliminates the electrical interferences.

However, there are several disadvantages for the optical biosensors, for example:

a. The most severe problem is the stability of the sensor where, in most cases, the indicator phase can be washed out or consumed. Also, the biologically active component lacks long-term stability.

b. If the cell is not well designed, interference from the ambient light will take place.

c. In developing a sensor, it is necessary to immobilize as many reagents as possible so that munipulations of the measurement can be simple. Losses in the sensitivity of many indicators are encountered when they are immobilized. This limits the use of many, otherwise valuable, indicators.

d. Optical fibers that can be used to transmit light in the UV, like quartz, are very expensive.

d. Application of Fiber Optic Biosensors

Optical biosensors are expected to have the features of both the selectivity of the biological system together with the advantages of the spectroscopic methods for the transducer. They have been used to determine enzyme activity, glucose, penicillin, urea, and many other metabolites. Fluorescence immunoassay has been reported and active research is still underway in all fields of optical bioassay.

Immobilizing all reagents on the tip of the fiber will result in the highest selectivity possible because the species generated will alter the spectral properties of the attached layer. The light transmitted through the fiber will hit this indicator layer and penetrate into it a distance (D) given by

$$D = \frac{\lambda}{2\pi(n_1^2 \sin^2 a - n_2^2)^{1/2}}$$

where D is always less than λ.

Hence, the signal obtained is a characteristic of the reaction taking place at the tip and is independent of the bulk solution.

4. Fiber Optic Biosensors for Hydrogen Peroxide

Hydrogen peroxide has great significance in the analysis of a wide variety of biological samples. For example, many enzyme reactions result in the generation of hydrogen peroxide in amounts proportional to the substrate concentration. Thus, a biosensor based on the detection of hydrogen peroxide will have many applications.

Spectroscopic methods for hydrogen peroxide determination are numerous. These include spectrophotometry, fluorescence, and chemiluminescence (CL). However, several problems that limit the use of many of these methods for biosensor development exist.

For instance, to the best of our knowledge, there is no suitable substance that can be used for reversible spectrophotometric determination of H_2O_2. This is because the oxidized colored substance can not be reversibly converted into the original form without the use of some other methods which involve redox chemistry. This problem necessitates that the dye be in the soluble form, otherwise, the sensor can only be used for a single measurement.

In case of fluorescence detection of hydrogen peroxide, another problem is encountered where the best fluorometric procedures (3,4) involve the production of a fluorescent dimer. For example, p-hydroxyphenylacetic acid is one of the best fluorometric reagents for the detection of hydrogen peroxide. When this compound is immobilized on the tip of the fiber optic, the dimer formed, in the presence of hydrogen peroxide and peroxidase, will also be in the immobilized state which results in a very long fluorescence life time. Also, reagent consumption limits reproducibility. Thus, the fluorometric substance should be included in the reagent phase.

Self-contained optrodes based on fluorescence measurement can be successful if they were constructed to respond to fluorescence quenching by oxygen or other quenchers. Quenching of the fluorophore does not result in a structural change and regeneration of the fluorophore is possible after removing the quencher by simple rinsing. Encouraging results were obtained using this approach (Fig. 2). However, this configuration does not eliminate interferences from other quenchers present in the sample to be analyzed.

The last possibility which will be discussed here is the chemiluminescence detection of hydrogen peroxide. CL is known to be one of the most sensitive techniques, with very minimal instrumentation requirements

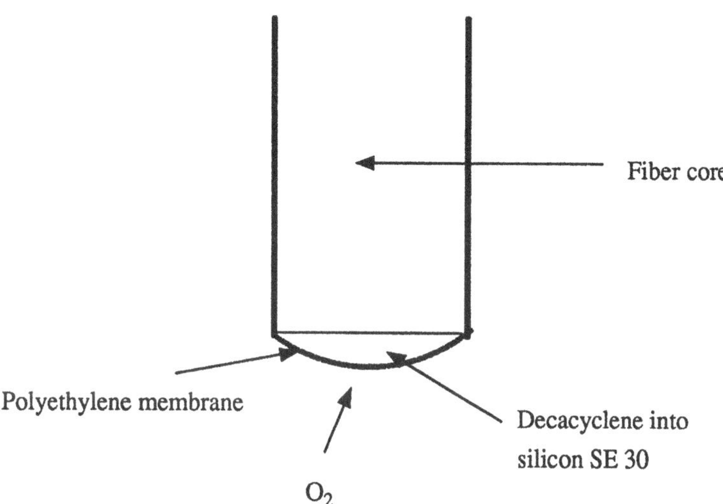

Figure 2. Representation of a peroxide sensor.

(Fig. 3). There are several CL methods for the determination of hydrogen peroxide. The most important of these are the luminol and the peroxyoxalate reactions (Table 1 summarizes the results obtained for hydrogen peroxide determination).

From the simplicity point of view, the peroxyoxalate system is preferred over

Table 1: Comparison Results of the Luminol and Peroxyoxalate CL Systems for Hydrogen Peroxide Determination[a]

Method	liner range	RSD
Luminol[b]	$1.2x10^{-4}M-2.4x10^{-8}M$	2.6
Peroxyoxalate[c]	$8x10^{-4}M-8x10^{-9}M$	3.0

[a] using cetyltrimethylammonium bromide surfactant.

[b,c] studies were conducted at pH 7.2

the luminol reaction because of three main reasons. First, there is no pH mismatch between the enzymatic and the peroxyoxalate reactions. Second, the need of a cooxidant (e.g., peroxidase) is eliminated. The third reason is the insolubility of the peroxyoxalate and the fluorophore in aqueous medium which allows successful incorporation of these substances into some polymer matrices. In addition to these advantages, it is well known that the peroxyoxalate reaction is at least 25 times more efficient than the luminol reaction.

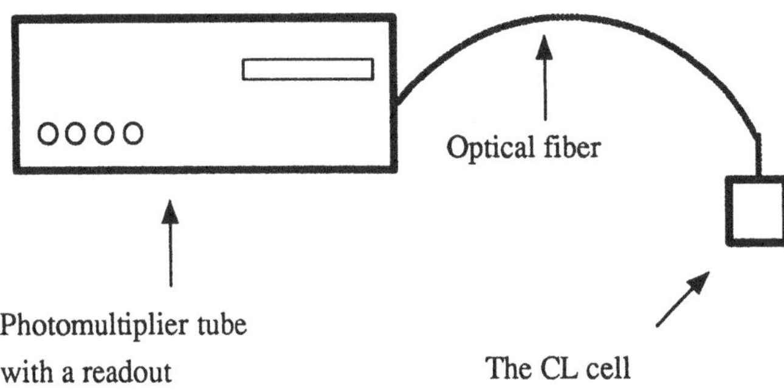

Figure 3. Experimental setup of CL based biosensor.

For these reasons, it seems reasonable to conduct some further studies on the system so that a real self-contained peroxide probe can be developed. However, considerable reagent consumption, at high substrate concentration, would certainly result in a reduced signal as the probe is used. Studies based on this approach are underway.

5. The Use of Surfactants in Optrode Development

Catonic surfactants were found to enhance the CL signal of the luminol reaction (Table 2) and overcome the pH mismatch between the enzymatic and the CL reactions (5). Also, the solubility of the peroxyaxalate was enhanced in the presence of cationic surfactants microemulsion (6). However, it should be pointed out that Tween surfactants always give a positive reaction with both systems as well as any H_2O_2 based system. This is, probably, due to the presence of an appreciable peroxide content in these surfactants. Thus, this type of surfactants should be excluded from any procedures that involve the direct or indirect determination of hydrogen peroxide.

Table 2 - The Effect of Surfactants on the CL Intensity of the Luminol Reaction

Surfactant	Average CL intensity (n=5)[a]
Cetyltrimethylammonium bromide	100
Myristyltrimethylammonium bromide	62
Lauryltrimethylammonium bromide	17
Cetylpyridinium chloride	19
Brij® - 35	19
No surfactant	15

[a] Relative CL intensity in arbitrary units normalized to 100

A rather interesting behavior of the peroxyoxalate CL system is that, in the presence of Tween surfactants, the reaction occurs in the absence of hydrogen peroxide and the fluorophore. This means that, if the Tween surfactants are pure as claimed, the change in the viscosity of the solvent eliminates the energy transfer step and direct CL is observed.

6. pH Based Biosensors

An example of this type of biosensors is urea which, in the presence of urease, is converted into ammonium and bicarboante according to the following equation

$$H_2N{-}C({=}O){-}NH_2 + 2\,H_2O + H^+ \xrightarrow{\text{urease}} 2\,NH_4^+ + HCO_3^-$$

The production of ammonium ions changes the pH of the reagent phase resulting in a change in the spectral properties of a pH indicator.

Urease, as well as bromothymol blue were successfully immobilized on a preactivated Immunodyne membrane. This sensor is very simple (Fig. 4) where only a membrane with coimmobilized urease and indicator is required.

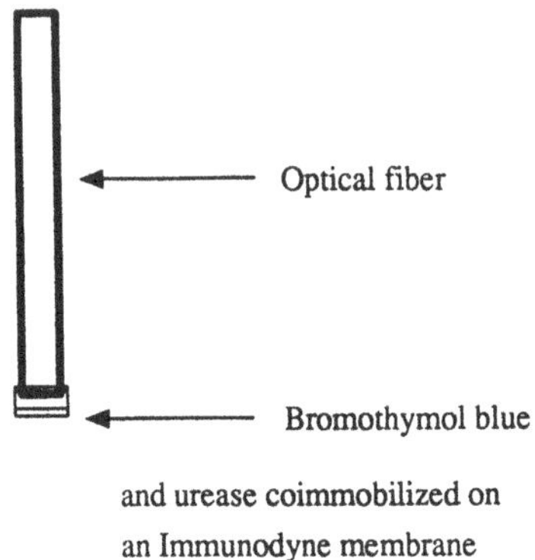

Figure 4. A schematic of the urea biosensor.

This approach can be adapted to other reactions that involve a pH change (e.g., penicillin/penicillinase reaction). However, a major problem was encountered where the immobilized indicator was not very sensitive towards minor pH changes. The sensitivity loss of many indicators and substances, when immobilized, is a real problem which faces optrode development. This handicap can be overcome by the use of certain immobilization media that can dissolve the substrate of interest. This approach is under investigation.

ACKNOWLEDGMENT

The financial assistance of the LEQSF (Grant RD-B-17) is gratefully acknowledged.

REFERENCES

1. G. G. Guilbault, Handbook of Enzymatic Analysis, Dekker, New York, 1977.
2. W. R. Seitz, CRC Critical Reviews in Analytical Chemistry, 19, 135(1988).
3. G. G. Guilbault, D. Kramer and E. Hackley, Anal. Chem., 39, 271(1967).
4. G. G. Guilbault, P. J. Brignac and M. Juneau, Anal. Chem., 40, 1256(1968).
5. M. S. Abdel-Latif and G. G. Guilbault, Anal. Chim. Acta, 221, 11(1989).
6. M. S. Abdel-Latif and G. G. Guilbault, Anal. Chem., 60, 2671(1988).

21

Fiber Optic Chemical Sensors (FOCS): An Answer to the Need for Small, Specific Monitors

Kisholoy Goswami, Stanley M. Klainer, Dileep K. Dandge and Johnny R. Thomas
FiberChem, Inc.
1181 Grier Drive, Suite B
Las Vegas, Nevada 89119, USA

1. What is a fiber optic chemical sensor?

Of the various emerging techniques, chemical (or biochemical) sensing with optical fibers is the most interesting. A fiber optic chemical sensor (FOCS) is a device with preselected chemical and/or physical properties attached to the distal end. The unique position of FOCS stems from the following advantages: (i) analytical operation can be performed remotely; (ii) no reference signal is required; (iii) it is immune to electromagnetic interferences (EMI); (iv) the sensing is done in situ and in real time; (v) inexpensive, high quality fiber optics are readily available; and (vi) the sensor can be deployed in hostile environments. In essence, FOCS is an integrated system consisting of the components as shown in the block diagram.

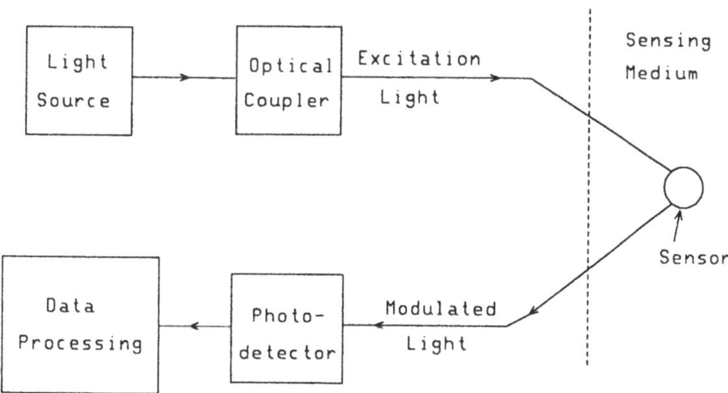

Figure 1: Block diagram of a fiber optic chemical sensor system.

2. How does a FOCS work?

In a fiber optic chemical sensor (FOCS), light rays are guided back and forth along transparent fibers of glass or plastic or a suitable dielectric medium. This light transmission through optical fibers is possible because of the total internal reflection phenomenon [1] as shown in Figure 2.

Total internal reflection of light occurs at the interface between two transparent optical materials having different refractive indices. Two conditions, however, have to be met for total internal reflection:

a) Light rays should travel from the optically dense material to an optically light medium, and
b) The incident angle with the normal to the interface should be greater than a critical angle.

If the refractive indices of air, the fiber optic core, and the clad are N_0, N_1 and N_2 respectively, then the critical angle, Φ_c, will be defined as $\Phi_c = \text{Sin}^{-1} N_2/N_1$.

Essentially, the FOCS system consists of a fiber coated with species specific chemistry whose interaction with a target analyte is measured by a miniature spectrometer. The spectroscopic principles forming the basis for FOCS measurements are: (a) refractive index, (b) absorption, (c) fluorescence, (d) reflection, and (e) scattering. Interaction of the analyte with the sensing reagent produces a change in the above-mentioned spectroscopic parameters. The readout device electronically converts light flux into voltage. Modulation in the voltage reading directly correlates with the analyte concentration.

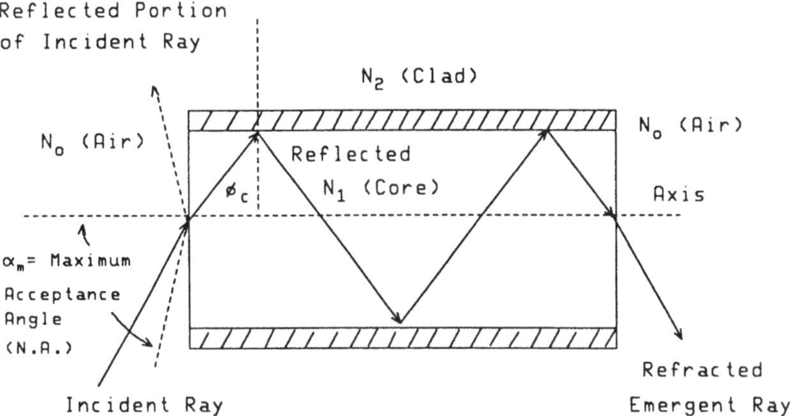

Figure 2: Light rays propagate in a fiber optic via total internal reflection.

In the following pages, an overview of fiber optic chemical sensors with respect to evolution in the instrumentation and sensor design will be provided. This will be followed by certain applications, where our own research work will be cited.

3. Instrumentation:

As shown in Figure 1, the principal components of FOCS systems consist of light source, fiber, optical coupler, sensor, detector, signal processor and associated electronics. Not too long ago, lasers were almost exclusively used as the light source. However, the current trend is to use incandescent sources or light emitting diodes (LED).

Incandescent sources (e.g. tungsten - halogen lamp) provide a wide distribution of wavelengths and the use of appropriate filters for wavelength selections makes this source very versatile. Light emitting diodes are becoming popular because of their low cost, long lifetime and miniature size.

For sensing applications, step index multimode fibers are employed. Inexpensive optical fibers covering most of the UV/visible and near-infrared region are available. The core diameter of the fiber can be anywhere from 125 μ to 1000 μm. Plastic fibers are also used in sensing applications, although these fibers sometimes exhibit undesirable luminescence.

The optical coupler separates the excitation light from the inbound signal. In a bifurcated fiber system this special feature is not required. However, in a single-strand FOCS system this isolation is essential. This can be done with a dichroic mirror, a beam splitter or a perforated mirror. The dichroic mirror has special optical coatings which allow the transmission of one wavelength band with the concurrent reflection of a second wavelength band.

In a typical fiber optic chemical sensor system, excitation light from an appropriate source is launched into the fiber. The excitation beam interacts with the sensing reagent and the target analyte to produce a measurable return light signal. Although most frequently fluorescence appears to be the returning signal, other techniques like absorption, scattering, refraction or reflection are also employed as the measurement techniques.

Figure 3 shows the configuration of a fiber optic spectrometer. This is a person-portable instrument developed in our laboratories. Light from a 12 watt tungsten-halogen lamp is filtered and collimated. The excitation light is then transmitted through a dichroic mirror placed at 45° and is launched into the fiber optic. The returning signal, after emerging out of the fiber, impacts upon the dichroic mirror and is reflected at 90° toward the detector.

Any component of the scattered excitation signal is prefiltered at this point. This beam then passes through another filter and is focused onto a silicon photodiode. The processed signal is then displayed digitally as volts.

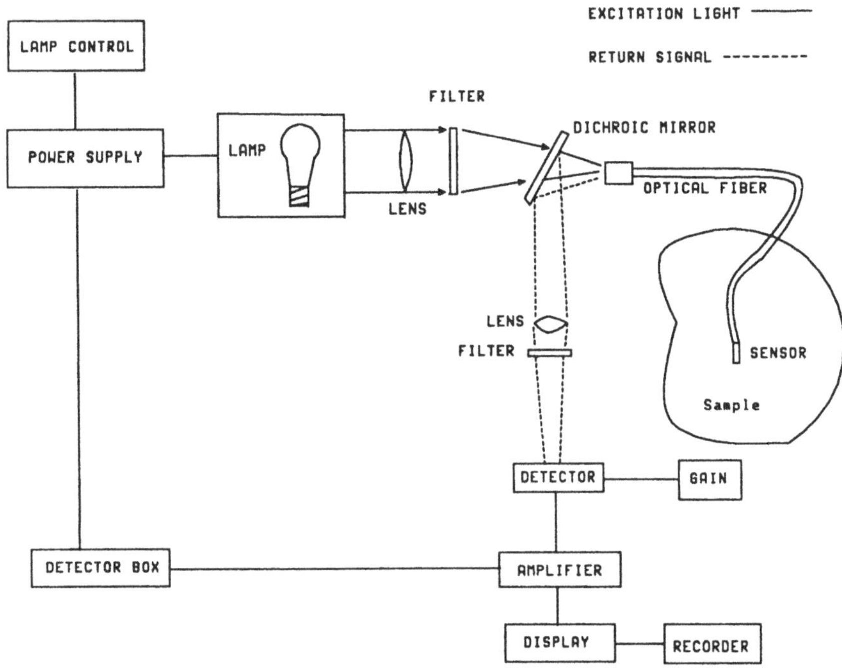

Figure 3: Salient features of a fiber optic chemical sensor system.

4. Sensor Configuration:

The design of the FOCS can have variations. To date, the most widely used FOCS design has been to put a reagent that specifically and sensitively interacts with the analyte of interest at the tip of the fiber. Fibers in the 100 to 600 μm diameter range are used most often. These have very small surface areas at their tips (7 x 10^{-5} to 3 x 10^{-3} cm^2) and it is difficult to provide enough chemistry at the end of the fiber for reliable measurements, i.e., good signal-to-noise ratios.

Several approaches have been used to place enough chemistry at the tip of the fiber to overcome the surface area limitations. These approaches include: (1) applying surface amplification techniques [2], that use a unique type of covalent immobilization; (2) imbedding the chemistry into a membrane [3], or polymer placed at the tip of the fiber; (3) attaching large surface area, porous glass fibers [4] or porous glass beads [5] to the tip.

The sides of the fiber, for all practical purposes, cannot be used because the light does not reach the outer surface of the clad, or, in cases where the clad is removed, the light comes out the sides and cannot be collected effectively. It has been found, however, that when the sensing reagents are coated on the side of a fiber optic whose clad has been removed, a measurable effect occurs in the evanescent wave region [6]. This effect can be used to identify and quantify a particular species.

The evanescent wave does not penetrate very deep into the clad. This is a function of the thickness of the sensing material, the angle of the incident light and the refractive indices N_1 and N_2. Proper selection of these parameters assures that light is optimally transmitted through the fiber, but it limits the allowable thickness of the reactive surface because only the depth to which the light penetrates can be interrogated. Several researchers are trying to develop immunological FOCS based on this technology [7].

In special situations, where the target analyte is a volatile species, reservoir FOCS (Figure 4) with gas permeable membranes have been used [8]. The sensing reagent is used in the solution form, and, therefore, the amount of material can be precisely controlled, assuring excellent sensor-to-sensor reproducibility.

To use the reservoir cell effectively, it is necessary to collect as much of the signal as possible. One way of doing this is to employ non-imaging optics (NIO), specifically the Winston cone. The NIO technology is based on research into solar concentrators [9]. Rather than follow

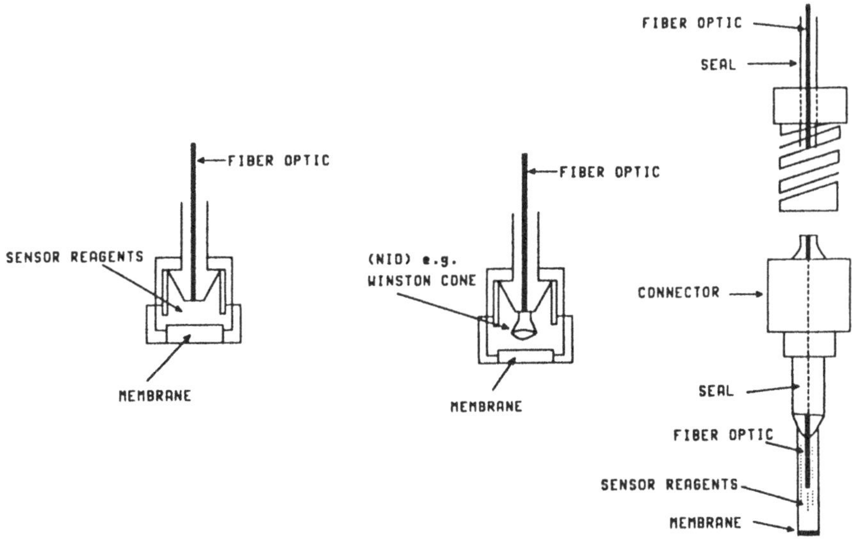

Figure 4: Reservoir FOCS Designs

the historical path of imaging optics, which depend on spatial coherence of transmitted rays, the NIO is optimized for power throughput. Figure 4 also shows a sample representation of the NIO device.

5. Types of Spectroscopic Measurements:

As mentioned before, a wide variety of techniques, such as fluorescence, refraction/reflection, absorption, scattering, energy exchange, etc., can be used for FOCS measurements. As the technology develops, it is expected that FOCS based on surface enhanced Raman and infrared vibrational spectroscopy will emerge.

Fluorescence is an inherently sensitive technique capable of measuring low analyte concentrations. The simplest type of fluorescence sensor measures fluorescence at a single wavelength. The appearance of a very small amount of light against a dark background results in a very sensitive measurement. An example is a pH sensor based on fluoresceinamine covalently linked to cellulose [10]. Fluoresceinamine is used as the pH-sensitive dye [11] because its fluorescence characteristics change in the middle of the pH range (4-8). In this sensor, the fluorescence intensity is increased as the acid form of the immobilized dye is transformed into the base conjugate.

The reduction in fluorescence intensity (or quenching) is another basis for remote sensing of analytes. We have developed an oxygen sensor [8] based upon the quenching of ruthenium trisbipyridyl emission. A reservoir cell has been utilized.

The trisbipyridyl complex of ruthenium can be excited between 430 and 490 nm and its emission peak appears at 610 nm. This compound exhibits a very large Stokes' shift and this makes the clean separation of the excitation and emission signals possible. The first excited triplet energy of 217 kJ/mole, and lifetime of 685 ns, make this complex a very interesting choice. It is reported that in oxygen-saturated aqueous solutions at room temperature, lifetime of $Ru(bpy)_3^{2+}$ decreases from 685 ns to 220 ns, suggesting that it can be used as an efficient oxygen sensor [8].

Integration of the fluid medium sensor chemistry into fiber optic technology is a very formidable task. We have attempted to simplify the sensor fabrication by using the reservoir cell as shown in Figure 4. The same design can be used for monitoring other dissolved gases (like CO_2, SO_2) in water, provided an appropriate gas permeable membrane is utilized. We have used teflon as the oxygen permeable membrane.

Figure 5 shows the typical response of the oxygen sensor. The starting point corresponds to "zero" oxygen.

Figure 6 depicts a linear response of the sensor as concentration of dissolved oxygen was varied. The sensor is reversible, although it takes about an hour to achieve the initial fluorescence intensity because of slow gas permeation through the membrane.

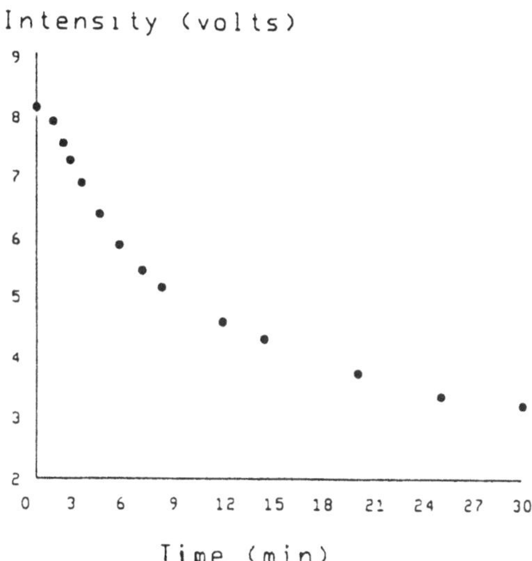

Figure 5: Response curve for the oxygen sensor when concentration of dissolved oxygen is 40 ppm.

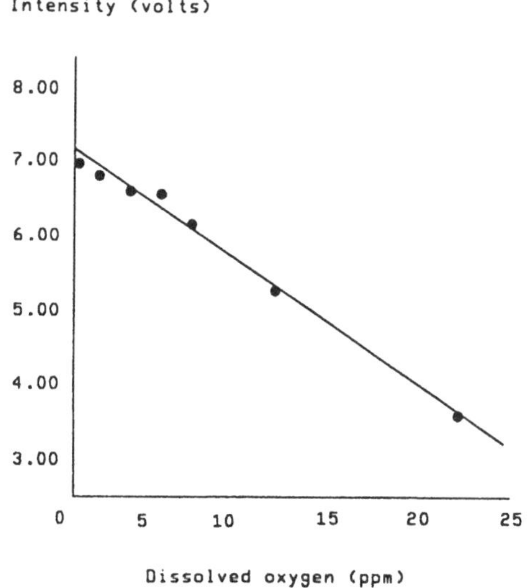

Figure 6: Linear response of the sensor for dissolved oxygen in water.

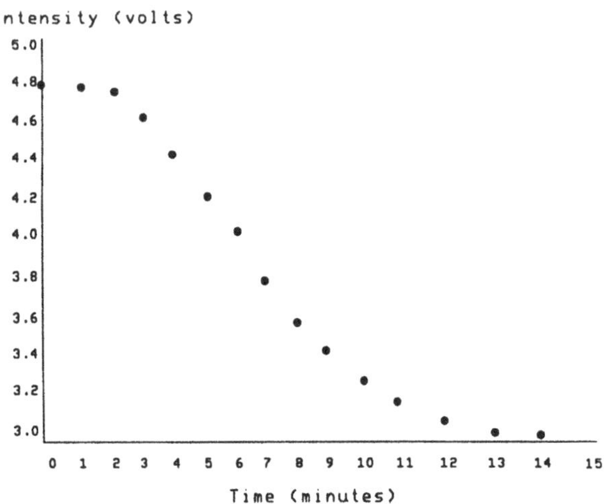

Figure 7: Response curve for the carbon dioxide sensor.

A FOCS for measuring carbon dioxide has also been developed and tested. Carbon dioxide dissolved in water exists in equilibrium with different species as shown below:

$CO_2(gas) + H_2O = CO_2(aq)$

$CO_2(aq) + H_2O = H_2CO_3$

$H_2CO_3 = H^+ + HCO^-_3$

Since a change in medium pH results as a consequence of CO_2 dissolution, this principle can be applied for measuring CO_2 in water. Dyes are available whose fluorescence properties are changed as the pH of the medium varies. Hydroxypyrenetrisulfonic acid-trisodium salt is such a pH-sensitive dye [12]. The hydrogen ion (H^+) sensitive fluorophore is isolated from the environment by using a membrane which only allows CO_2 to permeate through, but not protons. A reservoir cell (Figure 4) is employed for this purpose. The dissolved CO_2 within the reservoir cell then reacts with water and results in a drop in pH. This pH drop alters the fluorescence intensity.

Under the current state of development, polydimethylsiloxane-polycarbonate membrane has been employed for CO_2 permeation. Figure 7 shows the typical response of our diffusion controlled CO_2 sensor in a medium purged with CO_2 for 20 minutes. The response time appears to be about 5 minutes. Response time is being defined here as the time required for 90% of the signal change to take place.

Figure 8 shows the linearity of response for the CO_2 sensor. Experiments were done by dissolving precisely measured amounts of CO_2 in water. Both the oxygen and carbon dioxide sensors are intended for measuring dissolved gases in sea water.

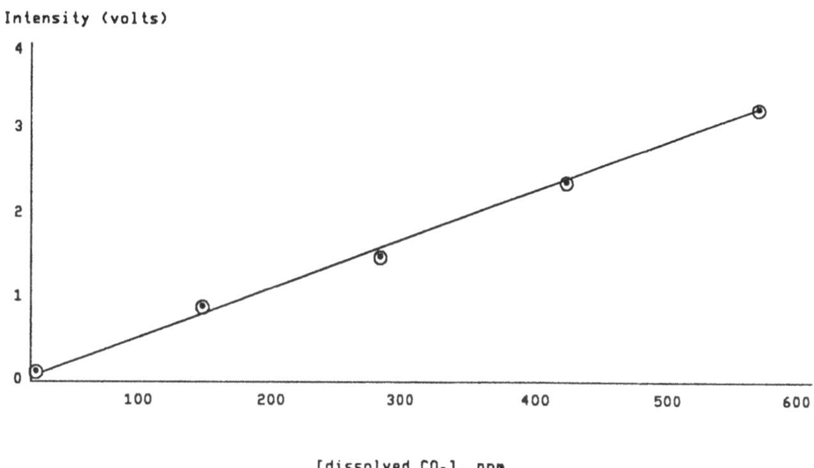

Figure 8: Linear response of the carbon dioxide sensor.

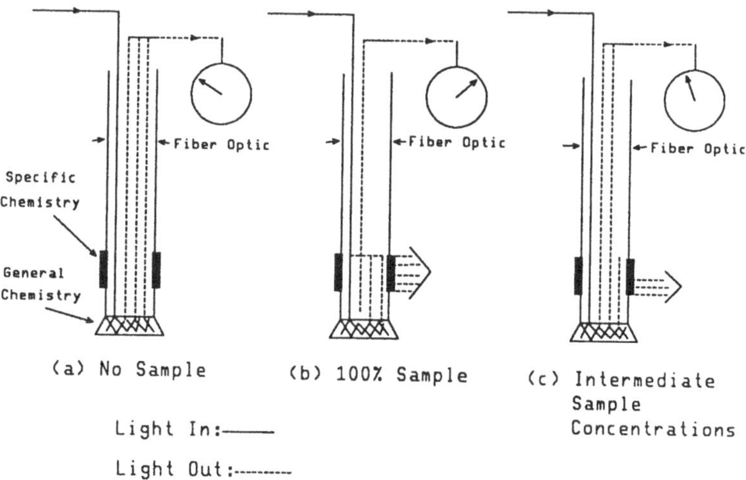

Figure 9: How a refractive index FOCS works.

Refraction can be utilized for making FOCS measurements as exemplified by the gasoline sensor [13]. In these types of measurements, the amount of light refracted changes as the analyte interacts with the coated surface. This FOCS consists of a bare fiber optic core with a thin clad of the sensing compound attached to its outer circumference near the distal end. In one design, the sensor has a fluorescent tip formed with an immobilized dye. An excitation signal is transmitted through the fiber tip and the fluorescence emission is used as a constant intensity light source of different wavelength than the incoming light. This is detected as the return signal. It is also possible to put the excitation source and the detector at the opposite ends of the fiber. A change in the refractive index of the medium surrounding the fiber alters its transmission characteristcs and results in a variation in the amount of light that reaches the detector. This is shown in Figure 9.

If the coating on the side of the fiber is closely matched to the index of refraction of the target molecule, specific and sensitive measurements are possible. In order to work properly, however, the side coat must have two (2) characteristics:

a) It must closely match the refractive index of the target compound.

b) It must have a highly specific affinity to the species of interest.

The latter is necessary because (i) the fiber optic index-matched system is not an accurate refractometer and cannot distinguish between compounds with close refractive indices and (ii) the refractive index of mixture, is an average of the species present and without preselection of the compound of interest the data would not be interpretable. The side coat preferentially concentrates the species of interest on the fiber thus enhancing its response vis-a-vis the other species present.

Here is how the sensor works. In the absence of gasoline, the returning light has a high intensity because air (or water) has a smaller refractive index than the core and thus acts as a clad. Under these circumstances, all of the light is propagated through the fiber. When gasoline is present, it is attracted to the high affinity material coated on the surface of the core, and there is an increase in refractive index at the surface of the core. As the refractive index of the clad changes and approaches that of the core, light leaks out the sides. The return signal decreases proportionately to the amount of gasoline present, due to the reduction in the fluorescent light, until it goes to zero.

Figure 10 shows the response of the FOCS to gasoline vapor and liquid. The width of the peaks in this figure have nothing to do with response time but only indicate the length of time the FOCS was in a particular medium. It can be seen that liquid gasoline does extinguish the signal and that the FOCS is completely reversible with response times of <5 sec. when going from air to liquid gasoline or the reverse. The reversible nature of this sensor indicates that only a physical interaction is taking place between the coating and the gasoline. The fact that laboratory data show that this FOCS responds to gasoline, and only slightly to kerosene and jet fuel, substantiates the specific affinity of the coating to key gasoline components. This sensor responds to gasoline in the vapor form or to neat liquid forms, as well as to gasoline dissolved in water.

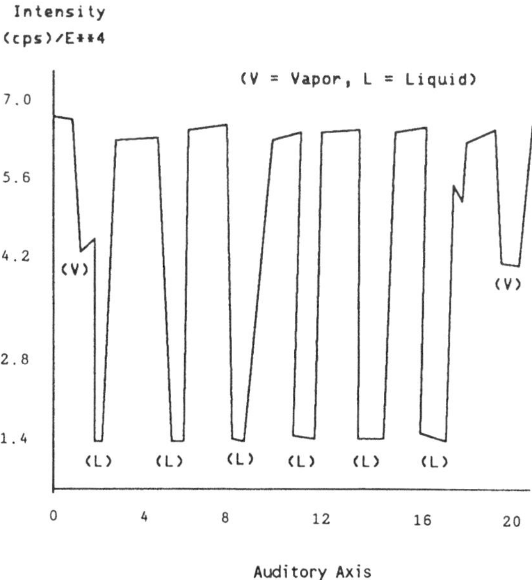

Figure 10: Reversibility of gasoline FOCS (computer trace of actual spectrum).

CONCLUSION:

The area of fiber optic chemical sensors is rapidly growing. The most important application of FOCS would be in monitoring. Some of the specific fields are medical, environmental, process control, military, space, and industrial safety. The anticipated low cost, ruggedness, and remote sensing capability will make FOCS system a desirable technology.

REFERENCES

1. Snyder, A.W. and Love, J.D. (1983), Optical Waveguide Theory, Chapman and Hall, New York, P.9.

2. Munkholm, C., Walt, D., Milanovich, F., and Klainer, S. (1986), Polymer modification of fiber optic chemical sensors as a method of enhancing fluorescence signal for pH measurement, Anal. Chem., 58: 1427.
3. Duportail, G., and Weinreb. A. (1983), Photochemical changes of fluorescent probes in membranes and their effect on the observed fluorescence values, Biochim. Biophys. Acta, 171: 736.
4. Macedo, P., Litovitz, T., Lagakos, N., Mohr, R., and Meister, R. (1984), Optical sensing apparatus and method, U.S. Patent #4,443,700.
5. Heitzmann, H. (1985), Optical sensor with beads, U.S. Patent #4,557,900.
6. Tai, H., Tanaka, H., and Yoshino, T. (1987), Fiber-optic evanescent-wave methane gas sensor using optical absorption for the 3.392-μm line of a He-Ne laser, Opt. Lett., 12: 437.
7. Block, M., Hirschfeld, T. (1986), Apparatus including optical fiber for fluorescence immunoassay, U.S. Patent #4,582,809.
8. Goswami, K., Klainer, S.M. and Tokar, J. M. (1988), Fiber optic chemical sensor for the measurement of partial pressure of oxygen. SPIE Proceedings, 990: 111.
9. Welfort, W.T. and Winston, R.A. (1978), The Optics of nonimaging concentrators: Light and Solar concentrators, Academic Press, New York.
10. Peterson, J., Goldstein, S., Fitzgerald, R., and Buckhold, D. (1980), Fiber optic pH probe for physiological use, Anal. Chem., 52: 864.
11. Saari, L. and Seitz, W. (1982), pH sensor based on immobilized fluoresceinamine, Anal. Chem., 54: 821.
12. Munkholm, C., Walt, D., and Milanovich, F. (1988), A fiber optic sensor for CO_2 measurement, Talanta, 35: 109.
13. Klainer, S.M., Goswami, K., LeGoullon, D., Dandge, D.K., Thomas, J.R., Simon, S.J., and Eccles, L. (1988), Monitoring of gasoline vapor and liquid by fiber optic chemical sensor (FOCS) technology, Symposium Proceedings, 1st International Waste Site Investigation, Las Vegas, 25.

22

Polymeric Indicator Substrates for Fiber Optic Chemical Sensors

W. RUDOLF SEITZ, YUNKE ZHANG, ZHANG ZHUJUN, AMY SOMMERS, CHEN JIAN, RICHARD RUSSELL AND DONALD C. SUNDBERG Department of Chemistry University of New Hampshire, Durham, New Hampshire

1. INTRODUCTION

We are interested in the development of chemical sensors based on immobilized chemical indicators coupled to a spectrometer through fiber optics. Indicators may be immobilized by attaching them to a solid support or confining them behind a barrier which is permeable to analyte but not to the indicator. Many systems are based on polymers. One facet of our research has involved the development of new polymer systems for use with fiber optic chemical sensors.

In this manuscript we will initially outline some of the requirements for polymer systems to be used in fiber optic chemical sensors. This will be followed by a review of some of the polymer systems that have been used by others. We will then describe some of our results with four different systems, poly(vinyl chloride), cellulose triacetate, poly(vinyl alcohol) and poly(ethylenimine).

2. POLYMER REQUIREMENTS

Polymers used in fiber optic chemical sensors may be divided into two categories. One category includes polymers that are discrete continuous phases. A good example is the silicone polymers that have been used in optical oxygen sensors (1-4). The other category involves polymers that are porous, and, therefore, present a large surface area to the sample where indicator and analyte can interact. Examples include poly(acrylamide) (5) and porous glass (6).

Discrete phase polymers are subject to several requirements. They need to be transparent to the wavelengths used for sensing. Their optical properties have to be constant when in contact with the sample. Ideally, the polymer should be clear if the measured parameter is fluorescence. If the measured parameter is absorbance or reflectance, however, scattering is desirable since it redirects incident light back towards the detection system.

In principle, indicator could be immobilized on the surface of a discrete phase polymer. However, unless the polymer surface is roughened or the polymer is rendered porous by some appropriate treatment, the amount of indicator that can be immobilized on the surface is impractically small for spectroscopic measurements. Instead, the indicator needs to be incorporated directly in the discrete phase polymer. This can be accomplished by covalently bonding the indicator to the discrete phase polymer. Alternatively, if the indicator is compatible with the polymer, it may remain in the polymer even while in contact with sample.

In discrete phase polymer systems, the analyte must be mobile in the polymer in order to interact with indicator. The discrete phase polymer "extracts" the analyte from the sample.

Porous polymer systems also need to be transparent at the wavelengths required for the optical measurement. If the dimensions of the heterogeneity are signicantly less than the wavelength of the radiation used for the optical measurement, the porous polymer will be clear. Alternatively, if there are separate domains in the polymer which differ in refractive index, light will be scattered at the interfaces and the polymer will be opaque. This interferes with fluorescence measurements but can be helpful for absorbance and reflectance measurements because scattering can redirect the incident light toward the detection system.

The pores of the polymer should be large enough to permit easy access to the analyte. However, it is desirable to be able to control their size so that larger species that might otherwise interfere can be excluded.

In all systems it is desirable to have some degree of control of the amount of indicator that enters the substrate since this affects sensitivity and can also influence the shape of the response curve. If the amount of indicator is small, it may be necessary to use greater source intensities to acquire a signal that is large enough to measure with adequate precision. This will lead to accelerated rates of photodegradation which limit sensor lifetime.

It is also advantageous to be able to control the amount of substrate since this affects the amount of indicator and the response time.

3. OTHER WORK

Polymeric supports for indicators for fiber optic chemical sensors have been considered in the extensive review by Wolfbeis (7). A variety of polymers have been used as indicator substrates. Only the most popular and versatile ones will be considered here.

Silicones have been widely used in sensors for detecting oxygen and carbon dioxide. Because they are hydrophobic they exclude liquid water. They are highly permeable to oxygen and carbon dioxide as well as water vapor. A variety of formulations are available. Some involve two components, the polymer and a "hardener", which crosslinks the polymer to form a flexible solid. Others involve a single component. Exposure to ambient water vapor causes the polymer to crosslink and form a solid.

Oxygen sensors have been prepared by dissolving or suspending indicator in the polymer prior to solid formation (1-4). This allows for control of the amount of indicator in the solid. The amount of substrate can also be controlled by dispensing a known volume of silicone.

In oxygen sensors, silicone can be considered to be extracting oxygen from the sample. Because oxygen is more soluble in silicone polymers than in water, the polymer is preconcentrating oxygen enhancing the sensitivity of the sensor.

In carbon dioxide sensors, silicone polymers are used as barriers which are permeable to carbon dioxide but prevent direct contact between an aqueous sample and an aqueous filling solution containing bicarbonate and a pH sensitive indicator (4,8). The filling solution is most frequently confined behind a silicone membrane, but can also be dispersed as droplets within the silicone polymer.

Most other common indicator substrates involve materials where interaction takes place at a surface. Cellulose was used as a substrate for covalent indicator immobilization in early work (9). Poly(methylmethacrylate) particles have served as a substrate for immobilizing hydrophobic organic indicators in the work of Narayanswamy and co-workers (10). The immobilization procedure involves contacting the substrate with a solution of indicator in a volatile organic solvent and then allowing the solvent to evaporate leaving a solid residue on the substrate surface. The cellulose and the poly(methylmethacrylate) particles are not porous. High surface area results from small particle size. Indicator phases prepared using these substrates have been highly scattering and are, therefore, well suited for absorbance and reflectance measurements.

Ion exchange materials have been used as substrates for "electrostatically "immobilizing hydrophobic counterions (11,12). A combination of electrostatic and hydrophobic interactions holds the indicator on the surface. The procedures involve stirring the ion exchanger in a solution containing a known amount of indicator until all the indicator is on the substrate. This allows for convenient control of the amount of the indicator. The first studies demonstrating the effect of indicator amount on optical sensor response were performed using this approach (11).

Porous glass provides several attractive features as an immobilization substrate. Because it has a high surface area, large quantities of indicator can be immobilized on a small amount of substrate. Using silane reagents it is possible to introduce a great variety of functional groups to a glass surface, making it a versatile substrate from the perspective of available immobilization chemistries. Porous glass is commercially available as particles with a variety of pore sizes and particle sizes. Single beads of porous glass have been glued to the end of a single optical fiber (13). However, this is a tricky operation, because the adhesive tends to be drawn into the glass, blocking contact with the sample. A more elegant approach is to prepare the controlled pore glass directly on the end of the fiber (6). The initial step is to attach glass of the appropriate composition to the end of an optical fiber. This is heated to induce separation into two phases, which differ in solubility. The glass is then treated to dissolve the more soluble phase resulting in a highly porous material.

Although procedures based on porous glass are attractive from several perspectives, they do not allow for ready control of the amount of indicator. In principle, this can be accomplished by controlling the conditions of the reactions required to activate the glass surface and covalently couple it to an indicator. However, it is extremely difficult to reproducibly control the area and the activity of the surface.

Poly(acrylamide) has also received considerable attention as an indicator substrate. The procedure involves reacting acrylamide with N,N-methylenebis(acrylamide) (BIS) in the presence of initiators. The resulting polymer may be clear or cloudy depending on the percentage of crosslinking reagent (14). The porosity of the poly(acrylamide) gel can be systematically varied by appropriate choice of initial concentrations (15). This is widely exploited in poly(acrylamide) gel electrophoresis, an essential technique for molecular biology. Poly(acrylamide) has also been used to entrap macromolecules such as enzymes in a solid matrix permeable to smaller molecules. Unlike porous glass which is rigid, poly(acrylamide) is firm but flexible and swells in contact with water.

Several approaches can be used to immobilize indicators to poly(acrylamide). In favorable cases, notably phenol red which has been widely used in optical pH sensors, the unmodified indicator couples directly to the polymer (16). The amount of indicator can be controlled by adding the appropriate initial quantity before the polymer is formed. Another approach is to covalently modify the indicator so that it has an acrylamide group which incorporates directly into the polymer (5). This also allows for ready control of the amount of indicator in the polymer.

Poly(acrylamide) is also amenable to sensor preparation using dipcoating procedures (5). The initial step is to modify the end of an optical fiber so that it contains acrylamide groups. These fibers are dipped into a polymerizing mixture of acrylamide, BIS and indicator and is slowly withdrawn such that a small amount of material adheres to the end of the fiber. The actual amount of substrate on the fiber depends on the rate at which the fiber is withdrawn and the viscosity of the mixture. Because amounts tend to be small, this procedure is most suitable for applications where small size is more important than longterm stability. Dipcoating is attractive from a commercial perspective because several sensors can be prepared in parallel.

4. POLY(VINYL CHLORIDE)

Poly(vinyl chloride) (PVC) by itself is rigid and impermeable at room temperature. However, addition of a plasticizer lowers the glass transition temperature, resulting in a material that is flexible at room temperature. Diffusion coefficients in plasticized PVC are on the order of 10^{-8} cm^2/sec, about 3 orders of magnitude less than in water. Therefore, hydrophobic analytes can be extracted from water into plasticized PVC where they can react with an indicator to form an optically detectable product.

PVC is most familiar to analytical chemists as a membrane material widely used in ion selective electrodes. Neutral ionophores are incorporated into the membrane so that it selectively transports the ion to be sensed. Membranes are typically prepared by solvent casting using compounds such as dioctyl phthalate (DOP) as plasticizers.

The PVC used in membranes for ion selective electrodes is prepared by emulsion polymerization, which results in a product containing residual surfactant. It is now recognized that the residual surfactant is essential for ion-selective electrode membranes because it renders the membrane permeable to the lipophilic counterions formed by complexation between the ion to be determined and the neutral ionophore in the membrane.

We were interested in using plasticized PVC as the substrate for optical detection of trace levels of 2,4,6-trinitrotoluene (TNT) and other polynitroaromatics in groundwater (17). These compounds react with primary and secondary amines to form a colored product which is readily detected optically. However, color development is slow requiring hours to detect ppm levels and two weeks to get observable color for 10 ppb TNT. Hence, our need was for an amine containing membrane that would be optically and chemically stable for weeks in contact with water.

Membranes were prepared by solvent casting from tetrahydrofuran (THF). Amines were incorporated into the membrane by dissolving them in THF along with PVC and the plasticizer, dioctyl phthalate.

Initial experiments were performed with emulsion polymerized PVC. However, it was found that this membrane becomes cloudy after being in contact with water for a few hours. The residual surfactants in the PVC act as sites for water nucleation. Water accumulates in the membrane forming domains that differ in refractive index from plasticized PVC. This causes the membrane to appear cloudy. Because their optical properties change with time, membranes prepared using emulsion polymerized PVC are unsuitable for optical measurements.

Bulk polymerized PVC is prepared using pure vinyl chloride. This material does not contain residual surfactant. We have kept membranes prepared from bulk polymerized PVC in contact with water for as long as two months and not observed any cloudiness. These membranes were prepared from Geon 143, a bulk polymerized PVC available from B.F. Goodrich, using 0.40 mLs of DOP as the plasticizer per gram of PVC. Increasing the plasticizer level results in membranes that are susceptible to cloudiness in contact with water.

The second problem was to incorporate a primary or secondary amine into the membrane. A procedure has been reported for covalently bonding primary amines to PVC containing 1.8% carboxyl groups (18). Unfortunately, however, this material is unsuitable as a medium for optical measurements because the carboxyl groups act as sites for water nucleation causing membranes to rapidly become cloudy. Therefore, we chose to look for an amine that would be sufficiently compatible with PVC so that it would remain in the membrane even when contact with water. Initially we attempted to modify common plasticizers so that they would contain amine groups. However, before we were successful in developing such a compound, we learned of commercial polyoxyalkyleneamines available from Texaco Chemical Company. The material that we found to be most suitable for our purpose has the tradename Jeffamine T403 and the structure shown below:

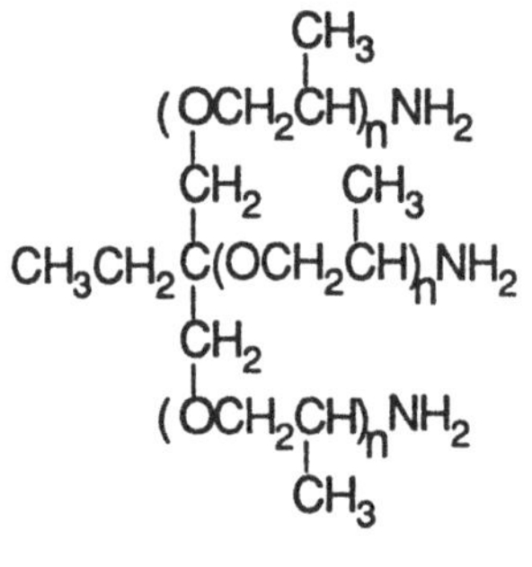

$$\begin{array}{c} (OCH_2CH(CH_3))_nNH_2 \\ | \\ CH_2 \\ | \\ CH_3CH_2C(OCH_2CH(CH_3))_nNH_2 \\ | \\ CH_2 \\ | \\ (OCH_2CH(CH_3))_nNH_2 \end{array}$$

The average molecular weight is 403. The sum of the three "n" values is between 5 and 6, and the primary amine content is 6.1 mmol/g.

Jeffamine T403 can actually serve as a plasticizer for PVC. However, because high concentrations of Jeffamine T403 are subject to rapid leaching in water, we found that it was better to incorporate DOP into membrane formulations to serve as the primary plasticizer.

Membranes prepared to contain Jeffamine T403 are subject to slow loss of amine in contact with water. For example, membranes prepared to have an initial nitrogen contents of 1.24 and 0.44 wt-% were found to have nitrogen contents of 0.17 and 0.26 wt-%, respectively, after being exposed to water for 46 days. Membranes prepared to have a lower initial amine content are much more stable to amine loss. Indeed, membranes prepared to have an initially higher amine content actually wind up with a lower amine content after several weeks. This means that high amine concentrations must somehow enhance the rate of amine loss. We believe that membranes that have high initial levels are subject to phase separation of the amine from the other components of the membrane.

Although our primary application involved absorption measurements, we also attempted to prepare fluorescent membranes by including a variety of lipophilic fluorophors in the solution used to prepare the membrane (19). However, it was consistently found that the fluorescence was weak or not observable at all. Plasticized PVC is not a good medium for fluorescence. This we attribute to quenching due to the external heavy atom effect associated with the chlorine atoms on PVC. For the same reason, chlorinated hydrocarbons are routinely avoided as solvents for fluorescent measurements.

The membrane formulation that we have developed has many other potential applications to optical sensing based on absorption besides the detection of polynitroaromatics. Covalent bonding to the primary amine functions on Jeffamine T403 can provide a means for increasing the affinity of an indicator for the PVC membrane relative to water. For example, in our attempts to develop a fluorescent membrane, we prepared a fluorescein isothiocyanate/ Jeffamine T403 conjugate which had a high affinity for the membrane.

5. CELLULOSE TRIACETATE

We have recently started to work with plasticized cellulose triacetate membranes. As with PVC, membranes are prepared by solvent casting. Plasticizer and polymer are dissolved in an organic solvent, usually cyclohexanone or tetrahydrofuran. Evaporation of the solvent leaves a flexible membrane which remains clear in contact with water. Like PVC, plasticized cellulose triacetate is a discrete phase which can extract hydrophobic compounds from water. The advantage of cellulose triacetate is that it is better medium for fluorescence than PVC. We have successfully prepared fluorescent membranes by dissolving a variety of fluorophors in the solution used for solvent casting. Our goal has been to detect polynitroaromatics and nitramines based on fluorescence quenching. However, these membranes are potentially useful for a variety of other optical sensing applications.

6. POLY(VINYL ALCOHOL)

We have also been interested in developing porous polymer substrates for optical sensing applications. Most of our work has involved poly(vinyl alcohol) (PVOH) crosslinked with glutaraldehyde. Initially, we investigated PVOH because it is transparent in the ultraviolet. While working with glutaraldehyde crosslinked PVOH, we realized that it offers several unique advantages as a substrate for immobilizing indicators for optical sensors. Since the characteristics of this material have already been described in the literature (20,21), we will briefly recapitulate them here with a few additional tidbits not already reported.

The procedure for preparing sensors based on PVOH involves the following sequence. First, indicator is covalently coupled to PVOH. A large quantity of PVOH is added to water at room temperature, such that the PVOH is hydrated but much of it does not actually dissolve. This material is covalently coupled to indicator and separated by filtration. The reactions that we have used to immobilize indicator are discussed below. After immobilization a small amount of indicator/PVOH conjugate is dissolved in water, and indicator absorbance is measured to determine the amount of indicator immobilized per gram of PVOH. At this point the amount of indicator can be adjusted, either by diluting with unreacted PVOH or by repeating the immobilization procedure with an additional batch of indicator. The next step is to dissolve the indicator/PVOH in water at elevated temperatures. Most our work has involved solutions that contain 5% (w/w) PVOH. It is possible to work with concentrations as high as 10% but these solutions are extremely viscous making it difficult to remove air bubbles.

PVOH is crosslinked by adding glutaraldehyde and HCl. The HCl catalyzes the reaction between PVOH and aldehyde to form an acetal linkage. The rate of this process depends on the concentration of acid. This makes it possible to choose an HCl concentration such that crosslinking is slow, and there is time to manipulate the PVOH/indicator/glutaraldehyde mixture as a liquid before it solidifies. This allows time to transfer a known volume of liquid to the end of an optical fiber or a fiber bundle where it can solidify in situ.

The procedure described above offers the important advantage that it allows independent and reproducible control of both the amount of indicator and the amount of substrate in the sensor. This makes it possible to vary these parameters in a systematic way and to design a sensor for a particular application. This has been demonstrated using covalently immobilized fluoresceinamine as an indicator for pH (20).

There are several reagents that can be used to modify PVOH so that it can covalently bond to indicators. However, all of our work has involved cyanuric chloride. The structure and reactions of cyanuric chloride are shown below:

$$\text{Cyanuric Chloride} + R_1OH \longrightarrow (OR_1)\text{-dichlorotriazine} + HCl$$

Cyanuric Chloride

$$(OR_1)\text{-dichlorotriazine} + R_2NH_2 \longrightarrow (OR_1)(NHR_2)\text{-chlorotriazine} + HCl$$

It reacts with amines, alcohols and thiols. In water, the three chlorides differ in their reactivity. The first chloride reacts at 0 degrees C, the second at room temperature, and the third at elevated temperatures. This allows for control over the reaction.

Indicator immobilization with cyanuric chloride is a two-step process involving sequential reaction with the indicator and then with PVOH or vice versa. Although the results that we have reported in the literature have involved reacting cyanuric chloride first with PVOH and then with indicator, we feel the alternative procedure is preferred, provided a clean indicator/cyanuric chloride conjugate can be prepared. The initial reaction between the indicator and cyanuric chloride can be performed in organic media avoiding hydrolysis of cyanuric chloride as a side reaction. The indicator/cyanuric chloride conjugate can be separated and purified to confirm that it has the expected structure, before it is reacted with PVOH.

Table 1 lists indicators that we have attempted to immobilize using cyanuric chloride. In all cases but one we have succeeded. The failure, however, is instructive, pointing out some of the hazards associated with our procedures. Attempts to immobilize morin have led to polymeric products that have been only weakly fluorescent or have not fluoresced at all in the presence of Al(III) which normally forms a strongly fluorescent complex with morin. One approach was to

TABLE 1

INDICATORS IMMOBILIZED ON PVOH

Indicator	ANALYTE
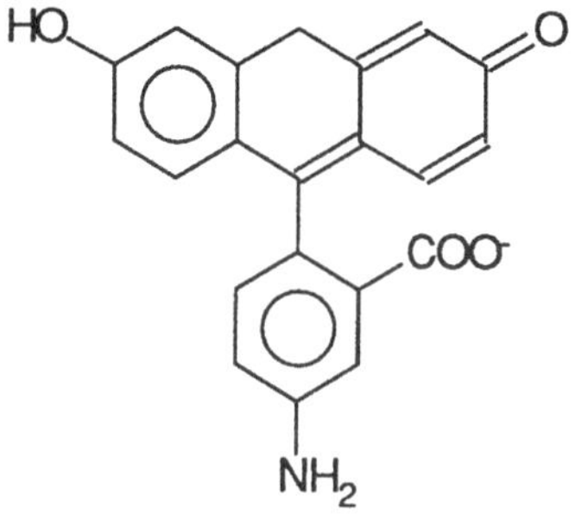 Fluoresceinamine	pH
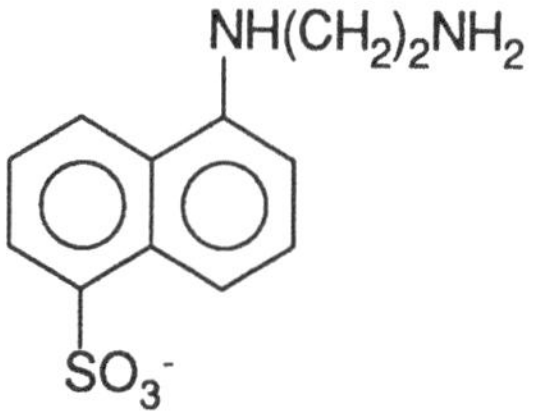 DA+	Cationic Surfactants
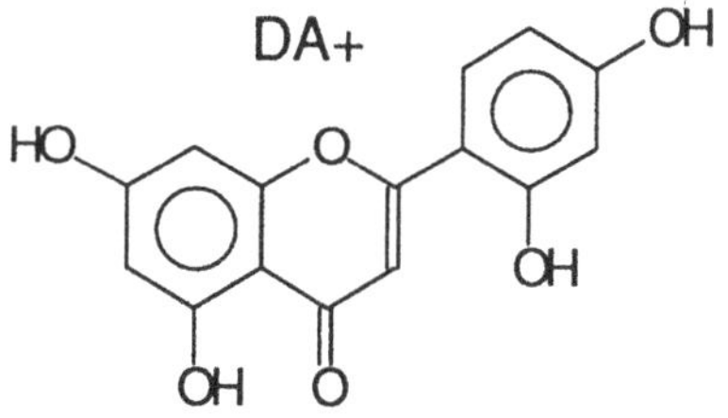 Morin	Al(III)
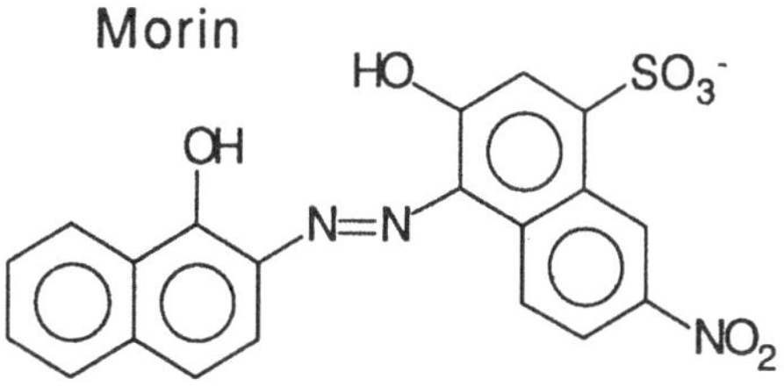 Eriochrome Black T	Mg(II)

prepare a morin/cyanuric chloride conjugate. The problem is that when this compound is combined with PVOH, it tends to react with the other -OH groups on morin rather than the -OH groups on PVOH, leading to a nonfluorescent product. Starting with cyanuric chloride activated PVOH and reacting it with morin was also unsuccessful. Although the dissolved PVOH/morin conjugate had the desired fluorescent properties, crosslinking was accompanied by a large decrease in fluorescence.

Successful use of a cyanuric chloride as an immobilization reagent is subject to certain limitations. If the initial step in immobilization is preparation of a cyanuric chloride/indicator conjugate, it is necessary that only one site on the indicator react. If cyanuric chloride can react with the indicator at more than one site, the cyanuric chloride/indicator conjugate will tend to react with itself when PVOH is added and the temperature is increased.

If cyanuric chloride is initially reacted with PVOH, then it must react more rapidly with indicator than with PVOH. Otherwise, the cyanuric chloride activated PVOH will react with itself when indicator is added and the temperature is increased.

Despite these limitations, PVOH is the only substrate that allows for independent control of the amounts of indicator and substrate and thus offers the opportunity to engineer sensor chemistry for a particular application.

7. POLY(ETHYLENIMINE)

Although it offers important advantages, PVOH is also subject to some serious limitations as an indicator substrate. Because alcohols are relatively unreactive, PVOH is not as versatile an indicator substrate as some other materials. Also, because the procedure requires the addition of HCl, it can not be used to immobilize reagents that are unstable in strongly acidic media, e.g. enzymes. Therefore, we are attempting to develop analogous procedures using poly(ethylenimine) (PEI) crosslinked with dimethyl adipimidate (DMA), a reagent that is used to crosslink proteins. The reaction is shown below:

$$(\text{-}CH_2CH_2NH\text{-})_n + \underset{\text{DMA}}{\begin{matrix} HN & & NH \\ \| & & \| \\ C & (CH_2)_4 & C \\ | & & | \\ CH_3O & & OCH_3 \end{matrix}} \xrightarrow[\text{pH 7-9}]{} \begin{matrix} (\text{-}CH_2CH_2N\text{-})_n \\ | \\ C{=}N \\ | \\ (CH_2)_4 \\ | \\ C{=}N \\ | \\ (\text{-}CH_2CH_2N\text{-})_n \end{matrix}$$

PEI

At pH 7, PEI can be crosslinked under conditions such that it takes several minutes for a solid gel to form. However, the resulting gel is runny and lacks the firmness of glutaraldehyde-crosslinked PVOH. When crosslinking occurs at higher pH, solid formation is faster and the gel is firmer.

PEI differs from PVOH in that the amine groups on PEI can be protonated. As the pH is reduced, the extent of protonation increases. Electrostatic repulsion between positively charged sites on the PEI causes the PEI to adopt an extended conformation. This effect is believed to account for the pH effect on the mechanical properties of crosslinked PEI. It will also be an important effect for sensor applications since it will cause pH dependent swelling of the gel.

ACKNOWLEDGEMENTS

Financial support for this research was provided by the U.S. Army Toxic and Hazardous Materials Agency through the U.S. Army Cold Region Research and Engineering Laboratory (Contract DACA89-86-K-0007) and by the National Science Foundation through Grant CHE85-02061.

REFERENCES

1. Cox, M. E., and Dunn, B. (1985). Detection of oxygen by fluorescence quenching, Appl. Opt. , 24 : 2114

2. Wolfbeis, O. S., Weis, L. J., Leiner, M. J. P., and Ziegler, W. E. (1988) Fiber-optic fluorosensor for oxygen and carbon dioxide, Anal. Chem. , 60 : 2028

3. Kroneis, H. W., and Marsoner, H. J. (1983). A fluorescence-based sterilizable oxygen probe for use in bioreactors, Sensors and Actuators , 4 : 587 (1983)

4. Bacon, J. R., and Demas, J. N. (1987). Determination of oxygen concentrations by luminescence quenching of a polymer-immobilized transition-metal complex, Anal. Chem. , 59 : 2780

5. Munkholm, C., Walt, D. R., Milanovich, F. P., and Klainer, S. M. (1986). Polymer modification of fiber optic chemical sensors as a method of enhancing fluorescence signal for pH measurement, Anal. Chem. , 58 : 1427

6. Zhou, Q., Shahriari, M. R., Kritz, D., and Sigel, G. H. Jr. (1988). Porous fiber-optic sensor for high-sensitivity humidity measurements, Anal. Chem. , 60 : 2317

7. Wolfbeis, O. S. (1988). Fiber optical fluorosensors in analytical and clinical chemistry, in Molecular Luminescence Spectroscopy: Methods and Applications-Part II (S. G. Schulman, ed.) Wiley Interscience, New York, pp. 182-187

8. Munkholm, C., Walt, D. R., and Milanovich, F. P. (1988). A fiber-optic sensor for CO2 measurement, Talanta , 35 : 109

9. Saari, L. A., and Seitz, W. R. (1982). pH sensor based on immobilized fluoreseinamine, Anal. Chem. , 54 : 821

10. Kirkbright, G. F., Narayanswamy, R., and Welti, N. A. (1984). Fiber optic ppH probe based on the use of an immobilised colorimetric indicator, Analyst , 109 : 1025

11. Zhujun, Z., and Seitz, W. R. (1984). A fluorescence sensor for quantifying pH in the range from 6.5 to 8.5, Anal. Chim. Acta , 160 : 47

12. Zhujun, Z., and Seitz, W. R. (1985). An optical sensor for Al(III), Mg(II), Zn(II) and Cd(II) based on electrostatically immobilized 8-hydroxyquinoline sulfonate, Anal. Chim. Acta , 171 : 251

13. Fuh, M. S., Burgess, L. W., Hirschfeld, T., Christian, G. E., and Wang, F. (1987). Single fibre optic fluorescence pH probe, Analyst , 112 : 1159

14. Hicks, G. P. and Updike, S. J. (1966). The preparation and characteerization of lyophilized polyacrylamide enzyme gels for chemical analysis, Anal. Chem. , 38 : 726

15. Fawcett, J. S., and Morris, C. J. O. R. (1966). Molecular-sieve chromatography of proteins on granulated polyacrylamide, Separation Sci. , 1 : 9

16. Peterson, J. I., Goldstein, S. R., Fitzgerald, R. V., and Buckhold, D. K. (1980). Fiber optic pH probe for physiological use, Anal. Chem. , 52 : 864

17. Zhang, Y., Seitz, W. R., Grant, C. L., and Sundberg, D. C. (1989). A clear, amine-containing poly(vinyl chloride) membrane for in situ optical detection of 2,4,6-trinitrotoluene, Anal. Chim. Acta , 217 : 217

18. Ma, S. C., Chaniotakei, N. S. and Meyerhoff, M. E. (1989). Response properties of ion-selective polymeric membrane electrodes prepared with aminated and carboxylated poly(vinyl chloride), Anal. Chem. , 60 : 2293

19. Zhang, Y., and Seitz, W. R. (1989). Single fiber absorption measurements for remote detection of 2,4,6-trinitrotoluene, Anal. Chim. Acta , 221 : 1 (1989)

20. Zhujun, Z., Zhang, Y., Wangbai, M., Russell, R., Shakhser, Z. M., Grant, C. L., and Seitz, W. R. (1989). Poly(vinyl alcohol) as a substrate for indicator immobilization for fiber-optic chemical sensors, Anal. Chem. , 43 : 202

21. Wangbai, M., Zhujun, Z., and Seitz, W. R.(1989). Poly(vinyl alcohol) based indicators for optical pH and Mg(II) sensing, in Chemical Sensors and Microinstrumentation , (R. W. Murray et

al., eds.), American Chemical Society, Washington, DC, pp. 273-282

23

The Use of Metal Island Films to Support Radiative Surface Plasmons as a Method of Transducing Interfacial Events

RENO F. DEBONO, M. THOMPSON, A.L. MALLON AND M.J. SCAINI Chemical Sensors Group, Department of Chemistry, University of Toronto, Ontario, CANADA, M5S 1A1

ABSTRACT

Surface plasmons(SP) are charge density waves which involve the oscillation of surface electron density at the metal interface. The use of SP as a method of signal transduction for biosensor development has been shown to be feasible with a Kretschman or a grating configuration. However, neither of these configurations lend themselves to miniaturization for in vivo sensing. An alternative approach has been employed here based on the observation that the visible absorption spectrum of small metallic particles is dominated by the SP resonance of the valence electrons. The resonance conditions depend on the size and shape of the metal particle and the local environment in which the particles are embedded. Preliminary experiments indicate that the absorption spectra of thin silver island films are sensitive to deposition and annealing conditions due to changes in the size and shape of the deposited islands. The effects of immersing these deposited films into different solvents and solutions indicates that a significant perturbation of the absorption curves occurs, inferring a perturbation of the surface plasmon resonance conditions. If this local environment is functionalized to provide a degree of chemical selectivity, then subsequent binding of an analyte should result in a change in the optical absorption spectrum which could provide the basis of transduction scheme for a biosensor.

INTRODUCTION

Metals can be modelled as a plasma of mobile conduction band electrons associated with a fixed lattice of positive ions. If a fluctuation in the electron density occurs then electrons will flow from a region of high electron density to a region of low electron density. This net movement of electrons generally overshoots the equilibrium point producing an oscillation of electron density which decays with time. Electron density oscillations which occur at the metal surface and propagate in the plane of the surface are referred to as a surface plasmons(SP) [1].

An oscillating electric vector which is perpendicular to the surface can induce a discontinuity in the electron density, initiating a charge density oscillation. If the incident electric field frequency matches the frequency of the surface plasmon then energy is coupled into this charge density oscillation, increasing its amplitude and producing a intense electromagnetic field which is localized at the metal surface. SP's cannot be excited by direct optical illumination of a smooth metal surface because energy and momentum conservation can not be obtained simultaneously. By the law of reciprocity these surface plasmons can only relax via non-radiative processes, hence the subclass of non-radiative surface plasmons. To generate SP at the smooth metal surface, prism[2] and grating[1] couplers have been used to increase the momentum of incident photons. This phenomenon physically manifests itself as a decrease in the reflected intensity of the incident radiation.

The use of non-radiative SP's as the basis of a biosensor has been shown to be feasible with a Kretschman[3-5] or a grating configuration[6] but neither of these configurations lend themselves easily to miniaturization for in vivo sensing. An alternative approach suggested here utilizes the presence of a curved boundary to allow direct excitation of a radiative surface plasmon by incident radiation. This requires metal particles which are much smaller than the wavelength of visible light.

Mie theory predicts that the absorption coefficient of a metal particle is related to the dielectric constant(ε_o) of the material which it is embedded in by equation 1.

$$K = \frac{18\pi C\varepsilon_o^{3/2}\ \varepsilon_2}{\lambda((\varepsilon_1 + 2\varepsilon_o)^2 + \varepsilon_2^2)} \qquad (1)$$

Where C is the volume concentration of the metal particles and $\varepsilon_1 + i\varepsilon_2$ is the dielectric constant of the bulk metal. If the local environment is functionalized to provide a degree of chemical selectivity, then subsequent binding of an analyte could cause a change in the local dielectric environment which would subsequently affect the optical absorption spectrum of the metal particle.

PROCEDURES

Glass wafers were cut to dimensions of 0.9 x 3cm from plain borosilicate microscope slides of thickness 1 mm. These wafers were then sonicated in a 1% aqueous solution of sodium dodecylsulphate detergent for 30 minutes, rinsed with water, soaked in chromic acid for 10 minutes, extensively washed with water and then oven dried for 20 minutes. Wafers were cleaned on the day of deposition.

Thin silver island films were prepared by thermal evaporation of 99.99% pure silver from a molybdenum boat located 29 cm below the glass wafers. Silver was deposited at less than 5 Å/sec at room temperature in a vacuum of 1×10^{-6} Torr. The thickness was monitored using a quartz-crystal oscillator. Note that the thickness reported should be considered as a relative quantity indicative of the mass of silver on the surface. Wafers were stored in a dark dust-free environment until used.

Annealing was carried out either at 100 °C or 250 °C by placing the wafer in an upright position in a 25 ml Pyrex erlenmeyer flask.

UV/V absorption spectra were recorded on a HP 8451A diode array spectrophotometer. The reference scan involved inserting a blank glass wafer into a cuvette which either was empty or contained the same solution into which the silvered wafer was to be immersed. The UV/V spectra were recorded such that the wafer was essentially perpendicular to incident beam.

RESULTS AND DISCUSSION

Silver island films were used for the following reasons: 1)silver has the sharpest and strongest SP resonance of all the metals 2)it is a much stabler system than colloidal solutions which tend to aggregate over time 3)a higher localized concentration of the metal particles can be obtained 4)easier to handle than colloidal solutions.

Thin homogeneous film growth is encouraged by fast deposition rates, but in order to create a system capable of supporting radiative surface plasmons silver island formation must be promoted. This is achieved by using slow deposition rates below 5 Å/sec. A series of wafers were coated with silver to examine the effect of thickness. The results are summarized in figures 1 to 3.

The peak position showed a strong correlation with the amount of silver which was deposited (fig. 1). As the thickness increased the peak position shifted from 420nm to 700nm while the full width at half height(FWHH) increased from a minimum of 100nm to over 400nm. The peak absorption of these films (fig. 2) show Langmurian behaviour. There is an increase in the absorbance from 7 Å to 20 Å after which it then levels off and stays constant from 20 Å to 100 Å after which the absorbance increases. The absorption curves in figure 3 are indicative of transitions from isolated hemispherical islands at 7 Å, to elongated islands at 31 Å, to thin homogeneous film behaviour at 122 Å. The shift of peak position to longer wavelengths with increasing thickness suggests that bridging may be occurring between the different islands.

The thicker films which were a transparent purple tended to yellow after sitting for over two weeks at room temperature. This suggested that some rearrangement of the silver structure was occurring with time and heating could speed up the process and allow a simple method of optimization[8]. To examine this a series of silvered wafers ranging in thickness from 7 Å to 215 Å were heated, a UV/V spectrum was run: 1)before annealing 2)after the wafer had been annealed at 100 °C for 5 min and allowed to cool and 3)after the wafer was annealed for a further 5 minutes at 250 °C and allowed to cool. These spectra are shown in figure 4 for a 122 Å thick silver wafer.

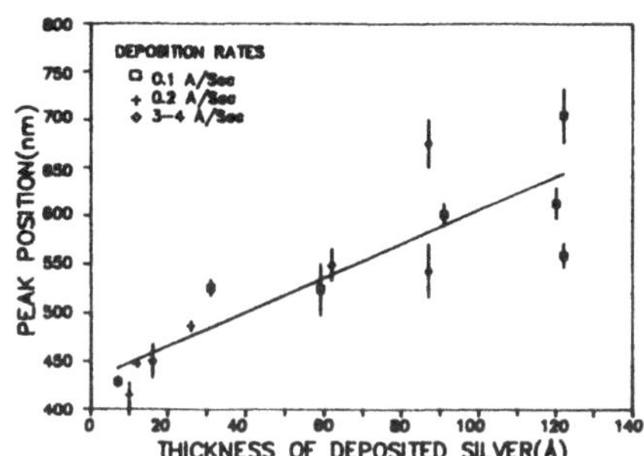

FIGURE 1. Effect of the amount of deposited silver on the peak position.

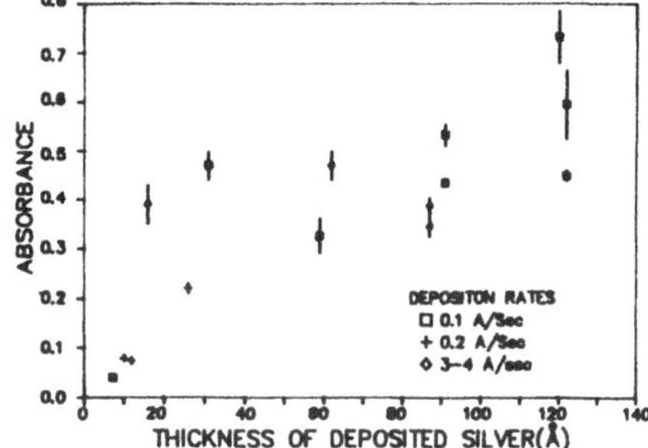

FIGURE 2. Effect of the amount of deposited silver on peak absorbance

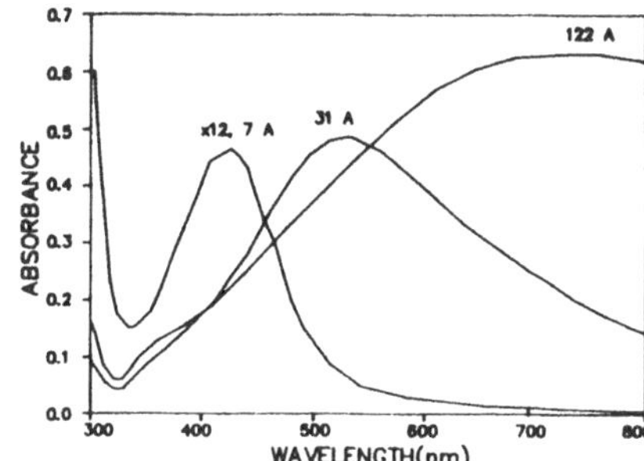

Figure 3. UV/V absorption curves of silvered wafers with different amounts of silver.

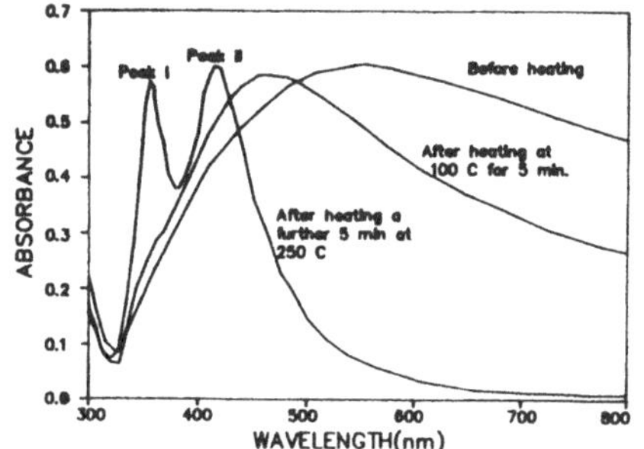

FIGURE 4. Effect of annealing on a 122 Å thick silver film

For samples which had less than 16 Å of silver no change in peak position was observed, but a decrease in peak intensity with increased heating resulted. Heating samples which were of greater thickness at a 100 °C for 5 minutes caused the peak to sharpen up and move to lower wavelengths. Heating for an additional 5 minutes at 250 °C caused the peak to split into two peaks which were centered at approximately 358nm(Peak I) and 420nm(Peak II) (see fig.4), possibly indicating two distinctive size distributions. This has yet to be confirmed using electron microscopy.

Initial experiments which involved immersion of the non-annealed wafers into water, 0.1M KCl, and hexane, showed enhancements or decreases in absorbance. These results will not be presented here in order to allow presentation of preliminary bovine serum albumin(BSA) solution studies. Results are summarized in figure 5 and table 1. In all cases a 87 Å thick silvered wafer which had been annealed at 250 °C was used. The wafers were immersed into a solution of constant ionic strength(36mM sodium phosphate buffer) whose pH and BSA content had been adjusted as outlined in figure 5.

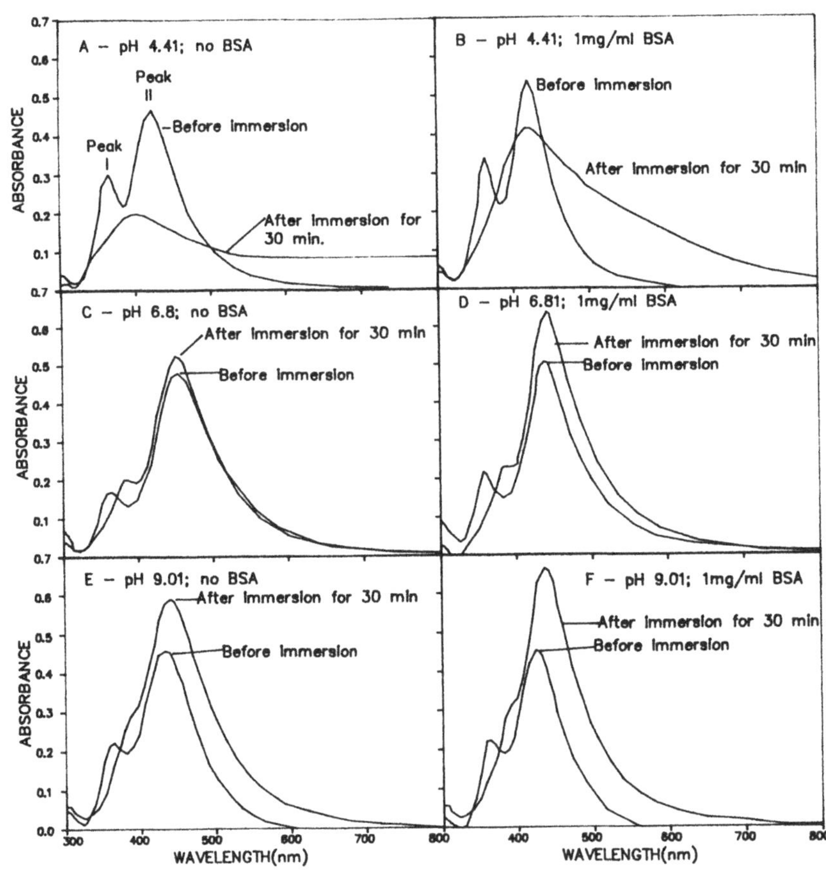

FIGURE 5. Effect of immersing 87 Å silver island films into 36 mM phosphate buffer at the pH's and BSA content outlined in each figure.

TABLE 1: EFFECT OF IMMERSING A 87 A THICK SILVER ISLAND FILM INTO A SOLUTION OF 36mM PHOSPHATE BUFFER AT VARIOUS pH'S AND WITH AND WITHOUT BSA

pH	No BSA Present			1mg/ml BSA Present		
	% Change in peak II maximum absorbance	Shift in position? of peak II	Peak I	% Change in peak II maximum absorbance	Shift in position of peak II	Peak I
4.41	− 58%	−22 nm	absent	−22%	0	absent
6.81	+ 8%	0 nm	merging	+ 25%	0	merging
9.01	+ 28%	+ 8 nm	merging	+ 46%	+12nm	merging

The dielectric constant for silver at 413nm is -4.3 + i0.23[9]. Inserting this value into the Mie equation one expects to see an enhancement in the absorption coefficient on going from a low dielectric environment of air (ε_o = 1) to a higher dielectric environment which has a dielectric constant less than 3, above this a decrease in the absorption coefficient would occur. This enhancement is observed when the absorption spectra of the silvered wafers in air and water (ε_o = 1.77) are compared in figures 5c-f. If albumin is adsorbed to the surface then the local dielectric constant would increase to a level of 2.25 which would result in a greater enhancement which is again observed when comparing figures 5c to 5d and 5e to 5f. Curiously when the pH is 4.01 a decrease in absorption is observed, it is highly unlikely that a protein layer has formed around the silver islands which has a dielectric greater than 3. This suggests that the simple dielectric model is not sufficient to explain this interaction. According to table 1 peak II exhibits a pH dependency which is accentuated when BSA is present at pH 6.81 and 9.01. At pH 4.41 peak II exhibits much more substantial reduction when BSA is not present.

CONCLUSION

The use of metal island films to support radiative SP does not require the use of couplers or parallel polarized light as in previous non-radiative SP based techniques. Preliminary studies indicate that radiative SP can easily be obtained by the direct illumination of silver island films by UV/V radiation. The SP resonance of these films can be optimised by annealing and are sensitive to their local environment. Simple UV/V absorption measurements of silvered wafers is able to provide interfacial information, this in association with the inherently small size of the metal islands will eventually allow its incorporation into an extrinsic or evanescently based multimode fiber optic system.

REFERENCES

1. H. Rather, Physics of Thin Films, 9, 145 (1979)
2. E. Kretschmann, Z. Physik, 241, 313 (1971)
3. M. T. Flanagan and R. H. Pantell, Electronic Letters, 20(23), 968(1984)
4. Bo Liedberg, C. Nylander and I. Lundstrom, Sensors and Actuators, 4, 299 (1983)
5. P. B. Danials, J. K. Deacon, M. J. Eddowes, and D.G. Pedley, Sensors and Actuators, 15, 11 (1988)
6. D. C. Cullen, R. G. W. Brown, and C. R. Lowe, Biosensors, 3, 211 (1987/88)
7. U. Kreibig and L. Genzel, Surface Science, 156, 678 (1985)
8. P. Boyer, J.L. Bijeon, J.P. Goudonnet, T. Inagaki and E.T. Arakawa, Surface Science, 217, 384 (1984)
9. P.B. Johnson and R.W. Johnson, Physical Review B, 6(12), 4370, 1972

24

Chemical Sensors Based on Photopyroelectric Transduction

M. S. HEIMLICH, U. J. KRULL, R. F. DEBONO, R. S. BROWN, Chemical Sensors Group, Dept.of Chemistry, University of Toronto, Erindale College, Mississauga, Ontario, Canada. L5L 1C6. (416)-828-5282

Chemical interactions at the gas/solid or liquid/solid interface can be studied by examining their characteristic absorption spectra. Upon reaching the excited state these systems may relax via radiationless de-excitation pathways, resulting in local heating. If the excitation source is pulsed at an appropriate frequency, thermal waves produced by a sub-monolayer coating of chromophoric material can be detected by using a pyroelectric material (PEM). The application of a temperature gradient across a PEM produces an electrical potential which can be monitored if both sides of the PEM are coated with a thin metal film. This forms the basis for a chemical sensor in which one side of the PEM is coated with a chemically selective chromophoric surface. The type of metal coating can be chosen to suit the chemistry being stabilized at the surface. This paper introduces the possibility of chemical sensor development involving stabilization of sulfur-terminated chemicals onto PEM's that are coated with gold and will provide results which demonstrate the potential of this transduction scheme.

INTRODUCTION

Electronic relaxation to the ground state can occur via several pathways. In addition to photon emission, one of the pathways is through radiationless de-excitation, which produces local heating (1). A pulsed excitation process can induce temperature fluctuations in the sample material, which results in the production of a thermal wave that propagates away from the region of excitation. In order to measure the temperature fluctuations, one requires a detector material which is sensitive to the small temperature changes that are produced by the sample.

PEMs generate an electric current as a result of a temperature differential across the thickness of the substance. The change in temperature (ΔT) induces a polarization in the PEM, producing a dipole moment in the direction of the temperature gradient.The result is a net voltage (V) across the PEM given by (2,3):

$$\Delta V(\omega) = \frac{P\,L}{\varepsilon}\,\Delta T(\omega) \quad (1)$$

$$\Delta V = \omega P A r\,\Delta T\,(1+\omega^2\tau_E^2)^{-1/2}, \quad \tau_E = r\,C \quad (2)$$

where ω is the angular frequency of the modulated incident radiation, P is the pyroelectric coefficient, L is the film thickness, ε is the film dielectric constant, A is the area of the film, r and C are the resistance and capacitance of the film and the electrical time constant of the detector output is given by τ_E.

Equation 2 indicates that the PEM can be considered in terms of an equivalent electrical circuit (Figure 1). In general, temperature changes on the order of 10^{-6} K can be detected. High impedance preamplifiers of low noise are required with these detectors, since the surface charge on the pyroelectric is on the order of 10^{-16} coulombs and the capacitance has a value of approximately 10 pF (3).

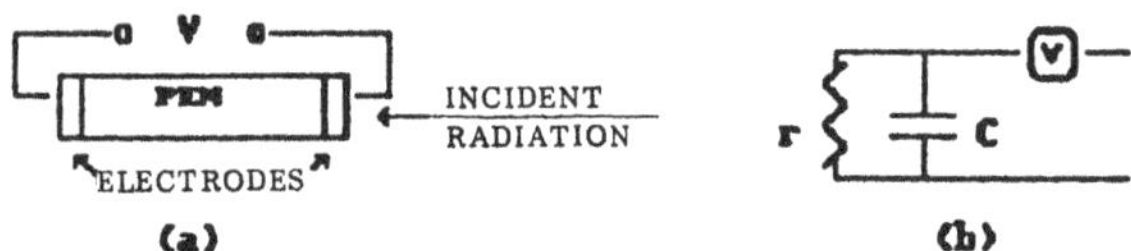

Figure 1. Pyroelectric detector (a) and equivalent circuit (b).

The function of PEMs is optimized when they are used as thin films. This property makes them ideal for spectroscopic absorption measurements that are generally difficult to achieve by conventional methods. Examples include samples having low optical density, high optical density, light scattering and specular reflection (4). Monolayer surface phenomena can also be studied using PEMs. Sensitivities of 10^{14} molecules/cm^2 have been achieved (5).

One of the advantages of PEMs is that they have linear response, across a large spectral bandwidth, to the thermal wave produced as a result of excitation. As a result, pyroelectric detection has been used for UV-visible (2,5,6), X-ray (7), and infrared absorption spectroscopic measurements (8).

By specifically using gold as the electrode metal on a PEM, it is possible to arrange for spontaneous deposition and self assembly of sulfur terminated molecules on to the electrode surface (9). Sulfur-gold interactions can be used to immobilize various chemical species, including some selective reagents, at the surface of a pyroelectric material in order to prepare a chemical sensor.

EXPERIMENTAL AND RESULTS

The PEMs were obtained from the Pennwalt Corporation (10). Sheets of 9 and 28 µm thick polyvinylidene fluoride (PVDF) film with 40 nm thick gold electrodes were used. Although smaller signals were obtained with the 28 µm film, the cell design and ease of handling dictated that this thickness be used for experimental purposes.

The cell was constructed from two pieces of Teflon, between which was sandwiched the PVDF film. One of the Teflon pieces had a 6 mm diameter hole to provide a working surface of PVDF film. Electrical contacts were made through the Teflon using thin aluminum wire and solder, and were connected to a shielded RCA phono jack.

The pyroelectric signal was fed to a Tektronix AM 502 amplifier using Belden low noise, 50 ohm coaxial cable. Data analysis was performed with a LeCroy 9400 digital oscilloscope with FFT option, or with an IBM-PC compatible microcomputer using an FFT algorithm and 16 bit analog to digital converter card.

The optical source used in the spectroscopic measurement was modulated mechanically since PEMs respond to changes in temperature. Frequency stability of the chopper was determined to be better than ± 0.2 Hz. A green He-Ne laser (543.5 nm, 1 mW) was used for single wavelength studies. Wavelength scans were done using a Cole-Parmer Quartz-Halogen Fiber-Lite source and an ORIEL grating monochromator.

The present experimental work was done to characterize the response of PVDF films as well as to determine if the system had the sensitivity and wavelength selectivity necessary for chemical sensor development using monolayer films.

Pyroelectric response as a function of optical intensity was measured using the He-Ne laser in conjunction with a set of neutral density filters and a Photodyne photometer. Figure 2a shows a linear response over the optical intensity range measured. The relationship between chopping frequency and signal is shown in Figure 2b. The response is linear within the range of the modulation unit.

The sensitivity of detection was determined in terms of surface area coverage, since monolayer phenomena were being investigated.

5 μl drops of 10^{-8} M eosin-5-isothiocyanate (EITC) in absolute ethanol were applied to the PVDF surface and measurements made after the application of each drop and evaporation of solvent. The effective surface coverage density given by one drop was approximately 10^{12} molecules/cm^2. The results of the experiment are summarized in Figure 3. After the EITC had been applied, the film was washed with water and dried by evaporation at room temperature. No change in signal was observed, indicating that the EITC was chemically stabilized on the electrode as a result of the sulfur-gold bonding.

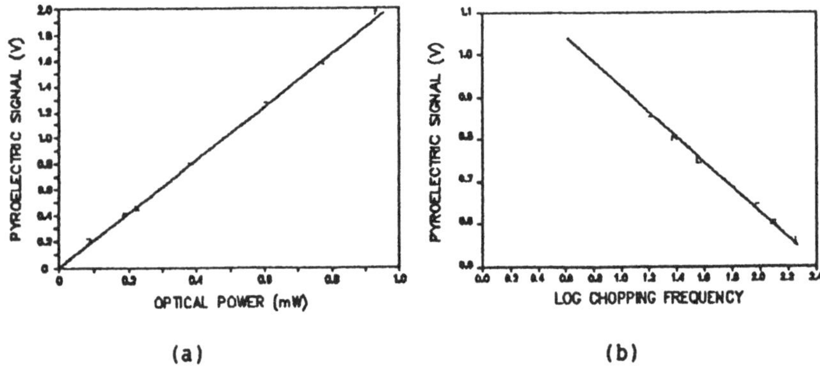

Figure 2. Pyroelectric signal as a function of optical power (a) and chopping frequency (b).

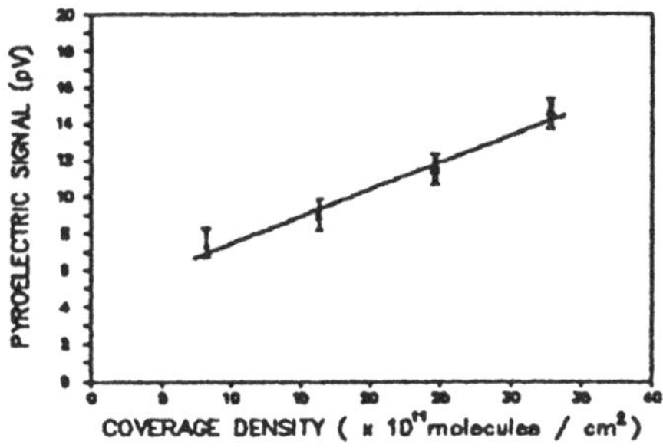

Figure 3. Submonolayer sensitivity of EITC

Wavelength scans were done to determine whether spectroscopic selectivity could be detected with the pyroelectric film. Scans were made of EITC (λ_{ex} = 525 nm, $\varepsilon \approx$ 83000 l mol^{-1} cm^{-1}) and fluorescein

- 5-isothiocyanate (FITC) (λ_{ex} = 495 nm, $\epsilon \approx$ 75000 l mol^{-1} cm^{-1}) and were normalized for the power spectrum of the Fiber-Lite. As a basis for comparison, spectra of EITC and FITC in solution were obtained using a single beam spectrophotometer. The spectral scans are shown in Figures 4a and 4b.

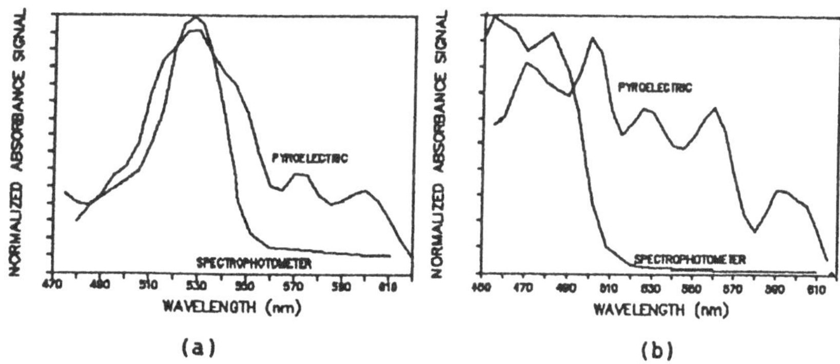

Figure 4. Spectral scans of EITC (a) and FITC (b).

DISCUSSION

Several materials are available for use as pyroelectric detectors. Triglycine-sulfate (TGS) is one of the more sensitive materials (p = 3 x 10^{-8} C cm^{-2} K^{-1}). However, it is hygroscopic, fragile and has a low Currie temperature of 49°C. Ceramics such as lead zirconate titanate (PZT) are strong, inexpensive and can be produced in large areas. La-modified $PbTiO_3$ (PLT) films have a pyroelectric coefficient of 5.3 x 10^{-8} C cm^{-2} K^{-1} (11). Plastic films like PVDF have poorer sensitivity (p = 3 x 10^{-9} C cm^{-2} K^{-1}), however, they can be produced in different shapes and are very inexpensive (3,5). The operating temperature range of PVDF is from -40°C to 100°C, making it highly versatile.

Figure 3 indicates that it is possible to achieve a sensitivity on the order of hundredths of a monolayer of EITC. A detection limit has not yet been established, however, detection of 0.005 of a monolayer of ammonia adsorbed on the silver electrode of a PVDF film has been possible (12).

The spectral scans of Figures 4a and 4b indicate that the pyroelectric signal is a function of the molecular absorption spectrum. Therefore, wavelength selectivity is available as a parameter for sensor development.

It has been observed that optical emission does not occur from fluorophores immobilized on gold surfaces (13). It is possible that the energy associated with photon emission is somehow converted to the generation of heat by a resonance coupling of the excited state dipole of the fluorophore with the conduction band of the metal. In such a case, the use of gold as an electrode surface on the PVDF would result in an increase in the pyroelectric signal. Therefore, the gold electrode would serve as both a surface suitable for chemical stabilization of sulfur-containing species and a pyroelectric amplifier for fluorophores.

Improvements that are being developed for this system include the use of PZT or PLT films to increase pyroelectric sensitivity, the placement of a charge amplifier near the cell to reduce noise and the introduction of a flow-through cell for measurement of dynamic vapour and solution samples.

CONCLUSIONS

The experimental results presented here show that chemical sensors can be based on a photopyroelectric transduction mechanism having submonolayer sensitivity and spectral selectivity. The design of such a device would incorporate the following general features:

1. Immobilization of one of a pair of complementary reactants on the electrode surface of the PEM. This provides a preconcentration of the analyte at the detector surface. Self-assembly of sulfur based systems onto gold are being examined, including the use of direct enzyme attachment to the gold electrodes via the sulfur moieties in the protein structure, as well as the binding of sulfur terminated lipids to the gold electrode, followed by incorporation of the enzyme to the lipid monolayer.

2. A reaction that produces a perturbation in the absorption spectrum of the material that is immobilized on the surface of the PEM. Detection of analyte is possible if the selective chemical reaction produces a change in the absorption spectrum of the receptor, or if the analyte introduces new spectral features.

3. The use of compact, yet intense optical sources. Testing of Super-Bright LEDs indicates that these sources may be feasible in some form of photopyroelectrically based fiber-optic spectrometer system by pulsing differently coloured LEDs at different frequencies. Chemometric data analysis would incorporate FFT spectral calculations and could be used for the development of sensor arrays (14).

REFERENCES

1. H. Coufal, A. Mandelis, Photopyroelectric Spectroscopy of Semiconductors, in Photoacoustic and Thermal Wave Phenomena in Semiconductors, North Holland, N.Y., 1987.
2. A. Mandelis, Chem. Phys. Lett., 108, 4, 388 (1984).
3. P. N. J. Dennis, in Photodetectors: An Introduction to Current Technology, Plenum Press, N.Y., 1986.
4. R. M. Miller, Termal Wave Spectroscopies - Where Do They Win?, in Springer Series in Optical Sciences, 58, Photoacoustic and Photothermal Phenomena, Springer-Verlag, London, 1988.
5. H. Coufal, Appl. Phys. Lett., 44, 1, p. 59 (1984).
6. H. Coufal and W. Knoll, Thin Solid Films, 160, 333 (1987).
7. H. Coufal, J. Stohr and K. Babershke, X-Ray Absorption Spectroscopy of Thin Films With A Pyroelectric Thermal Wave Detector, in Springer Series in Optical Sciences, 58, Photoacoustic and Photothermal Phenomena, Springer-Verlag, London, 1988.
8. M. Chirtoc, D. Dadarlat, I. Chirtoc and D. D. Bicanic, Photopyroelectric Spectroscopy of Water in the Near Infrared, in Springer Series in Optical Sciences, 58, Photoacoustic and Photothermal Phenomena, Springer-Verlag, London, 1988.
9. C. D. Bain and G. M. Whitesides, J. Am. Chem. Soc., 110, 5897 (1988).
10. Pennwalt Corp., Kynar Piezo Film Dept., P.O. Box 799, Valley Forge, PA 19482.
11. R. Takayama, Y. Tomita, K. Iijima and I. Ueda, J. Appl. Phys., 61, 1, p. 411 (1987).
12. H. Coufal, F. Trager, T. J. Chuang and A. C. Tam, Surface Science, 145, 504 (1984).
13. R. R. Chance, A. Prock and R. Silbey, Advances in Chemistry, 37, ED. I. Pregerene and S. A. Reil, Wiley, 1978.
14. R. Takayama, Y. Tomita, K. Iijima and I. Ueda, J. Appl. Phys., 63, 12, p. 5868, 1988.

25

Antibody-Based Biosensor for Continuous Monitoring

ANNE W. KUSTERBECK Bio/Molecular Engineering Branch, Naval Research Laboratory, Washington, D.C. 20375-5000

GREGORY A. WEMHOFF and FRANCES S. LIGLER Bio/Molecular Engineering Branch, Naval Research Laboratory, Washington, D.C. 20375-5000

1 INTRODUCTION

Bio-based systems may have a number of practical applications in the detection and monitoring of environmental hazards and therapeutic drugs. We present an overview of our preliminary investigations focusing on the development of a continuous flow antibody-based sensor.

2 PRINCIPLE OF OPERATION

The flow immunosensor relies on the reversibility of the antigen-antibody binding interaction. Schematically, antibody is covalently immobilized on a solid support of Sepharose 4B. The antigen-binding sites are saturated with a labelled antigen and the support placed in a column. The column is subjected to a continuous buffer flow and the compound of interest introduced to the buffer stream. Signal generation relies on the displacement of the tagged antigen from the antigen-binding sites by the free antigen in the stream and subsequent detection of the label downstream (Figure 1).

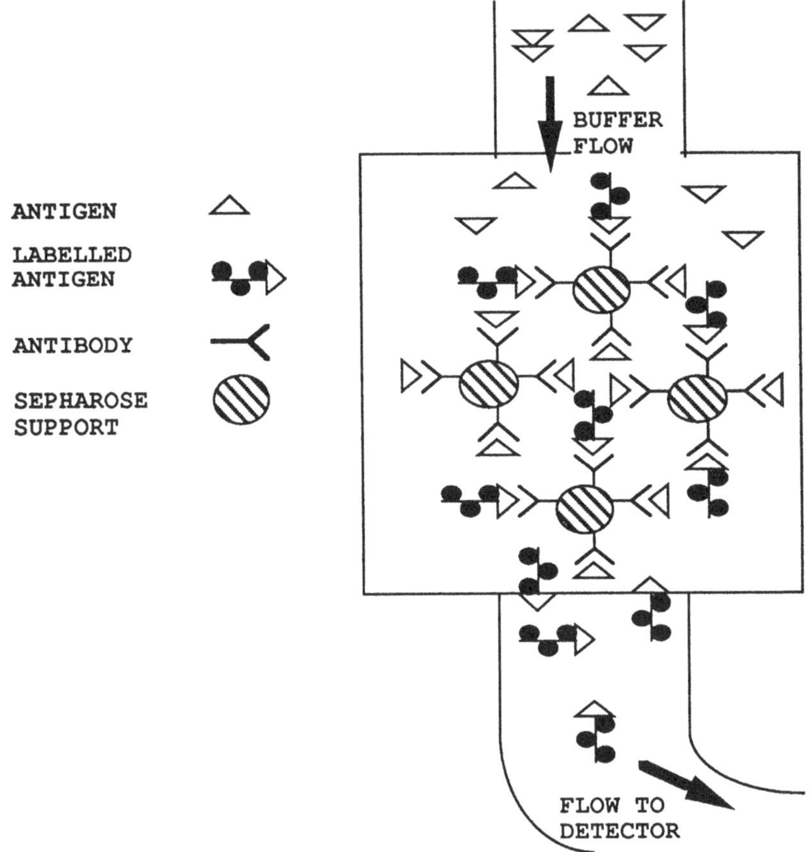

Figure 1 Principle of operation of the flow immunosensor

2.1 Experiments with the Model System

The model antigen selected to test the working parameters of the system was the hapten dinitrophenol (DNP). After coupling an anti-DNP antibody, Mab 51 (provided by Dr. Michael Steward, University of London), the antigen-binding sites were saturated with a labelled form of DNP. The label used in these studies was either ^{125}I or fluorescein. Samples of DNP-lysine were then introduced into the buffer stream and the column effluent was monitored for displacement of labelled antigen (Figure 2). Displacement was determined to be specific for the DNP molecule as lysine, bovine serum albumin, or glycine did not produce a signal when run on the column, even at molarities 10-fold higher (not shown).

3 CONCLUSION

Assays described as continuous are often flow injection systems which require incubation periods or the introduction of exogenous reagents (1-4). The methodology demonstrated here differs from previous approaches by performing the assay in a truly continuous flow environment with real-time results and no required reagent addition or mixing. The continuous flow immunosensor detects a labelled antigen while retaining the antibody on a solid support for reuse. The range of substances that can be detected using this system is conceptually limited only by the availability of a specific antigen-antibody pair.

ACKNOWLEDGEMENTS

We would like to acknowledge the contribution of Paul Charles for the synthesis of the tagged antigen, Dr. Michael Steward for the monoclonal antibody, and Dr. Reinhard Bredehorst for his helpful discussions. This work was supported by the Federal Aviation Administration, Contract No. DTFA03-83-A-00322 and the U.S. Customs Service.

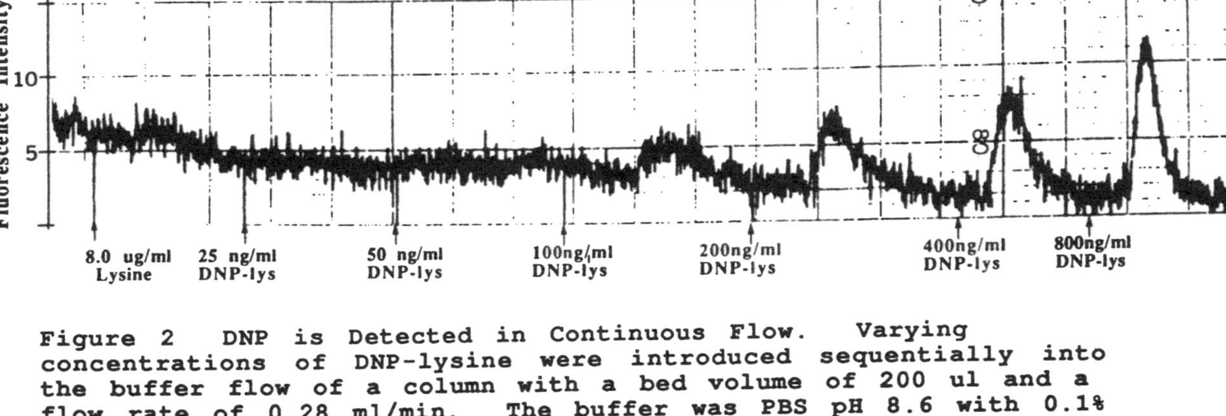

Figure 2 DNP is Detected in Continuous Flow. Varying concentrations of DNP-lysine were introduced sequentially into the buffer flow of a column with a bed volume of 200 ul and a flow rate of 0.28 ml/min. The buffer was PBS pH 8.6 with 0.1% v/v Triton X-100. The fluorimeter was a SpectraVision FD-300 equipped with an 8 ul flow cell. The excitation and emission wavelengths were 492 nm and 515 nm, respectively. High voltage was set at 900 V and the range set at 50. The strip chart recorder was set for a 50 mV input.

REFERENCES

1. B.A.Warden, K.Allam, A.Sentissi, D.J. Cecchini, R.W.Giese, Anal.Biochem. 162, 363-369 (1987).
2. U.Alwis, G.S.Wilson, Anal.Chem. 59, 2786-2789 (1987).
3. S.R.Lee, P.A.Liberti, Anal.Biochem. 166, 41-48 (1987).
4. H.A.Mottola, Anal.Chim.Acta 145, 27-39 (1983).

26

Rapid, Filtration-Based Immunoassays Performed with a Silicon Biosensor

MARIANN E. LUCAS, MARILYN F. HUNTINGTON, FRANCIS J. REGINA and JEFFREY M. BOLTS Allied-Signal Inc., Morristown, New Jersey

STEPHEN C. ALTER and MARK E. BALLMAN Environmental Technologies Group, Inc., Baltimore, Maryland

GREGORY L. KIRK Molecular Devices Corp., Menlo Park, California

1. INTRODUCTION

Immunoassays are considered to be among the most sensitive and specific methods of chemical analysis (1). However, even using automated immunoassay instrumentation, it has been difficult to perform sensitive immunoassays on the timescale of minutes. We will describe a rapid immunoassay system having an assay time of three minutes and a sensitivity of better than 1 ng of protein.

Our immunoassay system uses a Light Addressable Potentiometric Sensor (LAPS) (2) to monitor pH as a function of time at the surface of an affinity membrane. The sensor monitors changes in solution potential by measuring the corresponding changes in surface potential of an oxynitride-coated silicon chip, which is in contact with the solution. The system also uses two types of labelled antibodies: affinity-labelled antibodies to capture antigens on the surface of the membrane and enzyme-labelled antibodies to generate a measurable signal following the immunochemical capture reaction. The LAPS quantitates the membrane-bound complexes containing urease-labelled antibodies by monitoring the rate of pH increase resulting from the urease-catalyzed degradation of urea, Equation [1]:

$$NH_2CONH_2 + 2\ H_2O \xrightarrow{\text{urease}} 2\ NH_3 + H_2CO_3 \qquad [1]$$

Only immunocomplexes which contain both an affinity label (streptavidin) for membrane capture and an enzyme label (urease) for reaction catalysis will generate a detectable signal on the LAP sensor.

Two distinct immunochemical configurations have been demonstrated using the LAP biosensor. The fungal toxin T2 has been detected using a "displacement" immunoassay. In this assay, T2 in the sample cleaves a pre-formed, signal-generating immunocomplex which contains both an affinity-labelled T2 analogue and an enzyme-labelled antibody to T2. The signal is, therefore, inversely correlated with the concentration of T2 in the sample. In contrast, Staphylococcal Enterotoxin B, (SEB), is detected using a "sandwich" immunoassay. In this assay, the SEB protein in the sample forms a signal-generating immunocomplex in-situ by reacting with both affinity-labelled and enzyme-labelled antibodies in a reagent solution. The signal in this assay therefore increases as the concentration of SEB in the sample increases.

2. SILICON BIOSENSOR

2.1 Operation

The prototype Light Addressable Potentiometric Sensor used in this work consists of two distinct stations: a filtration station and a detection station. At the filtration station, a plastic "dipstick" supporting a biotinylated nitrocellulose membrane is inserted and secured in a plastic housing containing two circular holes. The sample and reagent solutions are pre-mixed and then applied to the membrane surface through these holes. A controlled vacuum is used to draw the mixture rapidly through the membrane. During filtration, antibodies and antibody complexes labelled with streptavidin are efficiently captured on the biotinylated membrane due to the high binding affinity of streptavidin and biotin.

The detection unit has two plungers which are designed to press the dipstick-mounted membrane against the LAPS silicon chip. The spacing of these plungers matches the spacing of the holes in the filtration unit, so that the plungers and silicon chip define between them a cylindrical volume centered over the spots of the membrane through which the sample and immunoreagents were filtered. The detection unit also contains a reservoir of phosphate buffered saline solution containing the enzyme substrate urea. When the dipstick is removed from the filtration station and inserted into the detection station, this reservoir contacts the membrane and the enzyme-catalyzed degradation of urea is initiated. The rate of change of pH is correlated with the amount of urease-labelled antibody immobilized on the membrane at the filtration spot. High sensitivity to urease, down to 40 picograms (3), results from the careful minimization of the volume of urea buffer to which the urease is exposed during detection. Indeed, the effective volume of the cylindrical reaction zone between the plunger and the silicon chip, located on either side of the membrane, is less than one microliter.

2.2 Theory

The sensor can measure pH changes as small as 5 microvolts per second at a 3 mm diameter spot on a nitrocellulose membrane. The LAPS measures interfacial pH as shown in Figure 1. A potentiostat controls the potential of the electrolyte with respect to ground. By adjusting the potential of the solution, it is possible to find a potential at which the silicon becomes reverse biased (Fig. 2),

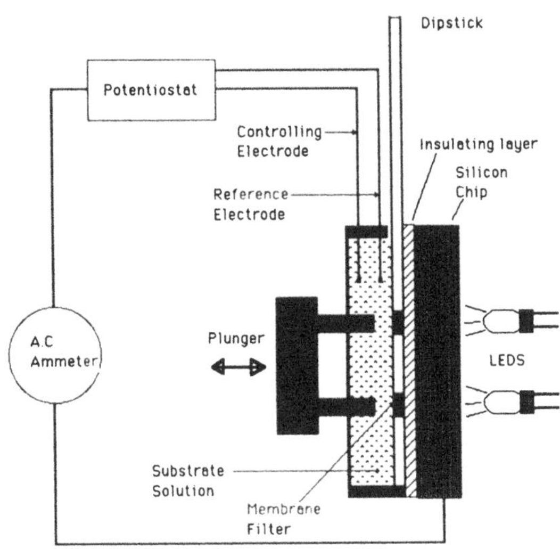

FIGURE 1 Schematic of a LAP biosensor.

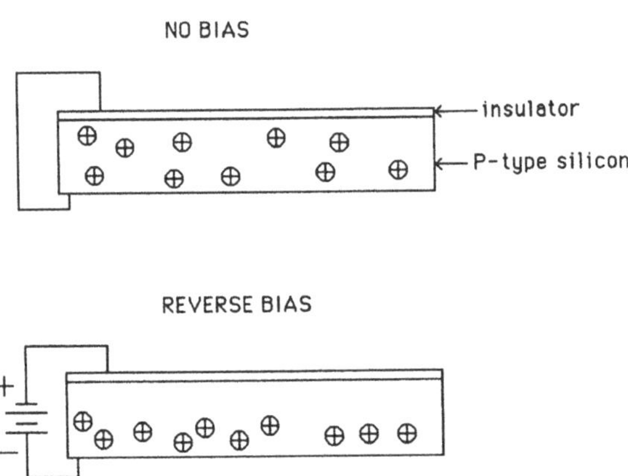

FIGURE 2 Formation of depletion layer of insulator.

and forms a depletion layer. This potential is marked by the onset of an alternating photocurrent resulting from the separation of hole-electron pairs in the depletion layer. The hole-electron pairs, in turn, are formed by absorption of light from the light emitting diodes (LEDs). The frequency of the alternating photocurrent is determined by the modulation frequency of the LED. No direct current passes through the insulating layer on the silicon chip and therefore no net electrochemistry is occurring at the insulator/electrolyte interface.

The potential at which a depletion layer is formed is a function of both the potential applied to solution and the surface potential at the insulator/electrolyte interface (Fig. 3). When an insulator such as silicon oxynitride is placed in aqueous solution, dissociation of protons from surface silanol and nitride groups results in the formation of a negative surface potential. The magnitude of this surface potential is a function of the degree of dissociation of these groups and is therefore dependent on the pH of the solution.

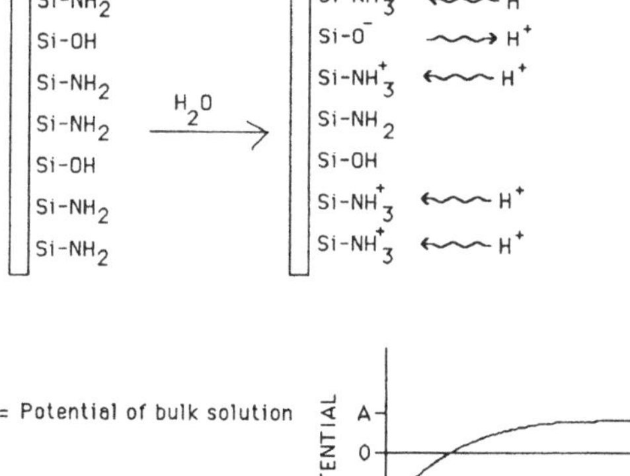

FIGURE 3 Surface potential at the insulator/electrolyte interface.

The light from the LEDs is collimated so that electron-hole pair excitation of the bulk silicon occurs only under the region of interest; therefore only the surface potential directly under the membrane test spot is monitored. Multiple sites can be measured with the same potentiostat simply by serially illuminating different regions of the silicon under the test membrane.

3. T2 ASSAYS

The trichothecene mycotoxin T2 (MW 466), is produced by fungi of the Fusarium species which can grow on grains used for human and animal consumption. A convenient analytical method for T2 would therefore be of great value in helping to assure the quality of various agricultural products.

We have developed a rapid assay procedure for T2 based on the LAP sensor and a displacement immunoassay configuration (Fig. 4).

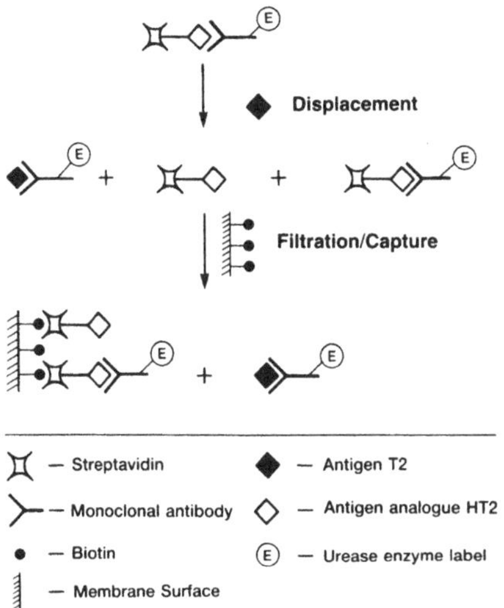

FIGURE 4 Displacement immunoassay configuration for T2 toxin.

The assay utilizes the HT2 toxin molecule (MW 424), which is a derivative of T2 toxin (Fig. 5). Although HT2 is recognized by

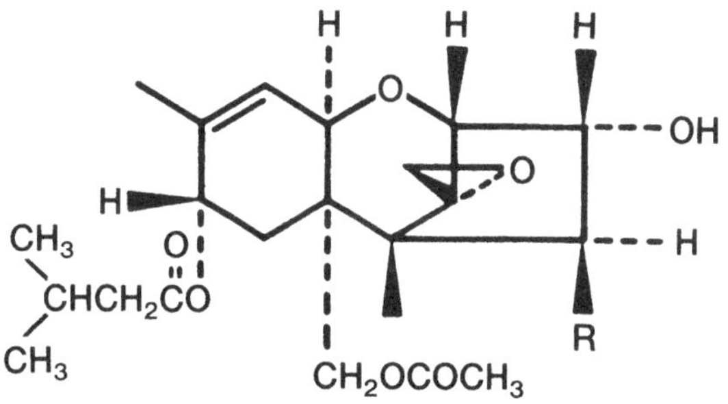

FIGURE 5 Structures of T2 toxin (R=$OCOCH_3$) and HT2 toxin (R=OH).

anti-T2 antibodies, it is less tightly bound than T2, and can be displaced from the antibody binding sites by T2 (4). This fact is exploited by the displacement assay configuration, in which T2 in a test sample displaces HT2 bound to anti-T2 antibody in a preformed immunocomplex. The immunocomplex is prepared in 200 μL of buffer solution A (see Table 1) by mixing 3 μg (50 pmol) of streptavidin-labelled HT2 with 40 ng (0.05 pmol) of urease-labelled antibody to T2. Addition of 100 μL of sample T2 to the complex causes displacement of the HT2-streptavidin from the antibody-urease conjugate, producing T2 complexed with antibody- urease conjugate and free HT2-streptavidin (displacement occurs in 90 seconds). The reaction mixture (300 μL) is then filtered through the membrane in 30 seconds. Antibody-urease conjugate bound to T2 sample is washed away by drawing 200 μL of buffer solution B through the membrane. Note that the pH of this solution is 6.5, approaching the optimum pH for urease activity (5).

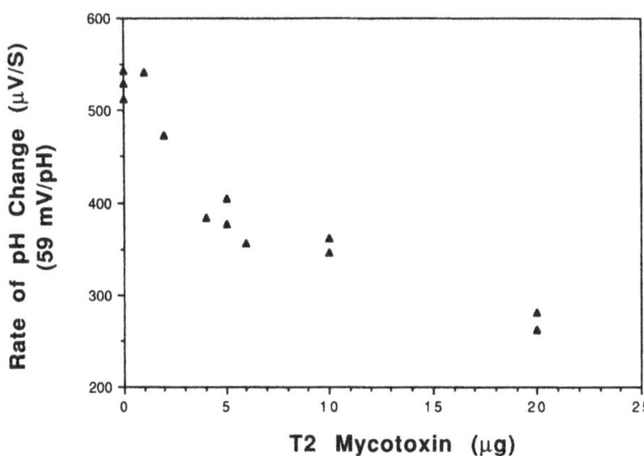

FIGURE 6 Plot of rate of pH change versus T2 toxin obtained using displacement immunoassay configuration.

TABLE 1 Components of Buffered Solutions

	A[1]	B
Sodium phosphate	10 mM	5 mM
Sodium chloride	120 mM	100 mM
Potassium chloride	2.7 mM	
Tween 20	0.05%	0.05%
BSA		1%[2]
Gelatin	0.1%	
pH	7.4	6.5

1. Solution A = PBS + Tween 20 + gelatin.
2. For SEB assays, 0.1% gelatin was substituted for 1% BSA in Solution B.

The displaced streptavidin-labelled HT2 and any remaining initial immunocomplexes containing streptavidin are both retained on the biotinylated membrane due to their streptavidin functionalities. The membrane is then transferred to the detection station of the biosensor and inserted into the substrate solution (buffer solution B containing 100 mM urea).

Figure 6 represents a dose response curve for T2 utilizing the above procedure. The vertical axis shows LAPS response (μV/s) and the horizontal axis gives amount of T2 in sample (micrograms). Increasing doses of T2 sample show a decrease in signal over the range 2 - 20 μg of T2. A concentration of less than 2 μg of T2 in 100 μL could also be detected in a total assay time of less than 3 minutes.

4. SEB ASSAYS

Staphylococcal Enterotoxin B (SEB), a protein of MW = 28400, is produced by certain strains of Staphylococcus aureus and is a major cause of food poisoning.

Our rapid assay procedure for SEB on the LAP biosensor employs a sandwich immunoassay configuration as shown in Figure 7. This assay exploits the fact that the SEB protein is large enough to accommodate the binding of two or more differently-labelled antibodies, resulting in the formation of an antibody-SEB-antibody immunochemical "sandwich" structure. A reagent mixture of 1 μg (7 pmol) of biotinylated antibody, 0.8 μg (1 pmol) of urease-labelled antibody and 1 μg (17 pmol) of streptavidin is prepared in 300 μL of buffer solution A. An immunochemical sandwich of SEB antigen with the two labelled antibodies is formed when 100 μL of SEB sample is added and mixed with this reagent (elapsed time approx. 15 seconds). The reaction mixture (400 μL) is filtered through the membrane. Uncomplexed components and free urease-labelled antibody are washed away by filtration of 500 μL of modified buffer solution B (see footnote 2 of Table 1). Total elapsed time to the end of filtration is 2 minutes. The membrane is then transferred to the detection station of the LAPS and inserted into the substrate solution: (buffer solution B containing 100 mM urea). The captured immunochemical sandwich, containing both streptavidin and urease labels, is detected by the sensor.

Figure 8 depicts a typical dose response curve for SEB, generated using the above procedure. The vertical axis shows LAPS response (μV/s), while the horizontal axis gives the amount of SEB (nanograms). The response to increasing doses of antigen is linear and increases over the range of 0 - 10 ng of SEB. An SEB concentration of 10 ng/mL is easily discernible from background in a total assay time of approximately 3 minutes. Interference due to Staphylococcal Protein A, which is also produced by Staph.aureus and has been shown to give false positive results in sandwich immunoassays (6), can be eliminated by including non-specific rabbit IgG (0.1%) in buffer solution A.

5. MATERIALS AND CONJUGATE PREPARATION

5.1 Materials

The following bioreagents were obtained from Sigma (St. Louis, MO): T2 toxin, HT2 toxin, urease, bovine serum albumin (BSA), phosphate buffered saline (PBS), rabbit polyclonal anti-SEB and SEB. Mouse IgG monoclonal anti-T2 was obtained from Hazelton Biologics (Lenexa, KS). m-Maleimidobenzoyl-N-hydroxysuccinimide (MBS) ester, streptavidin and N-hydroxysuccinimidobiotin (NHS-biotin) and bicinchoninic acid as BCA Protein Assay Reagent were obtained from Pierce (Rockford, IL). 2,2,2-trifluoroethane sulfonyl chloride was obtained from Fluka (Ronkonkoma, NY). Bio-Gel P-6 polyacrylamide

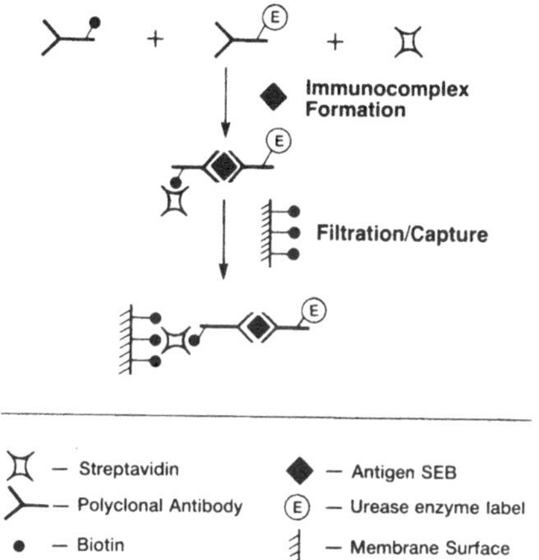

FIGURE 7 Sandwich immunoassay configuration for SEB.

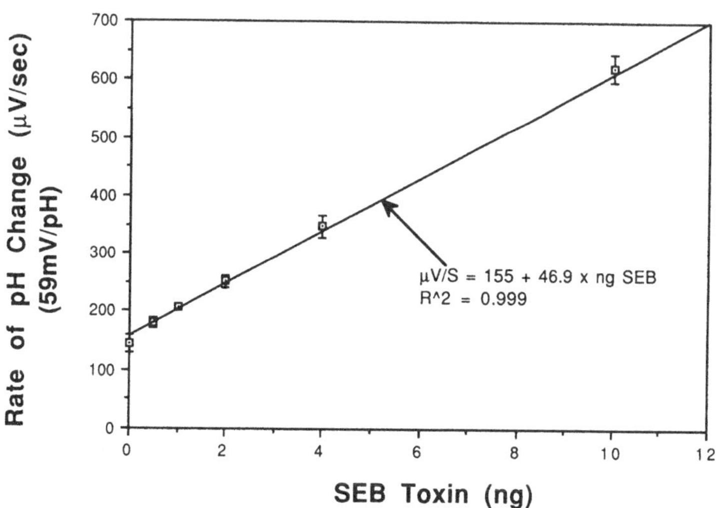

FIGURE 8 Plot of rate of pH change versus SEB obtained using sandwich immunoassay configuration.

gel was obtained from Bio-Rad (Richmond,CA). Biotinylated nitrocellulose membrane was prepared by Molecular Devices Corp. Solvents and salts were of standard reagent grade and were purchased from various commercial sources.

5.2 Conjugate preparations

Polyclonal anti-SEB was affinity purified over a column of SEB immobilized to cyanogen bromide activated-Sepharose 4B. Monoclonal anti-T2 was used as received. Biotinylated anti-SEB was prepared using NHS-biotin according to Hofman et al. (7). Protein concentrations of SEB stock solutions were determined using bicinchoninic acid (8) with bovine serum albumin as a standard.

Urease-labelled antibody was prepared by antibody activation with MBS ester prior to addition of urease (9), followed by purification over a column of Sephacryl S-300. Total protein concentration was determined by absorbance at 280 nm. The absorbance of a 1 mg/ml solution was estimated to be 0.84, based on an assumed 1:1 conjugation of urease ($A^{1\%}$ = 7.7 (10)) and antibody ($A^{1\%}$ = 14.0 (11)).

Streptavidin-labelled HT2 was prepared as follows: 4 mg (10 μmol) of HT2 toxin and 2.4 μL (30 μmol) of pyridine were added to 1 mL of nitrogen-purged dichloromethane. The mixture was cooled to 0°C, and 2.7 μL (25 μmol) of 2,2,2- trifluoroethane sulfonyl chloride was added. The reaction mixture was stirred under nitrogen for 2 hours at 0°C, then treated with consecutive washings (3X each) of ice water, 5% cold hydrochloric acid and water. The separated organic phase, containing the active ester of HT2, was dried over anhydrous sodium sulfate, filtered, and the filtrate was evaporated to dryness. The residue was re-dissolved in 100 μL of DMSO. 25 μL of the active ester of HT2 in DMSO was added to 1 mL of cold PBS containing 1 mg (0.02 μmol) of streptavidin. This reaction was allowed to stir for 16 hours at 0°C. The product, streptavidin-labelled HT2, was purified over a column (17 cm X 1 cm) of Bio-Gel P-6, eluting with PBS containing 0.02% sodium azide. Protein concentration was determined by absorbance at 280 nm, using $A^{1\%}$ as 40 (12).

6. DISCUSSION

In summary, a Light Addressable Potentiometric Sensor has been used to perform rapid and sensitive immunoassays for the detection of low and high molecular weight analytes. As little as 2 μg of T2 toxin or 1 ng of SEB may be detected in a 100 μL sample within 3 minutes. Two different immunoassay configurations have been demonstrated, both utilizing a combination of affinity-labelled and enzyme-labelled antibodies. In either configuration, the silicon-based LAPS detects pH changes caused by the reaction of an enzyme-labelled immunocomplex captured on an affinity membrane.

These results illustrate the general capability of our LAP biosensor to detect nanogram concentrations of protein within 3 minutes time. This can be compared to the commercially available LAPS-based assay for DNA that has 2 - 3 picogram sensitivity in 1 - 2 hours at 37°C (13). This large difference in sensitivity is expected due to differences in diffusion and binding rates. We have optimized the speed and sensitivity of our immunoassay system by, among other things, increasing antibody reagent concentrations and by performing the binding reaction steps in small fluid volumes.

It must be pointed out that the reagent concentrations and reaction timing must be carefully controlled in order to achieve good precision in these assays. These factors, together with the fluid handling, filtration and detection processes, are all amenable to automation.

To this end, we are currently developing a system in which the membrane filters are presented to the filtration and read stations in an automated and scheduled way by a tape drive mechanism (Fig. 9). A single spool of membrane filter tape could accommodate thousands of measurements. The sample stream is mixed with reagents and filtered through the membrane tape with accurate timing and flow rate, controlled by positive displacement automated pumps. A breadboard version of this system is currently under construction. It is expected that the final, automated LAP biosensor will be useful for any clinical, environmental and commercial applications requiring the rapid and convenient detection of low concentrations of chemical and biological analytes.

ACKNOWLEDGMENTS

This work was partially supported by the U.S. Army Chemical Research, Development and Engineering Center, Aberdeen Proving Ground, MD.

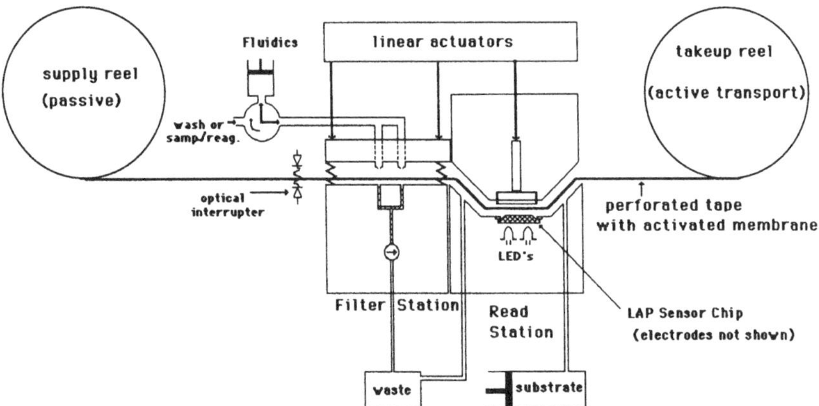

FIGURE 9 Schematic of an automated immunoassay reader system.

REFERENCES

1. Handbook of Experimental Immunology, Vol. I: Immunochemistry, (Weir, D.M., Ed.), Blackwell Scientific Publications, Palo Alto, CA (1986).
2. Hafeman, D.G. et al., (1988), Science, 240, 1182-1185.
3. For a detailed analysis of assay gain and sensitivity see: Bousse, L. et al., Sensors and Actuators, in press.
4. Hunter Jr., K.W. et al., (1985), Appl.Environ.Microbiol., 49, 168-172.
5. Sumner, J.B., (1951), The Enzymes, Vol. I, 886.
6. Hahn, I.F. et al., (1986), J.Immunol.Methods, 92, 25-29.
7. Hofman, K. et al., (1978), J.Am.Chem.Soc., 100, 3585-3590.
8. Smith, P.K. et al., (1985), Anal.Biochem., 150, 76-85.
9. Healey, K. et al.,(1983), Clin.Chim.Acta, 134, 51-58.
10. Gorin, G. and Chin, C., (1965), Biochim. Biophys. Acta., 99, 418.
11. Stevenson, G.T. and Dorrington, K.J., (1970), Biochem. J., 118, 703.
12. Chaiet, L. et al., (1963), Antimicrob.Agents Chemother., 3, 28.
13. Briggs, J. et al., (Feb. 1989), "A total DNA assay system," American Laboratory, 34-38.

27

The Silicon Microphysiometer: Detection of Biological Effects of Chemical and Biochemical Agents by Alterations of Cellular Metabolic Rate

J. Wallace Parce, George B. Sigal, Karen M. Kercso, and John C. Owicki, Molecular Devices Corporation, Menlo Park, California

1 INTRODUCTION

The silicon microphysiometer is a biosensor that measures the metabolic rates of cells by detecting the rate at which cells acidify their environment by the excretion of acidic metabolites such as carbon dioxide and lactic acid [1]. Although the instrument can be used for metabolic studies in cell biology, its applicability is much broader. For example, it can be used for *in-vitro* toxicology, for determination of chemotherapeutic efficacy, and to detect ligand-receptor interactions. The strategy behind the device is perhaps best conveyed by the following analogy.

A spider sitting in its web senses its environment largely by detecting vibrations in the web. These mechanical disturbances, which may signal the arrival of prey, predator, or mate, are transmitted to the spider from all parts of the web, because all of the web is mechanically coupled together. Pluck the web anywhere, and the disturbance ripples throughout the whole structure.

The biochemical pathways of a living cell correspond to the web. The intricate biochemical reactions that underlie the living state are richly coupled to one another, just as are the strands of silk in a web. The arrival of some stimulus causes changes in these pathways that are detected, spider-like, by the microphysiometer.

The strength of a disturbance as it propagates through the silk or biochemical web may vary widely from case to case. To detect faint disturbances, it behooves the spider to sit in a central location, where many strands of silk meet and no part of the web is too distant. It also benefits the spider to have a means of detecting extremely weak vibrations.

These issues of placement and sensitivity have counterparts in the microphysiometer. The metabolic processes of a cell, where energy is derived from food to power all the activities of life, are placed centrally from a biochemical viewpoint. It is difficult for something significant to happen to the cell without some alteration of energy expenditure. Sensitivity in the microphysiometer is provided by

Molecular Devices' proprietary biosensor technology, the Light Addressable Potentiometric Sensor (LAP sensor or LAPS).

2 THE LIGHT-ADDRESSABLE POTENTIOMETRIC SENSOR

The LAP sensor was described originally by Hafeman *et al.* [2], and only a brief discussion of the device will be given here. The LAP sensor potentiometrically detects the concentrations of ionic species that set the surface potential of the electrolyte/sensor interface. In this case the sensor surface is composed of protonatable silicon oxynitride, and the sensor measures pH.

Figure 1 is a schematic diagram of the LAP sensor. A potentiostat controls the potential of the electrolyte with respect to ground. By adjusting the potential of solution it is possible to find a potential Y at which the silicon becomes reverse biased and a depletion layer is formed beneath the insulator. The formation of the depletion layer is detected by the appearance of an alternating photocurrent in the AC ammeter. This photocurrent is the result of separation of hole-electron pairs in the electric field of the depletion layer. The hole-electron pairs are formed by absorption of light from the light emitting diode (LED). The frequency of the alternating photocurrent is determined by the frequency of modulation of the intensity of the LED. No direct current passes through the insulator and therefore no net electrochemistry occurs at the insulator/electrolyte interface.

The surface potential acts as a battery in series with the potentiostat, and so changes in surface potential can be detected as voltage changes in the potentiostat that are necessary to keep the silicon reverse biased. The silicon oxynitride surface behaves in a Nernstian fashion, that is, the surface potential changes by 61 mV per pH unit in the bulk solution at 37°C.

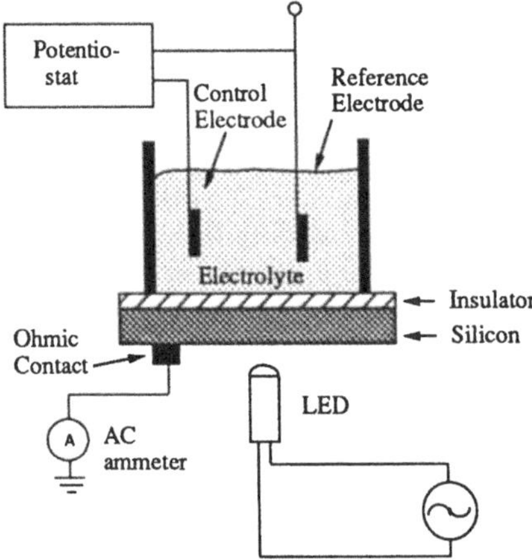

FIGURE 1 Schematic diagram of the LAP sensor.

3 OPERATION OF THE SILICON MICROPHYSIOMETER

Figure 2 is a block diagram of the silicon microphysiometer. Cell-culture medium is pumped by a syringe or peristaltic pump through a thermally regulated flow chamber containing cells and the LAP sensor. Upstream of the chamber are a degasser and valve.

Room-temperature medium passes through gas-permeable tubing in a degassing container held at 2/3 atmosphere; this prevents the formation of bubbles in the 37°C flow chamber due to outgassing. The valve, which may be an injection loop or shunt valve, is used to introduce test substances.

The flow chamber is shown in more detail in Figure 3. Adherent cells are typically grown on a microscope cover slip that is suspended 100 μm above the surface of the LAP sensor. Culture medium flows through a channel that is about 0.5 cm wide by 2 cm long (and 100 μm deep). Non-adherent cells can be retained gently in wells that are etched photolithographically into the surface of the sensor.

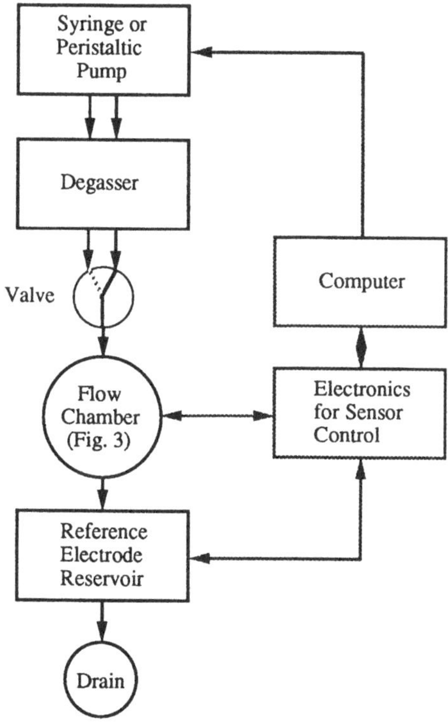

FIGURE 2 Block diagram of the silicon microphysiometer.

The cover slip is coated with a transparent conductive layer of indium-tin oxide, which permits it to serve as the controlling electrode. Downstream from the chamber is an Ag/AgCl reference electrode. The third electrical connection is made by grounding the base of the LAP sensor. The sensor electronics, pump, and data analysis are controlled by a personal computer.

Light from infrared light-emitting diodes is conducted sequentially to four sites in the chamber, each about 1 mm^2. An important feature of the LAP sensor is that pH is reported only from illuminated areas. Given that the density of cells in a confluent monolayer is about $10^5/cm^2$, each site detects the metabolic rate of about 10^3 cells in 100 nL.

The method for detecting metabolic rates is shown in Figure 4. Although cells constantly excrete acidic metabolites, the pH in the chamber can be kept constant at the physiologic value, 7.3 to 7.4, by the continual flow of fresh medium. When flow is temporarily interrupted (bars in figure), the acidic metabolites accumulate, and the pH decreases. The slope of a linear least-squares fit to the data then gives an acidification rate, which we identify as a metabolic rate. Medium with a low buffer capacity (about 1 mM) is used to accentuate the pH changes.

When the flow of medium is restored, the pH resets to the physiologic value. Typically flow is halted for 50 to 200 sec, during which time the pH drops 0.1 to 0.3 units. This is not harmful to the cells, and measurements have been done repetitively for as long as 90 hours.

We conclude by briefly describing two applications of the silicon microphysiometer, the first toxicological and the second involving ligand-receptor interactions.

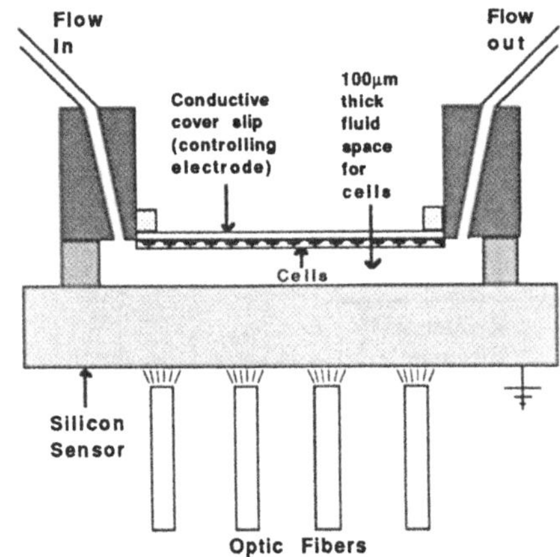

FIGURE 3 Cross-sectional view of the flow chamber.

4 RECOVERY FROM THE EFFECTS OF OCULAR IRRITANTS

There is a worldwide effort to develop *in-vitro* alternatives to the rabbit-eye or Draize [3] test for ocular irritancy. We have previously shown a strong correlation between *in-vivo* irritancy and the concentration of irritant that is sufficient to depress the metabolic rate of normal human epidermal keratinocytes in the microphysiometer [1]. This was a measure of the intensity of irritation immediately after a five-minute exposure. In addition to intensity, however, the duration of irritation is clinically important. That the microphysiometer can determine the kinetics of recovery from irritation is shown in Figure 5.

Keratinocytes were exposed to two irritants, dimethyl sulfoxide (DMSO) and ethanol (EtOH) at concentrations sufficient to reduce their metabolic rates by about 50%. This was 0.8 g/mL for DMSO and 0.2 g/mL for EtOH; EtOH is the stronger irritant. After the five-minute exposure, the metabolic rates of the cells treated with DMSO recover, while those for EtOH continue to decline. Such data suggest a relationship between *in-vivo* irritancy and recovery from toxic insult in the microphysiometer.

5 METABOLIC RESPONSE TO EPIDERMAL GROWTH FACTOR

Epidermal growth factor (EGF) is polypeptide that interacts with a receptor in the plasma membrane of cells in some tissues to regulate proliferation [4]. It is mitogenic for cultured normal human epidermal keratinocytes and is included in the culture medium at 10 ng/mL. When the cells are starved for EGF overnight, mounted into the microphysiometer, and exposed to 5 ng/mL EGF, the metabolic rate increases. Figure 6 shows this result, along with the results of control experiments in which an antibody against EGF was included at 1.25 μg/mL to abolish the response.

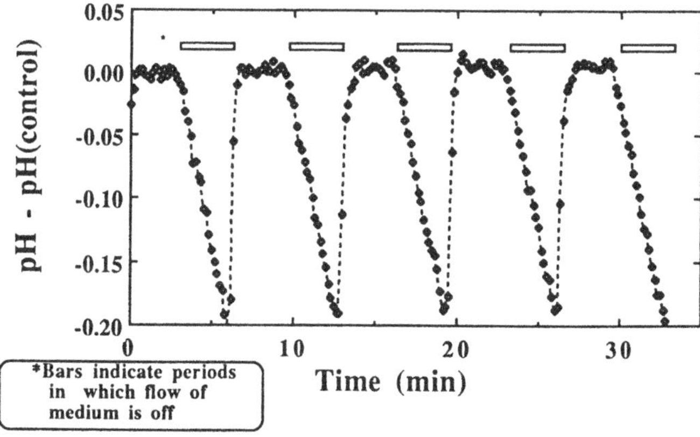

FIGURE 4 Detection of acidification rates with the microphysiometer.

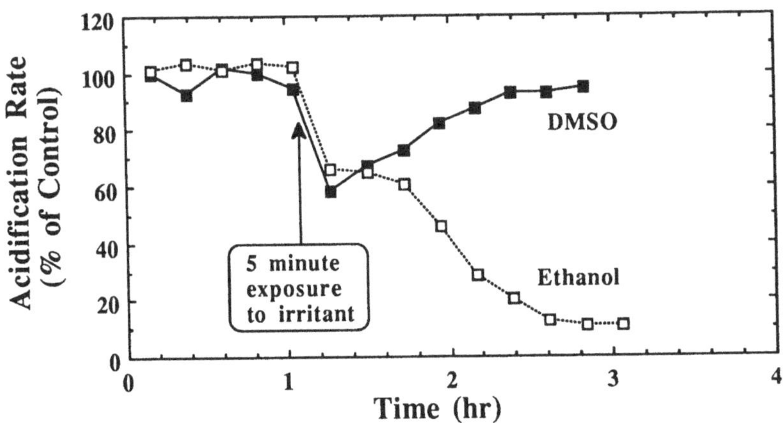

FIGURE 5 Recovery of keratinocytes from exposure to ocular irritants.

The transduction of the EGF binding signal involves protein phosphorylation by a tyrosine kinase. We have performed analogous experiments with representatives of most of the other important second-messenger systems for ligand-receptor interactions. The results are broadly similar to those for EGF, although the amplitudes and kinetics of the metabolic responses vary.

6 CONCLUSION

The silicon microphysiometer is a biosensor in the truest sense: it electronically transduces the response of living cells. Complementing other measures of metabolic activity, such as oximetry and microcalorimetry, it has the following novel or useful features:

Sensitivity. The metabolic rates of about 10^3 cells in 100 nL can be measured conveniently.

Non-invasiveness. The periodic excursions of pH (0.1 to 0.3 pH units) do not appear to harm or perturb the cells. We have kept cells alive in the microphysiometer with continual measurement of metabolic rates for as long as 90 hr.

Generality. Catabolic activity depends on a wide variety of biochemical processes, and we have shown that effects ranging from ligand-receptor interactions to cytotoxicity and viral infection can be detected by monitoring the acidification rate. This generality is a two-edged sword; to achieve specificity, it is crucial that biological or biochemical controls be implemented

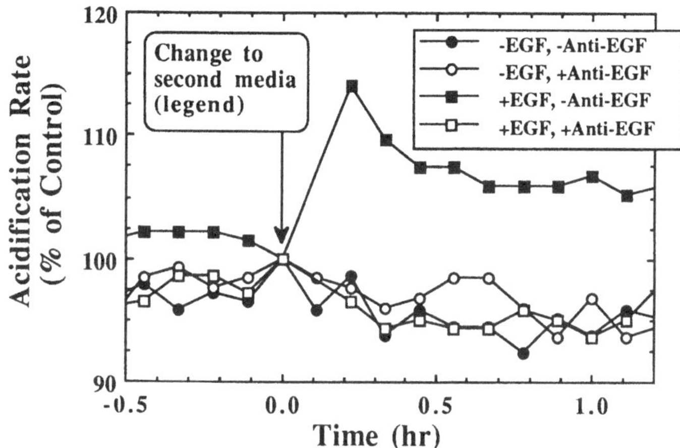

FIGURE 6 Metabolic response of human epidermal keratinocytes to epidermal growth factor.

Miniaturization and integration. The device is a product of silicon fabrication technology, and there are no significant barriers to improvements using these techniques. It should be possible to make the device much smaller, with the valves, pumps, and channels of the fluidics system implemented on the silicon wafer by micro-machining methods.

We expect the silicon microphysiometer to be useful in basic cell biology. Practical applications may include drug discovery, chemotherapeutic efficacy testing, *in-vitro* screening of ocular irritants, and the optimization of cell-culture media.

ACKNOWLEDGEMENTS

This work was supported in part by the U.S. Army CRDEC and DARPA, ARO contract DAAL03-86-0009 to MDC.

REFERENCES

1. J.W. Parce, J.C. Owicki, K.M. Kercso, G.B. Sigal, H.G. Wada, V.C. Muir, L.C. Bousse, K.L. Ross, B.I. Sikic, and H.M. McConnell, *Science*, in press (scheduled for the October 13, 1989 issue).
2. D.G. Hafeman, J.W. Parce, and H.M. McConnell, *Science*, **240**, 1182 (1988).
3. J.H. Draize, G. Woodard, H.O. Calvery, *J. Pharmacol. Exp. Ther.*, **82**, 377 (1944).
4. T.F. Deuel, *Ann. Rev. Cell Biol.*, **3**, 443 (1987).

28

Substrate-Supported Planar Membranes Containing Murine Antibody Fc Receptors: A Total Internal Reflection Fluorescence Microscopy Study

Claudia L. Poglitsch and Nancy L. Thompson, Chemistry Department, University of North Carolina, Chapel Hill, North Carolina, 27599-3290

1. INTRODUCTION

One method of obtaining information about the interaction of soluble ligands with membrane receptors is to use model cell membranes deposited on transparent planar substrates and techniques in fluorescence microscopy. Substrate-supported planar membranes have been used extensively in membrane biophysics and are also of interest in medical technology, optics and biosensor development (1-4). A technique in fluorescence microscopy that is particularly well-suited to supported planar membranes is total internal reflection (TIR) fluorescence microscopy (5) in which surface-bound fluorescent molecules are selectively excited by evanescent illumination. In this work, the equilibrium binding of monoclonal anti-(murine Fc receptor) Fab fragments and also of polyclonal murine IgG to Fc receptors in substrate-supported planar membranes constructed from mouse macrophage-related cell membrane fragments is investigated with TIR fluorescence microscopy.

2. CHARACTERIZATION OF ANTI-(Fc RECEPTOR) MONOCLONAL ANTIBODIES

Monoclonal antibodies specific for the murine macrophage Fc receptor $moFc_{\gamma}RII$ (6) were purified from the supernatants of cultured 2.4G2 hybridoma cells (7) by goat anti-(rat IgG) affinity chromatography using low pH elution. Two types of 2.4G2 antibodies were copurified

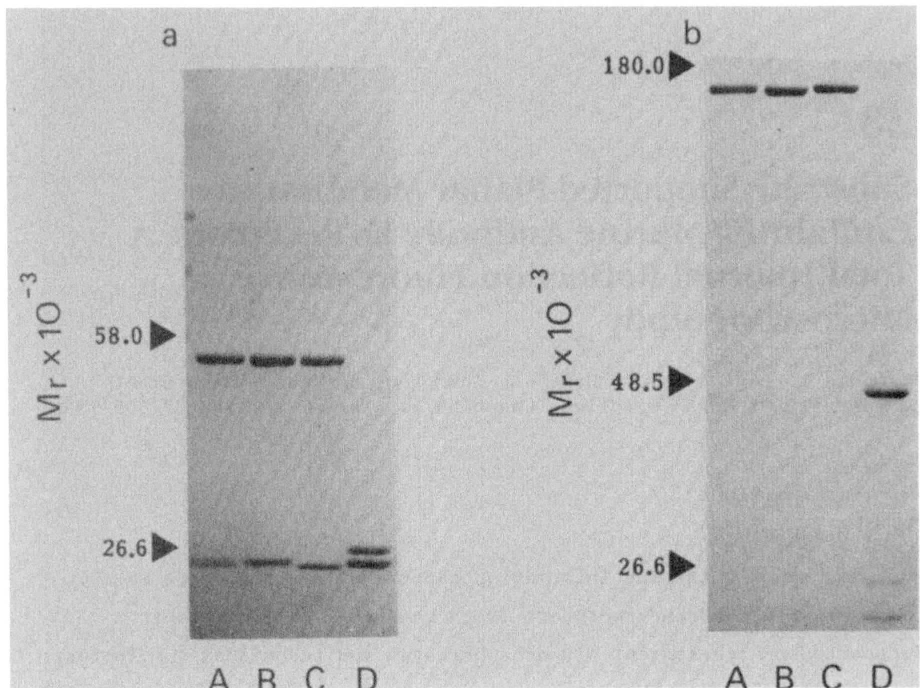

Figure 1. Sodium Dodecyl Sulfate Polyacrylamide Gel Electrophoresis of Intact 2.4G2 Antibodies and Their Fab Fragments. 10% acrylamide gels under (a) reducing and (b) nonreducing conditions were stained with Coomassie Blue: Lane A, 2.4G2 ±, bound by anti-(rat IgG); Lane B, 2.4G2-, not bound by MAR18.5, light chain 26 kD; Lane C, 2.4G2+, bound by MAR18.5, light chain 23kD; and Lane D, 2.4G2+ Fab.

(Fig. 1), consistent with the previously reported observation that 2.4G2 cells (a rat-mouse hybridoma) secrete one antibody with rat kappa light chains that binds to murine macrophage cell surfaces and one with murine light chains derived from the fusion partner that does not bind to macrophages (7). The two antibodies could be separated by affinity chromatography with the anti-(rat kappa light chain) monoclonal antibody MAR18.5 (cells from ATCC, American Type Culture Collection, Rockville, MD) and low pH elution. Enzyme-linked immunoassay confirmed that the bound and eluted (2.4G2+) but not the flow through (2.4G2-) antibodies contained rat kappa light chains.

TABLE 1 Fluorescence Immunoassay for 2.4G2+ Binding to J774A.1 Cells

	Intact IgG		Fab Fragments	
	1° assay	2° assay	1° assay	2° assay
2.4G2+	1.00 ± .11	1.00 ± .11	1.00 ± .14	1.00 ± .12
Rat IgG	0.12 ± .06	0.44 ± .05	0.02 ± .03	0.14 ± .06
2.4G2-	0.09 ± .06	0.14 ± .02	-	-
None	-	0.12 ± .08	-	0.12 ± .08

TABLE 1. The fluorescence arising from antibodies bound to single cells was measured with epifluorescence microscopy (8). The measured fluorescence was corrected for the background fluorescence from untreated cells (all data) and for the relative fluorescence yields of different labelled antibodies (1° assay). Shown are the mean and standard errors in the mean for 30-36 cells per antibody combination.

2.4G2+ Fab fragments were produced by papain digestion and purified by MAR18.5 affinity chromatography (Fig. 1). The specificity of intact 2.4G2+ antibodies and their Fab fragments for J774A.1 cells (ATCC), which are macrophage-related cells that express $moFc_{\gamma}RII$, was examined by two immunofluorescence assays. Cells were treated with tetramethylrhodamine-labelled intact and Fab fragments of 2.4G2 antibodies and rat IgG (1° assay) or with these antibodies (unlabelled) followed by tetramethylrhodamine-labelled anti-rat IgG $(Fab')_2$ (2° assay). The assays showed that 2.4G2+ but not 2.4G2- or rat IgG antibodies specifically bound to J774A.1 cells through their antigen-binding regions (Table 1).

3. SUBSTRATE-SUPPORTED PLANAR MEMBRANES CONTAINING Fc RECEPTORS

Substrate-supported planar membranes containing $moFc_{\gamma}RII$ were prepared from J774A.1 cells by a modification of previously published procedures for isolating J774A.1 membrane fragments (9) and for depositing membrane fragments of other cell types on planar substrates (10). J774A.1 cells were disrupted by nitrogen cavitation and the resulting homogenate was clarified by low force centrifugation.

Suspended membrane fragments were then pelleted by sedimentation, dissolved in a deoxycholate buffer, and dialyzed extensively against phosphate-buffered saline (PBS) to produce a solution of protein-containing liposomes. Fused silica substrates and glass microscope slides (1" x 1" x 1mm) were cleaned as described (8), and mounted together with a spacer (~ 100 μm). A 70 μl volume of J774A.1-derived liposomes was passed between the substrates and allowed to adsorb, and residual liposomes were removed by washing with PBS.

The properties of the supported planar membranes were investigated by labelling the membranes with the fluorescent lipid 1-acyl-2-[12-[(7-nitro-2-1,3-benzoxadiazol-4-yl)amino]dodecanyol]phosphatidylethanolamine. Epifluorescence microscopy indicated that the substrate was uniformly coated with fluorescent lipids within optical resolution and pattern fluorescence photobleaching recovery, performed as described (8), demonstrated that the fluorescent lipid lateral mobility was very low ($\leq 5 \times 10^{-12}$ cm^2/sec).

4. TOTAL INTERNAL REFLECTION FLUORESCENCE MICROSCOPY

The specific binding of tetramethylrhodamine-labelled 2.4G2+ Fab fragments to J774A.1-derived substrate-supported planar membranes was examined with fluorescence microscopy (11) adapted for TIR illumination (Fig. 2). Substrate-supported planar membranes were pretreated with bovine serum albumin (BSA) in PBS and then treated with 250 μl of

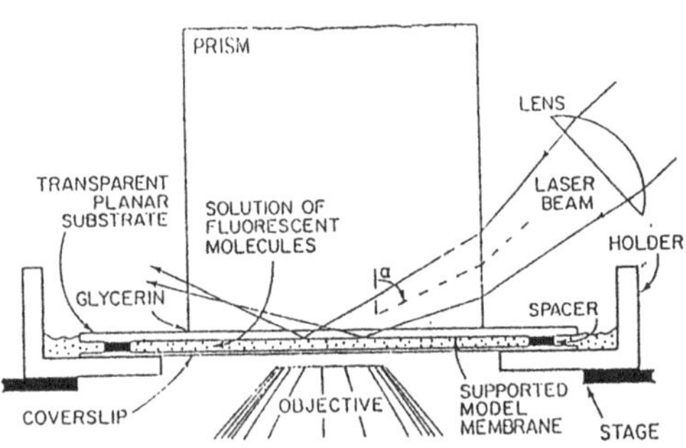

Figure 2. TIR Fluorescence Microscopy. A fused silica cubic prism is optically coupled to the membrane-supporting substrate with glycerin. An argon ion laser beam (514.5 nm and $1/e^2$ radius ~ 0.75 mm) is roughly focussed and totally internally reflected at the membrane /solution interface (incidence angle α = 75°; elliptically-shaped illumination, 20 μM x 200 μM; focal length of auxiliary lens, 80 mm). Surface-associated fluorescence excited by the evanescent field (depth ~ 900 Å) is collected by the microscope objective.

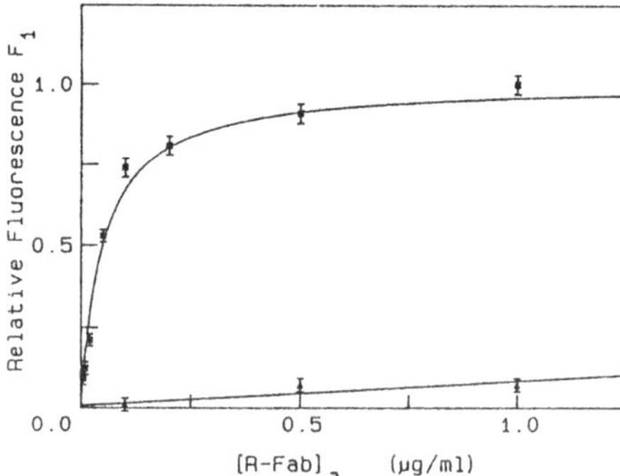

Figure 3. 2.4G2+ Fab Binding To Substrate-Supported Planar Membranes. Shown is TIR-excited fluorescence measured for Fc receptor-containing supported planar membranes in equilibrium with tetramethylrhodamine-labelled (■) 2.4G2+ and (▲) rat IgG fragments.

BSA solutions containing labelled 2.4G2+ or rat IgG Fab fragments. The fluorescence excited by the evanescent wave (F_1) as a function of the applied concentration of labelled Fab fragments, denoted by $[R\text{-}(2.4G2+\ Fab)]_a$ and $[R\text{-}(rat\ IgG\ Fab)]_a$, is shown in Figure 3. The measured fluorescence increased with $[R\text{-}(2.4G2+\ Fab)]_a$ to a saturation level whereas very little surface-associated fluorescence was detected for the same range of $[R\text{-}(rat\ IgG\ Fab)]_a$.

The concentrations of labelled Fab fragments remaining in solution after equilibration with the supported planar membranes were measured with epifluorescence microscopy by focusing the laser beam to a small spot (~ 0.7 µm radius) in the solution approximately 50 µm from the two adjacent membrane-coated surfaces. Fluorescence collection was restricted to the region of the focused spot by a pinhole placed at an intermediate image plane (12). The solution fluorescence was linear with $[R\text{-}(rat\ IgG\ Fab)]_a$ and also for the higher values of $[R\text{-}(2.4G2+\ Fab)]_a$ and was used as a calibration for the lower R-(2.4G2+ Fab) solution concentrations (data not shown). For $[R\text{-}(2.4G2+\ Fab)]_a < 200$ ng/ml the average solution concentration depletion was 22 ± 2 ng/ml. This value, together with the known sample volume (250 µl) and planar membrane surface area (2 in^2) implied that the density of bound R-(2.4G2+ Fab) was ≤ 60 molecules/μm^2. Assuming that the surface density of moFc$_\gamma$RII on J774A.1 cells was approximately 500,000 copies (13) distributed over 400 μm^2 (14), then the receptors were diluted ~ 20-fold in the substrate-supported planar membranes.

In the simplest case, the normalized surface-associated fluorescence (F_1, Fig. 3) measured as a function of the solution concentration of labelled 2.4G2+ Fab fragments, should be of the form

$$F_1 = \frac{K_1\ [\text{R-(2.4G2+ Fab)}]}{1 + K_1\ [(\text{R-2.4G2+ Fab})]} \qquad [1]$$

where K_1 is the association constant for 2.4G2+ Fab with $moFc_{\gamma}RII$. Consistent with Eq. 1, a plot of $F_1/[1 - F_1]$ was linear with zero intercept. The slope given by a least squares analysis yielded $K_1 = (9.6 \pm 0.4) \times 10^8\ M^{-1}$, which is consistent with the previously reported value for the binding of ^{125}I-labelled 2.4G2+ Fab fragments to J774A.1 cell surfaces (13).

The Fc-binding activity of $moFc_{\gamma}RII$ in the supported planar membranes was confirmed by examining the fluorescence of surface-bound R-(2.4G2+ Fab) fragments in the presence of unlabelled polyclonal murine IgG. Unlabelled murine IgG, but not IgG $(Fab')_2$ fragments, inhibited the binding of labelled R-2.4G2+ Fab fragments to planar membranes (Fig. 4). As expected, the concentration of murine IgG at which one-half of the bound R-(2.4G2+ Fab) was blocked increased with the concentration of R-(2.4G2+ Fab) (data not shown).

A possible mechanism for the inhibition shown in Figure 4 is one in which murine IgG completely blocks the binding of 2.4G2+ Fab fragments to $moFc_{\gamma}RII$. In this case, the inverse of the measured fluorescence normalized to its value in the absence of murine IgG is given by

$$F_2^{-1}\ [\text{Murine IgG}] = 1 + \frac{K_2\ [\text{Murine IgG}]}{1 + K_1\ [\text{R-(2.4G2+ Fab)}]} . \qquad [2]$$

The curve in Figure 4 was fit to the functional form of Eq. 2 with K_2 as a free parameter and with K_1 and [R-(2.4G2+ Fab)] equal to their experimentally determined values. The best-fit value of $K_2 = 2.6 \times 10^5\ M^{-1}$ is slightly lower than the value obtained for the binding of murine IgG to macrophage cell surfaces as measured by competitive

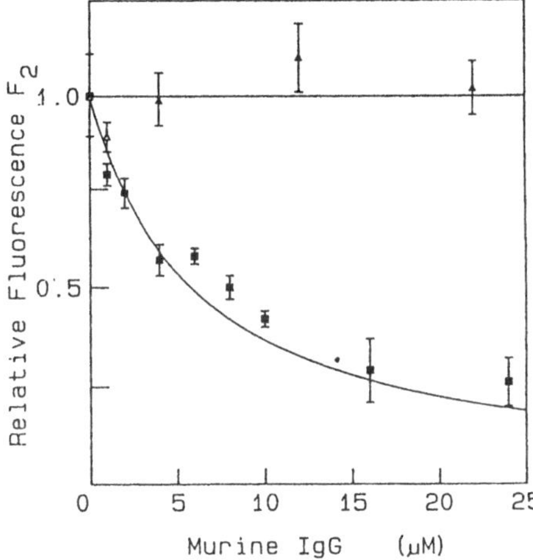

Figure 4. Association of Polyclonal Murine IgG With Supported Planar Membranes. Shown is the normalized fluorescence obtained with evanescent excitation and arising from R-(2.4G2+ Fab) bound to planar membranes as a function of the concentration of unlabelled polyclonal murine (■) intact IgG and (▲) IgG $(Fab')_2$ for $[R\text{-}(2.4G2+\ Fab)]_a$ = 50 ng/ml. The solid line for the intact IgG is the best fit of the experimental data to Eq. 2 and the bars represent standard errors in the mean of 9 measurements.

assays with radioactively-labelled ligands under nonequilibrium conditions (15).

5. SUMMARY

A relatively simple procedure for constructing substrate-supported planar membranes from isolated cell membrane fragments (10) has been adapted to macrophage membranes containing the murine IgG Fc receptor $moFc_{\gamma}RII$. The specific interactions of anti-$moFc_{\gamma}RII$ receptor antibodies and of murine IgG with reconstituted $moFc_{\gamma}RII$ have been quantitatively investigated with TIR fluorescence microscopy. Future applications may include measurement of the kinetics of IgG-$moFc_{\gamma}RII$ interactions by combining TIR illumination with fluorescence photobleaching recovery or correlation spectroscopy, investigating the possible clustering of IgG-$moFc_{\gamma}RII$ complexes by scanning fluorescence correlation spectroscopy, and examining possible changes in $moFc_{\gamma}RII$ conformation as characterized by fluorescence energy transfer in conjunction with measurements of the orientation distribution of the reconstituted $moFc_{\gamma}RII$ (1,11).

6. ACKNOWLEDGMENTS

We thank Jay C. Unkeless of Mt. Sinai Medical School and Betty Diamond of the Albert Einstein College of Medicine for 2.4G2 hybridoma cells, and Lois L. Wright of Burroughs Welcome Co. and Arthur G. Palmer of the Research Institute of Scripps Clinic for their contributions. This work was supported by NIH grant GM37145, NSF-PYI grant DCB8552986 and E.I. du Pont de Nemours & Co.

7. REFERENCES

1. N. L. Thompson, A. G. Palmer, L. L. Wright, & P. E. Scarborough (1988) Comm. Molec. Cell. Biophys. 5, 109.
2. H. M. McConnell, T. H. Watts, R. M. Weis, & A. A. Brian (1986) Biochim. Biophys. Acta 864, 95.
3. J. L. Tedesco, U. J. Krull, & M. Thompson (1989) Biosensors 4, 135.
4. J. F. Place, R. M. Sutherland, & C. Dahne (1985) Biosensors 1, 321.
5. D. Axelrod, T. P. Burghardt, & N. L. Thompson (1984) Ann. Rev. Biophys. Bioeng. 13, 247.
6. J. C. Unkeless, E. Scigliano, & V. H. Freedman (1988) Ann. Rev. Immunol. 6, 251.
7. J. C. Unkeless (1979) J. Exp. Med. 150, 580.
8. L. L. Wright, A. G. Palmer, & N. L. Thompson (1988) Biophys. J. 54, 463.
9. J. D.-E. Young, J. C. Unkeless, H. R. Kaback, & Z. A. Cohn (1983) Proc. Natl. Acad. Sci. U.S.A. 80, 1636.
10. T. H. Watts, A. A. Brian, J. W. Kappler, P. Marrack, & H. M. McConnell (1984) Proc. Natl. Acad. Sci. U.S.A. 81, 7564.
11. A. G. Palmer & N. L. Thompson (1989) Proc. Natl. Acad. Sci. U.S.A. 86, 6148.
12. A. G. Palmer & N. L. Thompson (1989) Applied Optics 28, 1214.
13. I. S. Mellman & J. C. Unkeless (1980) J. Exp. Med. 152, 1048.
14. H. R. Petty, D. G. Hafeman, & H. M. McConnell (1981) J. Cell. Biol. 89, 223.
15. D. R. Burton (1985) Mol. Immunol. 22, 161.

29

A Nicotinic Receptor Optical Biosensor

KIM R. ROGERS and MOHYEE E. ELDEFRAWI University of Maryland School of Medicine, Department of Pharmacology and Experimental Therapeutics, Baltimore, Maryland 21201

DAVID P. RICHMAN University of Chicago, Department of Neurology, Chicago, Illinois 60637

1. INTRODUCTION

Neurotransmitter receptor proteins are excellent candidates as sensing elements in biosensors because of their high affinity and selectivity for sepcific ligands. They can recognize families of chemicals of physiological, pharmacological and toxicological significance, that range from amino acids and peptides to therapeutics, drugs of abuse and toxicants. Although optic immunosensors which make use of total internal reflection fluorescence (i.e. evanescence) have been initially used in immunochemical biosensors (1,2), evanescent fluorosensors, with an appropriate indicator chemistry, can also provide a sensitive and stable transducer for a receptor-based biosensor (3). In this receptor-optical sensor, the incident light excites a fluorophore just outside the waveguide boundary (approximately 1000 Å), then a portion of the resultant fluoroescence becomes trapped and is transmitted back up the fiber. This technique is well suited to a receptor-based or immunochemical biosensor because the fluorescently-tagged ligand, or antibody bound to the receptor protein, which is immobilized at the fiber surface, can be monitored without interference from the ligand in bulk solution.

The nicotinic acetylcholine receptor (nAChR) binds several drugs and toxins of pharmacologic interest and has been implicated as the target of an autoimmune attack in the neurological disease myasthenia gravis (MG) (4). Myasthenics produce antibodies against their own skeletal muscle nAChR. Binding of these antibodies may block receptor function, speed receptor metabolism and/or induce complement-mediated membrane lysis; thereby decreasing the number of nAChRs and destroying postsynaptic folds (5).

The nAChR was selected for the first studies in the biosensor because the pure receptor is easily obtained in milligram quantities from *Torpedo* electric organ, its molecular properties have been elucidated (6) and its genes have been cloned (7). It is likely to be the first receptor to be produced by genetic engineering in quantities for commercial use.

METHODS

The nAChR was purified as previously described (6) and adsorbed on quartz fibers during a 12 h incubation in a solution (10 mM sodium phosphate buffer pH, 4.0) containing 50 μg/ml nAChR (3). Excess receptor was removed from the fibers by rinsing in 5 ml of 154 mM NaCl, 10 mM sodium phosphate, pH 7.4 (PBS).

α-Bungarotoxin (α-BGT) (Ventoxin, Frederick, MD) and mAB 132, the monoclonal antibody against the major antigenic site of the nAChR of *Torpedo* (8), were labelled with fluorescein isothiocyanate (FITC) as previously described (3). All fluorescence experiments were carried out using a fluorimeter designed and built at ORD, Inc. (North Salem, NH). The specific details have been previously described (9).

nAChR-coated fibers were placed into the fluorimeter and 5 nM FITC-α-BGT perfused over the receptor coated fibers at 0.2 ml/min. For drug displacement studies, the fibers were pretreated for 10 min with the competing ligand. For the "sandwich type" immunoassays, receptor coated fibers were incubated with mAb 132 (0.1 μg/ml) for 1 h, or MG sera (1:10 in PBS buffer) for 1 h then mAb 132 (0.1 mg/ml), 1 h prior to perfusion with FITC-goat anti-rat IgG (5 nM). For immunoassays using FITC-mAb 132, receptor coated or control (i.e. no receptor) fibers were perfused with 20 nM FITC-mAb 132. For species cross-reactivity studies, quartz fibers were incubated with the rat, human, rabbit or sheep IgG (1 mg/ml) for 1 h prior to washing and perfusion with 5 nM FITC-goat anti-rat IgG.

2. RESULTS AND DISCUSSION

FITC-α-BGT bound in a dose dependent manner with similar rates to both untreated quartz fibers and those coated with nAChR. However, at 5 nM FITC-α-BGT, nonspecific (i.e. nonreceptor) binding was completely eliminated by adding bovine serum albumin (BSA) to the assay buffer (Fig. 1)

The binding of α-BGT to the nAChR is a quasi-irreversible event, making it difficult to study competition displacement of its binding under equilibrium conditions. However, affinities of receptor agonists and antagonists are determined by measuring their effects on the association rate of α-BGT (10). Consequently, we used initial rates of association of FITC-α-BGT to nAChR-coated fibers to measure the relative affinities of a number of receptor ligands, which compete at the α-BGT binding site (Table 1). Both agonists and antagonist effectively blocked FITC-α-BGT binding to the nAChR, thereby reducing the rate of increase in observed fluorescence. The relative affinities of these cholinergic ligands were similar to those observed in purified membrane preparations (11).

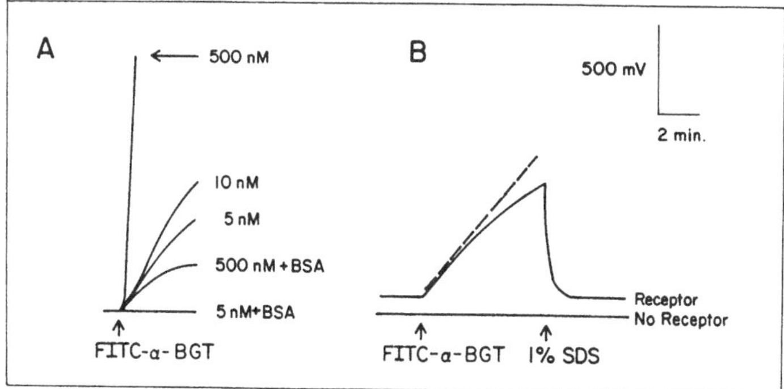

FIGURE 1 Binding of fluorescently labelled α-BGT to: A) Untreated quarts fibers in the presence and absence of BSA (0.1 mg/ml in PBS buffer), B) Untreated and nAChR-coated quartz fibers. FITC-α-BGT was introduced at 5 nM in PBS containing (0.1 mg/ml). (From Ref. 3).

Table 1. Inhibition by Receptor Ligands of the Binding of FITC-α-BGT to the nAChR on the Optic Fibers.

Drug		% inhibition of initial rate of fluorescence change
Agonists	Acetylcholine	61
	Carbamylcholine	42
	Nicotine	27
Depolarizing blockers	Decamethonium	52
	Succinylcholine	45
Competitive antagonists	d-Tubocurarine	87
	Pancuronium	76
	Naja α-neurotoxin (10 μM)	100

Unless otherwise specified, the drug was present at 1 mM in PBS containing BSA (0.1 mg/ml) and FITC-α-BGT (5 nM). Initial rate of fluorescence change in the absence of inhibitor =100%. The values are means of two experiments which varied by <10%. (From Ref. 3).

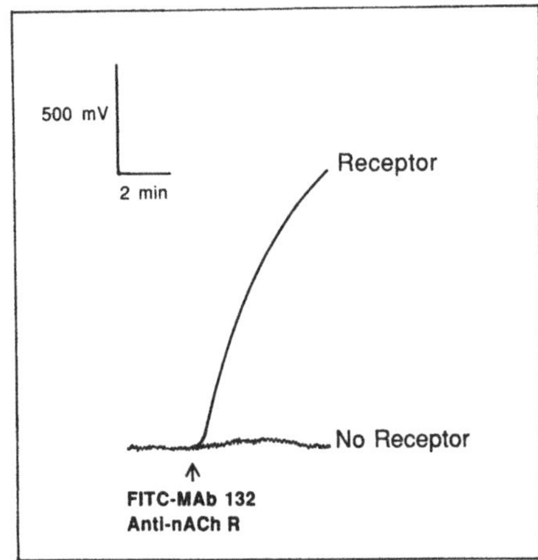

FIGURE 2 Specific binding of fluorescently-labelled mAb 132 to untreated (no receptor) or nAChR-coated fibers. Flow buffer was PBS containing mAb (5 nM) and BSA (0.1 mg/ml).

FITC-mAb 132 fluorescence was seen only when the nAChR was on the optic fiber (Fig. 2). Similar to results shown for FITC-α-BGT, non-

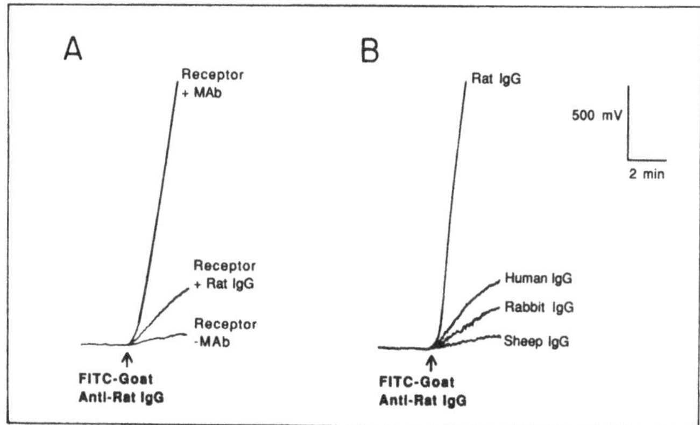

FIGURE 3 Binding of FITC-goat anti-rat IgG (5 nM) to A- quartz:receptor:mAb 132, quartz:receptor:rat IgG, or quartz:receptor; B- quartz: rat IgG, human IgG, rabbit IgG or sheep IgG.

specific binding of IgG to the untreated quartz fiber was eliminated by addition of 0.1 mg/ml BSA to the assay buffer. In a "sandwich type" version of this assay, mAb 132 which was bound to the adsorbed nAChR, was detected using FITC-goat anti-rat IgG (Fig. 3A). Nonspecific binding of rat IgG to the adsorbed nAChR, measured using FITC-goat anti-rat was 17% of the binding of mAb 132 to nAChR (Fig. 3A). Further, the binding of FITC-goat anti-rat to the receptor coated fiber was diminished by 96% in the absence of mAb 132 (Fig. 3A). The relative cross-ractivity of FITC-goat anti-rat antibody to IgG of other species was very low (Fig. 3B) with inter-species recognition for adsorbed immunoglobulins as 13, 6 and 2% for human, rabbit and sheep IgG, respectively.

Preexposure of the nAChR-optic fiber to MG sera, from 10 patients with large variations in their antibody titers (4) did not significantly inhibit binding of mAb 132 to the nAChR as visualized by FITC-goat anti-rat IgG (Table 2). The differences were less than those between controls and were unrelated to the anti-AChR titer. This result is possibly due to the low cross-reactivity between human muscle anti-nAChR antibodies and the *Torpedo* nAChR (12).

This study provides evidence that an optic sensor using FITC-α-BGT and nAChR adsorbed onto a quartz fiber, can detect ligands which bind to the receptor. Furthermore, this sensor can detect specific binding of a rat monoclonal antibody mAb 132 to the nAChR using FITC-mAb 132 or by means of a "sandwich type" assay using FITC labelled anti-rat IgG. The mechanism of the transduction is simple, the technique is sensitive and specific, and the signal depends only on the receptor-ligand binding event.

Table 2. Effects of Sera from Myasthenic Patients on the Fluorescence Signal Produced by Binding of mAb 132.

Patient#	Anti-nAChR Titer (nM)	% of mAb 132 binding for control A
Control A	----	100
1	8.48	125
2	22.00	119
3	1.44	94
4	2.16	106
5	0.08	106
6	9.70	88
7	124.00	131
8	3.23	106
9	0.00	100
Control B	----	88
11	35.00	106

ACKNOWLEDGMENT

This work was supported in part by DOD contracts No. DAAA-15-89-R-0031 (to M.E.E.) and DAAA-15-88-C-0026 (to ORD Inc.); NS15462 and NS21442 (to D.P.R.). The authors wish to thank Dr. James F. Howard (Univ. of North Carolina, Chapel Hill) for supplying the human sera and Dr. Amira T. Eldefrawi (Univ. of Maryland) for editing the MS and Mrs. Sharon Mills for word processing.

REFERENCES

1. T.B. Hirschfeld and M.J. Block, "Fluorescent Immunoassay Employing Optical Fiber in Capillary Tube," U.S. Patent 4,447, 546 (1984).
2. R.M. Sutherland, C. Dahne, J.F. Place and A.R. Ringrose, J. Immunol. Meth., 74, 253 (1984).
3. K.R. Rogers, J.J. Valdes and M.E. Eldefrawi, Anal. Biochem., (in press).
4. M.E. Seybold and J.M. Lindstrom, Ann. N.Y. Acad. Sci., 377, 292 (1981).
5. J.E. Rash, C.S. Hudson, E.X. Albuquerque, M.E. Eldefrawi, R.F. Mayer, W.F. Graham, T.J.A. Johnson and F.D. Giddings, Ann. N.Y. Acad. Sci., 377, 38 (1981).
6. M.E. Eldefrawi and A.T. Eldefrawi, Arch. Biochem. Biophys., 159, 362 (1973).
7. T. Claudio, M. Ballivet, J. Patrick and S. Heinemann, Proc. Natl. Acad. Sci. USA, 80, 111 (1983).
8. C.M. Gomez, D.P. Richman, P.W. Berman, S.A. Burres, B. Arnason and F.W. Fitch, Biochem. Biophys. Res. Commun., 88, 575 (1979).
9. T.R. Glass, S. Lackie and T. Hirschfeld, Applied Optics, 26, 2181 (1987).
10. S.G. Blanchard, V. Quast, K. Reed, T. Lee, R.V. Schimerlik, T. Claudio, C.D. Strader, H.H. Moore and M.A. Raftery, Biochemistry, 18, 1875 (1979).
11. J. Schmidt and M.A. Raftery, J. Neurochem., 28, 617 (1974).
12. C.M. Gomez, D.P. Richman, S.A. Burres and B.G.W. Arnason, Ann. N.Y. Acad. Sci., 377, 97 (1981).

Index

Printed and bound by CPI Group (UK) Ltd, Croydon, CR0 4YY
17/10/2024
01775700-0014